CURRENT DIRECTIONS IN RADIOPHARMACEUTICAL RESEARCH AND DEVELOPMENT

Developments in Nuclear Medicine

VOLUME 30

Series Editor: Peter H. Cox

The titles published in this series are listed at the end of this volume.

Current Directions in Radiopharmaceutical Research and Development

edited by

STEPHEN J. MATHER

Department of Nuclear Medicine,
St Bartholomew's Hospital,
London, UK

KLUWER ACADEMIC PUBLISHERS
DORDRECHT / BOSTON / LONDON

A C.I.P. Catalogue record for this book is available from the Library of Congress

ISBN-13: 978-94-010-7289-2 e-ISBN-13: 978-94-009-1768-2
DOI: 10.1007/978-94-009-1768-2

Published by Kluwer Academic Publishers,
P.O. Box 17, 3300 AA Dordrecht, The Netherlands.

Kluwer Academic Publishers incorporates
the publishing programmes of
D. Reidel, Martinus Nijhoff, Dr W. Junk and MTP Press.

Sold and distributed in the U.S.A. and Canada
by Kluwer Academic Publishers,
101 Philip Drive, Norwell, MA 02061, U.S.A.

In all other countries, sold and distributed
by Kluwer Academic Publishers Group,
P.O. Box 322, 3300 AH Dordrecht, The Netherlands.

Printed on acid-free paper

Softcover reprint of the hardcover 1st edition 1996

CONTENTS

FOREWORD - RADIOPHARMACEUTICALS FOR THE FUTURE

Keith E. Britton

The new radiopharmaceutical is the life blood of nuclear medicine (1). Whereas for radiology to progress, a newer, larger, more expensive, high technology machine is required, a new radiopharmaceutical with a conventional gamma camera provides a new investigation. However the increasingly unfavourable regulatory environment is responsible for over half the cost of the new radiopharmaceutical with the consequence of reducing the competitiveness of nuclear medicine. The promised increase in the cost of production of the molybdenum-99 for the Technetium-99m generator will aggravate this situation further.

The key question for the development of a new radiopharmaceutical is whether it is chance, serendipity or science, or all three. In the beginning were the physicists making new elements whose existence was deliberately useful - I-131, I-123, or by chance such as the finding that Thallium- 201 went to the guinea pig heart (2), after which it was rationalised that it was a potassium analogue with active transport into muscle. Physical properties of half life and suitability for mechanical imaging systems, and an understanding of the parent-daughter decay schemes led to the development of the Mo-Tc-99m generator, the basic work horse for nuclear medicine. More exotic generators for Iodine-132, Gold- 195m, Gallium-68 and others have not generally progressed. The development of positron emitting radionuclides and positron emission tomography has led to the increasingly used 18F-DG (deoxyglucose) for 'nuclear radiology' which is outdoing X-ray CT and MRI in identifying active tissue in lymph nodes less than the conventional 1 cm which is considered normal.

The rise of structure-activity relationships then dominated pharmaceutical development. Each compound had its own combination of charge, whether it is an electron donor or acceptor, its lipophilicity-hydrophilicity balance, its redox potential and pK, its chirality and isomerism. For example there was the view of Deutsch et al (3) that a technetium-99m labelled compound must not be reducible if it is to be retained in the heart. The development of Tc-99m MIBI (methoxyisobutyl isonitrile) was based on this theory, but its success was not because it contained Technetium in a ground state but because it is protein bound intracellularly. It's serendipitous use in tumour localisation: parathyroid, breast, myeloma etc led to the discovery that its intracellular residence depends on the absence of the P-glycoprotein, the G-protein that is responsible for multiple drug resistance, MDR, in many tumours (4). Indeed it's use in tumour imaging and in the assessment of MDR may exceed its initial cardiac intentions.

The development of a new hypoxic agent, HL91, by Amersham International follows the analysis of nitroimidazole whereby a compound is designed to reduce and re-oxidise but in hypoxia a second reduction step occurs fixing the hypoxic agent in the tissue. HL91 however was found to be an efficient hypoxic agent without the structure thought necessary for this double reduction step; it is now under clinical evaluation (5).

The active analogue approach whereby a set of compounds is synthesised so as to mimic features of a chosen natural compound has been successful. Initially it was based on the comparison of two dimensional structures. The development of MIBG by Weiland et al (6) by testing a thousand compounds has led to great benefits in the diagnosis and therapy of neural crest tumours. The use of I-131 MIBG therapy prior to surgery has been beneficial in allowing the child with neuroblastoma to continue to thrive and not lose any hair while making the tumour operable (7) as compared to chemotherapy. Here the power of the pharmaceutical industry over the radiopharmaceutical industry is preventing this important development being generally implemented in childhood neuroblastoma.

The active analogue approach includes the pharmacophore and leads to computer aided radiopharmaceutical design. The concept of a pharmacophore is to look at features common to a set of drugs or compounds binding to and acting on the same receptors, drugs which are responsible for recognition and transduction of the appropriate response. The likelihood of receptor binding with the active analogue depends on the arrangement of the molecules that look similar. The active analogue approach states that one needs to vary the shape of the ligand to test the shape of the receptor. In this way hopefully the common variables that lead to recognition and binding can be separated from the variables that lead to activation. This is required because one does not want to destroy or activate the system while it is actually being imaged. The pharmacophore approach emphasises the minimum volume requirements of the particular compounds in order to fit the particular shape of the receptor binding site. This process of molecular recognition is the basis of biological interaction: substrate with its enzyme, a hormone with its receptor, a drug with its metabolic site and an antigen with its antibody. It may be demonstrated that three dimensionally an enzyme acting on its substrate and an antibody acting with its antigen are very similar, indeed the interaction between these pairs are by the same sort of mechanism (8).

It is in three dimensions that the recognition process takes place and in this situation the match stick chemical formulae have to be seen to be merely as the backbone on which and around which an electron cloud is dispersed - a chemical ectoplasm representing the unique persona of the molecule. The comparisons of analogue molecules then become the comparisons of the negatively charged electron clouds around their chemical structures. In this it can be seen there are basically two classes of molecule in the recognition process - the binder and the bindee (1,9). Radiopharmacology is reduced to the concept of characterising a particular and specific binder molecule on the target cell or metabolic process and finding a highly avid, highly specific, non toxic, molecular bindee that can be radiolabelled and used to target in vivo the system that is under study.

Computer aided design takes the rules of quantum mechanics which can measure and calculate distribution of electrons, the geometrical relationships, the energies of the molecules, the electrostatic potential and their thermodynamic properties. The Schroedinger equation is used, which relates the energy, E, for a molecule in a specified nuclear geometry and wave form: Hw = Ew. From the wave function, w, the electron density map, H and electrostatic fields can be calculated (10). The basic information about the molecular structure needed for such calculations comes from chemistry, mass spectroscopy, crystallography, and magnetic resonance. These and other physical techniques are used to probe the molecule and measure the relationships of its constituents. Having characterised the molecule the specifications of appropriate analogues can be made and these bindees synthesised. Alternatively the structural and electron density requirements of a complimentary receptor molecule can be identified and the putative receptor, the binder, described. On this basis agonist and antagonist blocking bindee molecules can be designed.

The biological base of radiopharmacy then takes its place. What binders - molecules, receptors, systems, tissues are important to target. Are surface binders the best target - receptors antigens, transport G proteins etc, or should the internal systems of the cell be the goal - signal transduction enzymes, mRNA, cytosolic and oncoproteins, or in cancer and other proliferative disorders, the cell nucleus, oncogenes, supressor and stimulating genes.

The target binding surface of the cell has been well explored with a range of tumour associated and other antigens identified and used for pathological tissue characterisations (11). These include the exposure of myosin in myocardial infarction to antimyosin (12), the epithelial surface antigens hidden from blood such as the polymorphic epithelial mucins, PEM, exposed to blood by the architectural disruption of the malignant process with antibodies such as HMFG1, 2, SM3 for breast and ovarian cancer imaging (13, 14), or fixed surface colonic crypt antigens with PR1A3 antibody for colon carcinoma (15) or dispersed oncofoetal antigens such as carcinoembryonic antigen for many cancers (16).

There are at least 90 natural biologically active peptides in man including endocrine, paracrine and autocrine hormones, cytokines, and other active agents. Each has its receptor and/or gene protein leading to stimulation or inhibition of an aspect of intracellular function, particularly signal transduction of information from the cell surface to the nucleus. Such agents enter the cell directly or through transport proteins and engage nuclear protein and/or nucleotide sites to control gene expression. A small start in using a few of them as radiopharmaceuticals has been made: I-131 vasopressin (17), I-131 insulin (18), I-123 and In-111 octreotide (19, 20), I-123 vasoactive intestinal peptide (21), and I-123 and Tc-99m Interleukin II (22, 23) are examples, the first few pages of a great book to be written.

These peptide molecules whether based on the bindee properties of antibodies or analogues of known biological peptides may all be synthesised directly or by genetic engineering. The genetic engineering process also enables a "cartridge" for binding the chosen radionuclide to be attached e.g. for P-32 (24).

The optimal radionuclide for imaging has moved from I-131, to I-123, to In-111 and will settle with Tc-99m with its advantages of relative cheapness, ready availability and an increasingly understood chemistry. For therapy while I-131 remains the model, arguments for particular situations require long lived beta emitters such as Sr-89, P-32, and In- 114m; for other situations short-lived high energy beta emitters such as Y-90, or low energy such as Re-186, Re-188, Sm-153, with some gamma emission to allow imaging at the time of therapy.

The development of radiolabelled oligonucleotides for direct gene location and as an adjunct to gene therapy proving uptake in the desired target cell is the next wave. Conventional oligonucleotides are too susceptible to circulating nucleases and have been replaced by thiolated derivatives. These have disadvantages of avid protein binding in the circulation and may be replaced by peptide nucleotides, PNA, where the phosphodiester core is replaced by a dimensionally similar peptide on which the purines and pyramidines are arranged. Aptamers, mimic molecules of nucleotides with similar properties are also under investigation (25).

From the above discussion it can be seen that nuclear medicine is moving from its origins in the nucleus of the atom to investigation of the nucleus of the cell.

In this book the experts plot the path from the development of radiopharmaceuticals for the imaging of a particular function of an organ with high sensitivity but usually low specificity to tailor-made cell type specific and sensitive agents. The radionuclide of choice for imaging is Tc-99m and its chemical neighbour Rhenium-186/188 has therapeutic potential. The direct labelling of whole monoclonal antibodies with Tc-99m has given way to an indirect approach, either the labelling of a linker which is subsequently attached to the molecule of interest, or else the linker is attached first and the Tc-99m introduced later.

The binder bindee concept is fully exploited with a range of cell surface binders from radiolabelled steroids to agents for the various central nervous system receptors. The monoclonal antibodies and their fragments for cancer and non cancer detection are described as is the help that computer modelling can bring in designing specific molecules for particular receptors.

New directions include the assessment of tissue hypoxia, and radiolabelled oligonucleotides for imaging the cell nucleus. Smaller and smaller agents are sought for better tissue penetration such as peptide radiopharmaceuticals and genetically engineered single chain Fv constructs.

Technical matters are described including radioligand binding assays and microautoradiography of radiopharmaceutical distribution, which in turn can help with the microdosimetry of the chosen therapeutic radionuclides. To improve the availability of radiopharmaceuticals for positron emission tomography, long lived positron emitters for imaging are discussed.

This is an excellent compilation of radiopharmaceutical research and development. It not only points the way forward but gives the means of transport to ride into the future.

References

1. Britton KE. The development of new radiopharmaceuticals. Eur J Nucl Med 1990; 16: 373-385.
2. Bradley-Moore PR, Lebowitz E, Greene MW, Atkins HL, Ansari N. Thallium 201 for medical use. J Nucl Med 1975; 16: 156-160.
3. Deutsch E, Glavan KA, Sodd VJ, Nishiyama H, Ferguson DL, Lukes SJ. Cationic Tc-99m complexes as potential myocardial imaging agents. J nucl Med 1981; 22: 89-90.
4. Piwica-Worms D, Chiu ML, Budding M et al. Functional imaging of multidrug-resistant P-glycoprotein with an aganotechnetium complex. Cancer Res 1993; 53: 1-8.
5. Cook GJR, Barrington S, Houston S, Maisey MN, Fogelman I. HL91, a new Tc-99m labelled agent with potential for identifying tumour hypoxia : correlation with FDG PET. J Nucl Med 1996; 37: 87P-88P.
6. Weiland DM, Wu JL, Brown LE et al. Radiolabelled adrenergic neuroblocking agents: adrenomedullary imaging with 131-iodo benzylguanidine. J Nucl Med 1980; 21: 349-353.
7. Hoefnagel CA, de Kraker J, Valdes Olmos RA, Voute PA. 131-I-MIBG as a first-line treatment in high-risk neuroblastoma patients. Nucl Med Commun 1994; 15: 712-717.
8. Lerner RA, Tramontano A. Catalytic anibodies. Sci Am 1988; 3: 52-50.
9. Britton KE, Granowska M. The present and future of radiolabelled antibodies in oncology. Ann Nucl Med 1993; 7: 127-132.
10. Richards GR. Computer aided molecular design. IBC technical Services, London 1989.
11. Britton KE. The tissue characterisation of malignancy with radionuculide studies In: Radioactive Isotopes in Clinical Medicine and Research. 21st Bad Gastein Symposium. Bergmann H, Sinzinger M eds. Birkhauser, Basel 1995; 249-280.

12. Khaw BA, Strauss HW, Moore R et al. Myocardial damage delineated by Indium-111 antimyosin Fab and Technetium-99m pyrophosphate. J Nucl Med 1987; 28: 76-82.
13. Girling A, Bartkora J, Burchell J et al. A core protein epitope of the polymorphic epithelial mucin detected by monoclonal antibody SM3 is selectely exposed in a range of primary carcinomas. Int J Cancer 1989; 43: 1072-1076.
14. Granowska A, Britton KE, Mather SJ et al . Radioimmunoscintigraphy with Technetium-99m-labelled monoclonal antibody, SM3, in gynaecological cancer. Eur J Nucl Med ; 30: 483-489.
15. Granowska M, Britton KE, Mather SJ et al. Radioimmunoscintigraphy with Technetium-99m labelled monoclonal antibody, 1A3, in colorectal cancer. Eur J Nucl Med 1993; 20: 690-698.
16. Baum RP, Hertel A, Lorenz M et al. ^{99m}Tc-labelled anti-CEA monoclonal antibody for tumour immunoscintigraphy: first clinical results. Nucl Med Commun 1989; 10: 345-50.
17. Britton KE, Khokar AM, Brown NJG, Davison A, Slater JDH. A non-invasive test for receptor binding applied to nephrogenic diabetes insipidus. Postgrad Med J 1977; 53: 374-377.
18. Sinclair AJ, Signore A, Bomanji J et al. In vivo kinetics of I-123 labelled Insulin : studies in normal subjects and patients with diabetes. Nuc Med Commun 1987; 8: 779-786.
19. Ur E, Mather SJ, Bomanji J, Ellison D, Britton KE, Grossman AB. Pituitary imaging using a labelled somatostatin analogue in acromegaly. Clin Endocrinol 1993; 36: 147-150.
20. Krenning EP, Kwekkeboom DJ, Bakker WH et al. Somatostatin receptor scintigraphy with ^{111}In-DPTA-D-Phe and ^{123}I-Tyr^{3}-octreotide the Rotterdam experience with more than 1000 patients. Eur J Nucl Med 1993; 20: 716-31.
21. Vigolini I, Raderer M, Kurtaran A et al. Vasoactive intestinal peptide-receptor imaging for the localization of intestinal adenocarcinoma and endocrine tumours. New Engl J Med 1994; 331: 1116-121.
22. Signore A, Chianelli M, Ferretti E, et al. A new approach for in vivo detection of Insulitis in type 1 diabetes: activated lymphocyte targeting with I-123 labelled Interleukin 2. European Journal of Endocrinology 1994; 131: 431-7.
23. Chianelli M, Signore A, Sobnack R, Fitzberg AR, Britton KE, Mather SJ. 99m-Tc-Interleukin-2: A new radiopharmaceutical for the in vivo detection of lymphocytic infiltration. In: Nicolini M, Bandoli G, Mazzi V, eds, Technetium and Rhenium in chemistry and Nuclear Medicine 4. Padova: SG Editorali 1995: 551-555.
24. Neri D, Petrul H, Winter G, Light Y, Marais R, Britton KE, Creighton AM. Radioactive labelling of recombinant antibody fragments by phosphorylation using human casein kinase II and [y-^{32}P]-ATP. Nature Biotechnology 1996; 14: 485-490.
25. Hnatowich DJ, Mardirossian G, Fogarasi M. Properties of single-stranded phosphodiester and phosphothioate DNA labelled with Technetium-99m. J nucl Med 1995; 36: 103P.

LIST OF CONTRIBUTORS

Colin M. Archer
Healthcare Research and Development
Amersham International plc.
Amersham Laboratories
White Lion Road
AMERSHAM, Bucks., HP7 9LL
U.K.

Co-authors: Barabara Edwards and Nigel A. Powell

David Barlow
Department of Pharmacy
Kings College
Manresa Rd,
LONDON SW3 6LX
U.K.

Philip J. Blower
Department of Nuclear Medicine
Kent and Canterbury Hospital
Ethelbert Road
CANTERBURY, Kent CT1 3 NG
U.K.

Keith E. Britton
Department of Nuclear Medicine
St. Bartholomew's Hospital
LONDON EC1A 7BE
U.K.

Anthony P. Davenport
Clinical Pharmacology Unit
University of Cambridge, Box 110
Level 2, F&G Addenbrookes Hospital
CAMBRIDGE CB2 2QQ
U.K.

Co-author: Fraser D. Russell

Jonathan R. Dilworth
Department of Biological & Chemical Sciences
University of Essex
Wivenhoe Park
COLCHESTER CO4 3SQ
U.K.

Co-author: Suzanne J. Parrott

Robert D. Hancock
IBC Advanced Technologies
P.O. Box 98
AMERICAN FORK, UT 84003
U.S.A.

Donald J. Hnatowich
Department of Nuclear Medicine
University of Massachusetts Medical Center
55 Lake Avenue North
WORCESTER, MA 01655
U.S.A.

Hank F. Kung
Department of Radiology
Room 305
University of Pennsylvania
3700 Market St.
PHILADELPHIA, PA 19104
U.S.A.

Stephen J. Mather
Department of Nuclear Medicine
Imperial Cancer Research Fund
St. Bartholomew's Hospital
LONDON EC1A 7BE
U.K.

Suresh C. Srivastava
Radionuclide and Radiopharmaceutical Research Division
Brookhaven National Laboratory
Building 801
UPTON, NY 11973-5000
U.S.A.

Lorna M.D. Stewart
Applied Development Laboratory
Imperial Cancer Research Fund
Dominion House
59 Bartholomew Close
LONDON EC1A 7BE
U.K.

Alfons M. Verbruggen
Laboratory of Radiopharmaceutical Chemistry

University Hospital Gasthuisberg
Herestraat 49
B-3000 LEUVEN
Belgium

Michael J. Welch
Division of Radiation Sciences
Mallinckrodt Institute of Radiology
Washington University School of Medicine
510 S. Kingshighway Blvd
ST. LOUIS, MO 63110
U.S.A.

Co-authors: Joanna B. Downer and John A. Katzenellenbogen

Leonard I. Wiebe
Noujaim Institute for Pharmacological Oncology Research
Faculty of Pharmacy
University of Alberta
EDMONTON, Alberta
Canada T6G 2N8

Jamal Zweit
Joint Department of Physics
Institute of Cancer Research
The Royal Marsden Hospital
Downs Road
SUTTON, Surrey, SM2 5PT
U.K.

PREFACE

Radiopharmaceutical research has recently undergone a major change in direction. In past years it has been concerned mainly with the development of perfusion tracers, the biodistribution of which reflect the regional blood flow to areas of major organs such as the heart and brain. However, a major new direction of interest now lies in the development of receptor-binding radio-tracers which can be used to perform in-vivo characterisation of diseased tissues and it is likely that much of the future research in this field will follow this direction.

The difficulties in developing such tracers are considerable. The researcher must first identify a promising target for radiopharmaceutical development. High specific activity radioactive molecules must be designed and synthesised which will both bind to the target receptor with high affinity, and also have the physicochemical characteristics which will allow them to reach the target site in sufficient quantity while at the same time showing minimal uptake in non-target tissues.

Thus the knowledge base required for radiopharmaceutical development has now expanded beyond the limits of radiopharmaceutical chemistry to include aspects of biochemistry, molecular biology and conventional drug design. The portfolio of basic knowledge required to support current radiopharmaceutical development is changing and scientists working in this arena need to be trained in this regard. At the same time, the very latest developments in the field need to be communicated to the scientific community in order to stimulate the advancement of this exciting new direction of research.

With this in mind, the first of a new series of courses called "The First Easter School in Radiopharmaceutics" was recently held in Liverpool in the UK. The course was supported financially by the European Commission through their Training and Mobility of Researchers programme.

The aim of this 'Easter school' was to introduce advanced aspects of relevant topics to the radiopharmaceutical research community in an intensive one-week course. The course followed three principal themes: (i) Recent advances in radiopharmaceutical chemistry: (ii) Promising targets for radiopharmaceutical development: (iii) Tools and supporting technology. The course thus both informed the participants not only of the opportunities for research but also the means by which to pursue it.

Since the course was only able to cater for a limited number of participants, the contributions of most of the lecturers at the Easter School have been combined in this book in order to make the information more widely available. The content of the book mirrors that of the course and includes contribution in the fields of Radiopharmaceutical Chemistry, Targets for Radiopharmaceutical Development and Radiopharmaceutical analysis. Since regrettably not all of the lecturers were able to provide written chapters the discerning reader will notice a few notable gaps, particularly in the important fields of radiolabelled peptides research and radiohalogens. Hopefully these shortcomings will be addressed in a later edition.

Each of the contributors is recognised as an expert in their field. Many have world-wide reputations in the Nuclear Medicine community, although to save their embarrassment I will not mention their names! The names of some other authors will not be so familiar to many readers. In the rather cosy, closed world of Nuclear Medicine, we have much to learn from researchers in other fields and a number of the contributors were selected to provide a novel perspective.

This book should be of interest to everyone working in the Radiopharmaceutical and Nuclear Medicine communities. For those requiring only to be kept up-to-date with current developments, a browse through selected chapters, particularly those concerned with potential targets for development, will provide interesting reading. For those involved more at laboratory bench of radiopharmaceutical research, a detailed perusal of the texts and their associated bibliographies will ensure that they are as well-equipped as possible to make good progress in their chosen field.

In collating this volume I would like to thank my colleague, Mr Paul Maltby of The Royal Liverpool Hospital whose local knowledge and hard-work on the ground made the running of the Easter School possible. I would also thank my employers - Kings College, London and the Imperial Cancer Research Fund - and the Commission of the European Communities for their financial support.

Stephen J Mather
Editor

RADIOPHARMACEUTICALLY RELEVANT CHEMISTRY OF TECHNETIUM AND RHENIUM

Jonathan R. Dilworth and Suzanne J. Parrott

Introduction

The initial phase of the development of technetium-99m based imaging agents was of necessity heavily biased to the establishment of the basic coordination chemistry of the element. This led directly to the successful clinical use of a number of the so-called technetium essential agents for imaging *inter alia* major organs and bone. Now, some thirty or so years on there is need for a second generation of more specifically targeted agents, based on the use of bifunctional chelating ligands which bind both technetium and a biological molecule to direct the whole conjugate to specific binding sites *in vivo*. As Deutsch discussed recently [1a] this has resulted in a significant shift in emphasis from basic coordination chemistry to the biochemistry of the biological targeting system. However as the number and diversity of the biological targets increases it will doubtless be desirable to have a wider range of bifunctional chelates available, and coordination chemistry will still play an important role in the development of new imaging agents based on technetium.

The emphasis of this review is very much on the syntheses and structures of recently reported technetium complexes relevant to the development of new radiopharmaceuticals. It focuses primarily on classical chemical structural studies using the very long-lived, weak β-emitting technetium-99 isotope. A valuable comprehensive review of the known X-ray crystal structures of technetium complexes appeared in 1994 [1b], and attention is here focused on complexes which have been reported in the last two or three years and appear to have some potential relevance to radiopharmaceutics. Space does not permit complete coverage here, and we have attempted to illustrate the range of stereochemistries, oxidation states and overall charges available for the development of technetium and rhenium based radiopharmaceuticals. The details of the biological molecules used with the bifunctional chelates and their medical applications of the conjugates are dealt with elsewhere in this volume. The complexes have been somewhat arbitrarily classified according to the 'core' ligands (oxo-, nitrido-, diazenido- etc.) present, with further subdivisions based

S. J. Mather (ed.), Current Directions in Radiopharmaceutical Research and Development, 1–29.

on the nature of the co-ligands. A final section covers homoleptic complexes and lower oxidation state complexes without the multiply-bonded core ligands.

A comparatively recent and exciting development has been the proposed use of β-emitting isotopes of Re (^{186}Re and ^{188}Re) for therapy. A brief survey of relevant recent developments in rhenium coordination chemistry is also presented.

The Oxo Core

The oxo ligand forms the most common core for technetium-99m and rhenium based imaging and therapeutic agents. There are two main types: the mono oxo core $M=O^{3+}$ and the dioxo core MO_2^+, where M=Tc or Re. The co-ligands surrounding this oxo core determine the biodistribution, stability and the overall geometry of the complex. The typical oxidation state of technetium in these complexes is +5.

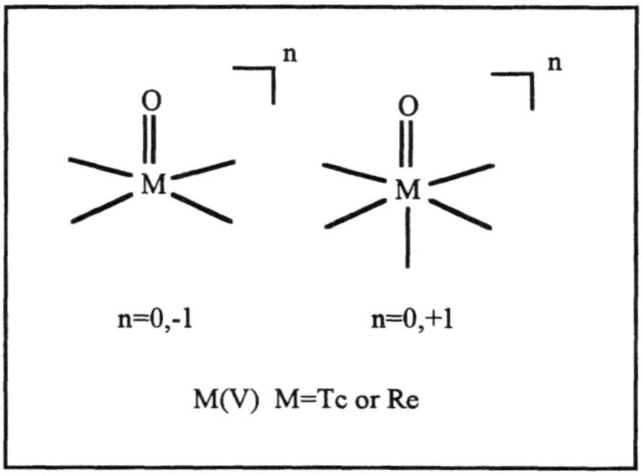

The Mono-Oxo Core

Some of the known polydentate ligand/TcO species together with representative structures are summarised in Table 1 at the end of this chapter, . The predominant geometry is square pyramidal, although some octahedral complexes are known. Positively charged square pyramidal complexes are very rare, instead of forming a positively charged 5-coordinate complex a nucleophilic ligand is accommodated *trans* to the oxo- group to yield a neutral, octahedral species. Synthesis of these complexes is typically directly from $[TcO_4]^-$ and a reductant, usually stannous chloride, is necessary for some systems. Tetradentate ligands provide the framework for a majority of technetium agents because the intrinsic chelate effect enhances complex stability. The coordination chemistry will be considered by ligand type commencing with the most common tetradentate N_2S_2 ligands then looking at the more recent developments made in the search for novel technetium complexes.

N_2S_2 SYSTEMS

A major class of radiopharmaceutically important complexes are based on the $[TcO(N_2S_2)]$ system. One example is [TcO(ECD)], Figure 1, which is currently being evaluated as a potential marker for cerebral blood flow [2]. Neutral [3,4] and anionic [5] $[Tc(V)O]^{3+}$ complexes of N_2S_2 ligands have been synthesised. The overall net charges and consequently the biodistribution of these complexes is determined by the ionisation of the two S-H and two N-H groups (either as amines or amides) of the ligand, Figure 1. The diamide dithiol ligand (DADT) forms complexes which are negatively charged due to the complete ionisation of the two S-H and two N-H groups [6]. The considerably lower pKa of amide ensures that the amide groups are deprotonated in preference to amine NH. Complexes of the bis(aminoethanethiol) (BAT) ligand are neutral and lipid soluble due to the ionisation of 2S-H and 1N-H groups on complexation. All of these N_2S_2 chelate complexes are isostructural and display a square based pyramidal geometry about the central technetium atom with the oxo group occupying the axial site.

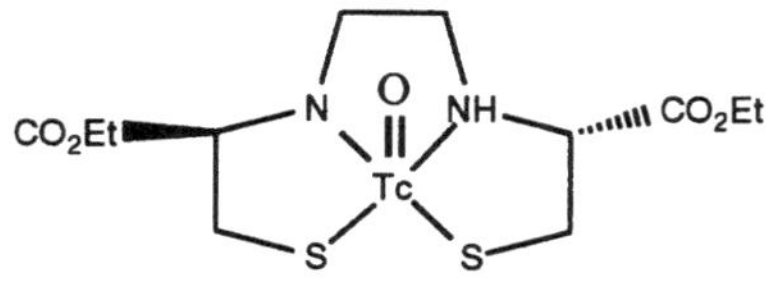

Figure 1

Since the report of these basic types of N_2S_2 ligands a very large number of variants have been synthesised [7,8,9]. One type is the amine amide thiol (AADT) ligand where the amino nitrogen is alkylated for potential conjugation to molecules of interest. Complexes of both ^{99}Tc, Figure 2, and Re have been characterised and were confirmed as having a penta-coordinate square pyramidal geometry [10].

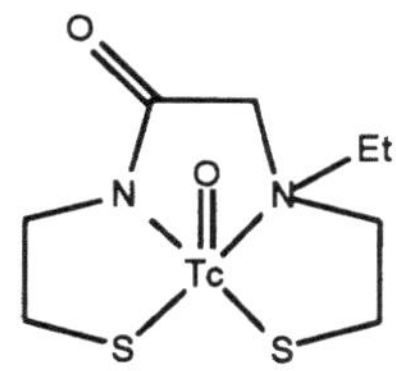

Figure 2

U-BAT is a ligand with two amine groups (one an arylamine) which have different pK_a values which allows control of the overall charge on the complex [11]. Comparison of the crystal structures of [TcO(U-BAT)] (**A**) and [TcO(OU-BAT)] (**B**), Figure 3, show the two complexes to be essentially isostructural. The N_2S_2 donor set is in the equatorial plane of the square based pyramidal geometry with the oxo group at the apex. The bond distances of Tc-N (2.184 and 2.074Å for **A** and **B** respectively) are consistent with amine-Tc bonding for **A** and Tc-imine bonding for **B**. Under appropriate conditions the two complexes can be interconverted. The retention times of these two species will not be significantly different so as to be able to observe this interconversion, however, the

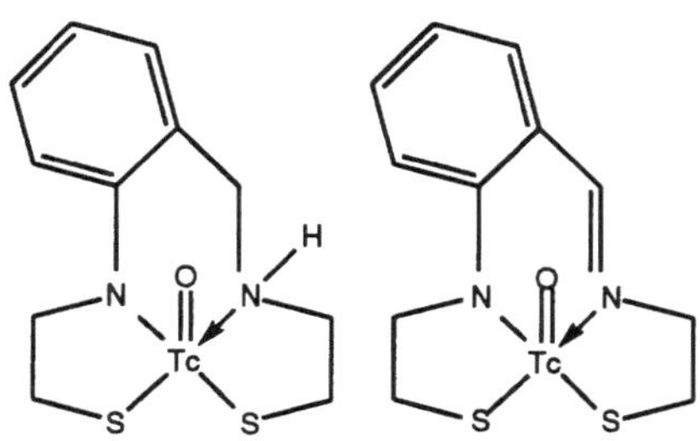

A B

Figure 3

in vivo stability could be different. Such oxidation reactions for coordinated amine ligands could occur for other ligand systems, one such example is the oxidation of PnAO on Ni(II) to an unsaturated imine [12].

Biodistribution of the first generation technetium based imaging agents relied on the size, shape or polarity of the complex. More recent developments, however, have focused on developing technetium complexes with improved organ specificity. This is achieved by the synthesis of complexes which contain biologically active molecules that will have specific uptake *in vivo*. There are three approaches for coordinating a biologically active molecule to technetium which are (i) direct labelling of the biologically active molecule, (ii) use of preformed chelates and (iii) post-conjugation labelling of the chelate ligand coupled to the biologically active molecule. The following consideration of these approaches is based on coordination chemistry, a more biological approach is given elsewhere in this volume.

Direct labelling of the biologically active molecule with technetium has proven successful for the labelling of proteins which have available SH groups which include monoclonal antibodies and fragments [13,14]. The disadvantage to this approach is that the coordination chemistry cannot be controlled or optimised as the identity and characteristics of the binding sites are not understood.

The use of preformed chelates whereby the metal chelate undergoes a process of conjugation to a biologically active molecule via an active group (usually an ester) on the chelate backbone is a more viable approach. The tetrafluorophenyl ester of MAG_3 has been used to prepare ^{99m}Tc-labeled IL2, Interleukin-2, for the detection of immune mediated diseases [15]. The advantage to this approach is that the ligand provides a stable, inert chelation of the metal and minimises non-specific binding of the metal. Figure 4 shows the structures of MAG_3 [16], DADT [5], MAMA [17] and HL15[18] complexes and the site of attachment of the targeting molecule is indicated.

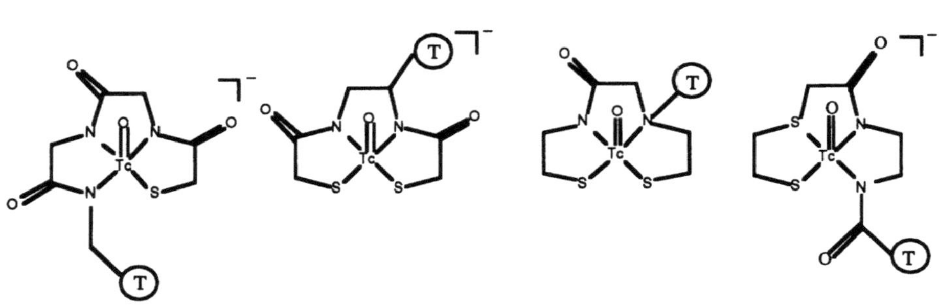

MAG3 DADT MAMA HL15

Figure 4

Post-conjugation labelling is achieved by the synthesis of a chelate ligand with the biologically active molecule attached prior to complexation with technetium [19]. A possible drawback to this approach is the possibility of non-specific, labile binding of the metal to the biologically active molecule.

A potential disadvantage of both conjugation approaches is that the metal chelates are bulky and the size and mass of the complex may impede the biological activity of the conjugated ligands and therefore the *in vivo* distribution. The challenge has been to label receptor-binding, low molecular weight peptides with technetium without loss of receptor binding affinity or specificity. An alternative strategy is to design a metal complex in which the overall shape and external substituents simulate a bioactive molecule and therefore allow specific targeting of the complex. Figure 5A shows the structure of progesterone and a proposed structure of a metal complex Figure 5B which is constructed so as to mimic the steroidal hormone.

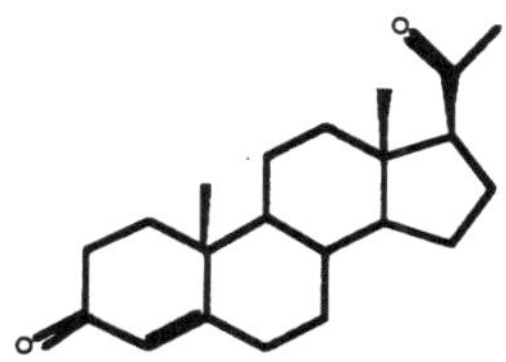

Figure 5A

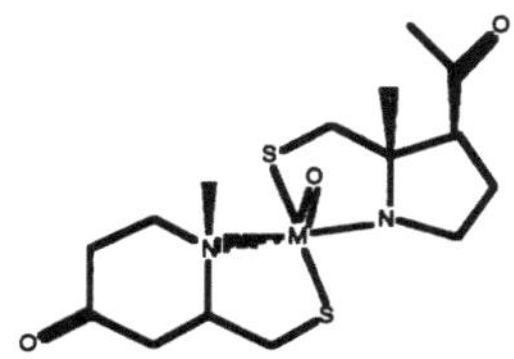

Figure 5B

Figure 6A shows the structure of estradiol and Figure 6B a technetium complex which represents the first steps towards a mimic of the hormone [20]. The ligand periphery incorporates a phenol group which is known to be essential for receptor binding. The complex was found to have quite low receptor-binding affinity (0.014%) which is probably due to the differences between the hormone and complex structures, however, this approach could lead to a new generation of imaging agents.

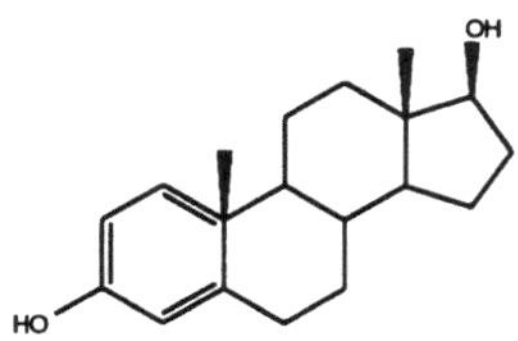

Figure 6A

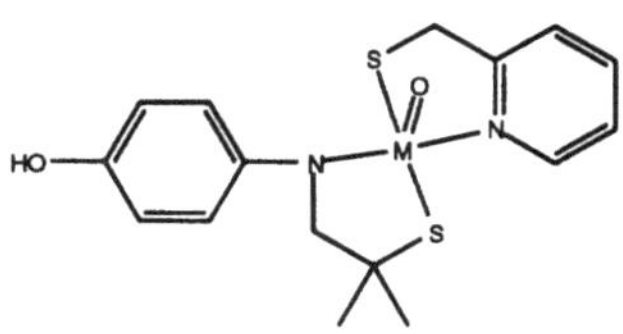

Figure 6B

A variety of rhenium N_2S_2 complexes have been reported and some of these have been referred to above [21]. Due to the difficulties in reduction of Re(VII) to Re(V), an intermediate such as Re-citrate is synthesised prior to reduction to the desired complex. The geometry surrounding the central metal atom is typically square pyramidal with the N_2S_2 ligand occupying the basal plane with the oxo ligand at the apex.

An exception to this was found in the structure of *syn*-[ReO(DL-ECH$_3$)] [22], Figure 7, which contains a N_2S_2 ligand with two carboxylic acid groups one on each side of the ligand and one of the carboxylic acid groups was found to have co-ordinated to the central rhenium atom resulting in the complex attaining an overall octahedral geometry. The carboxyl group is bound cis to the apical oxo ligand leaving the basal coordination plane to have the unusual configuration of NS_2O donor set. Such carboxyl ligation appears to be a common feature of ReO chemistry with such ligands. Conjugation of biologically active molecules to rhenium chelates has been used for specific targeting [7,23].

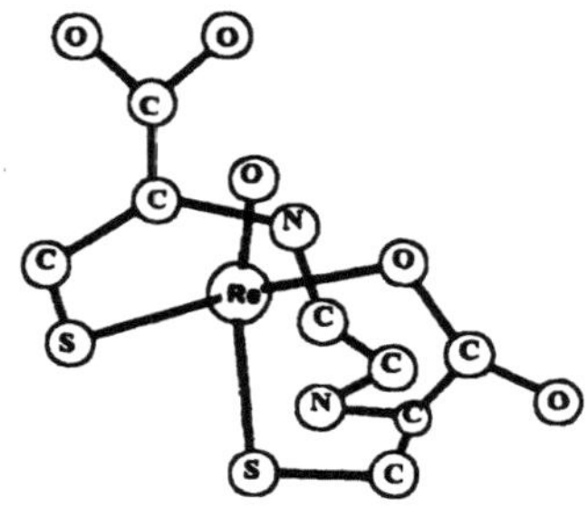

Figure 7

SCHIFF BASES

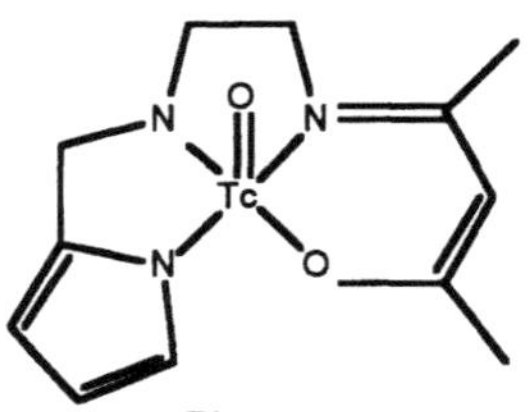

Figure 8

Technetium complexes of Schiff bases which are known are based on the N_3O [24] and N_2O_2[25] ligand framework. [TcO(MRP20)], Figure 8 , is an example of a N_3O complex. In both complexes the Schiff base coordinates in the basal plane with the oxo ligand at the apical site which results in the arrangement of the donor set attaining a square pyramidal geometry around the central technetium atom.

AMINOAMINEOXIMES

[^{99m}Tc-HMPAO] is a cerebral perfusion imaging agent for the evaluation of stroke [26] and is also used to label white blood cells [27]. The structure of the ^{99}Tc complex has been determined by X-Ray crystallography and the technetium geometry is analogous to [TcO(PnAO-1-(2-nitroimidazole))] discussed below [28]. [^{99m}TcO(d,l-HMPAO)] has been shown to be taken up into the brain and then converts to a more hydrophilic species that is unable to diffuse back out of the brain, resulting in significant brain retention [29]. The *meso* analogue undergoes this conversion at a much slower rate so consequently is able to diffuse out of the brain.

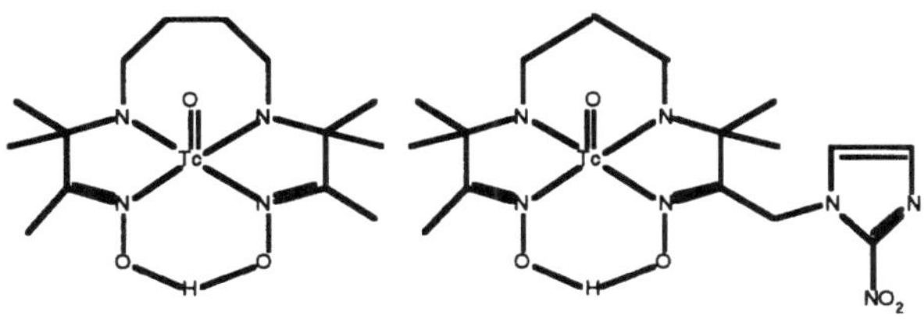

Figure 9A Figure 9B

The nitroimidazole complex, [TcO(PnAO-1-(2-nitroimidazole)] is currently being investigated for imaging hypoxic tissue [30]. The crystal structure of the ^{99}Tc complex was found to have a square-pyramidal geometry about the central technetium (V) atom with the oxo group occupying the apical position, Figure 9B. The plane of the nitroimidazole group is perpendicular to the plane of the four co-ordinated nitrogen atoms, the nitro group is *trans* with respect to the oxo core. The two amines and one oxime are deprotonated giving the complex an overall neutral charge. It has been suggested that the mechanism of uptake for nitroimidazole complexes is the reduction of the nitroimidazole group *in vivo* and subsequent trapping of the product in the hypoxic tissue. This can be contrasted with the technetium BnAO complex, Figure 9A, which has shown uptake into hypoxic tissue [31]. Surprisingly the technetium complex of the analogous nitroimidazole substituted ligand was found to have less uptake into hypoxic tissue than the complex of the unsubstituted ligand. Introduction of a second nitroimidazole substituent onto the ligand was found to reduce further uptake into the hypoxic tissue. The mechanism of uptake into hypoxic tissue remains unclear. The system is discussed in more detail elsewhere in this volume.

N_2S, N_2SO AND NS_3 SYSTEMS

The N_3S complex [^{99m}TcO(MAG$_3$)]$^-$ is widely used as a renal imaging agent [32]. The structure of the analogous ^{99}Tc complex reveals that the ligand adopts a square pyramidal geometry around the central technetium atom with the oxo-core occupying the apical position, Figure 10A [16]. The Tc(V) is above the sulphur and amide donor plane. The carboxylate group is not coordinated and is thought to be necessary for efficient renal clearance. A related complex is that of mercaptoacetyl diglycine ligand (MAG$_2$), [TcO(MAG$_2$)]$^-$, which has the donor set of S,N,N,O and the geometry around the central technetium atom is also square pyramidal with the oxo core at the apex, Figure 10B [33].

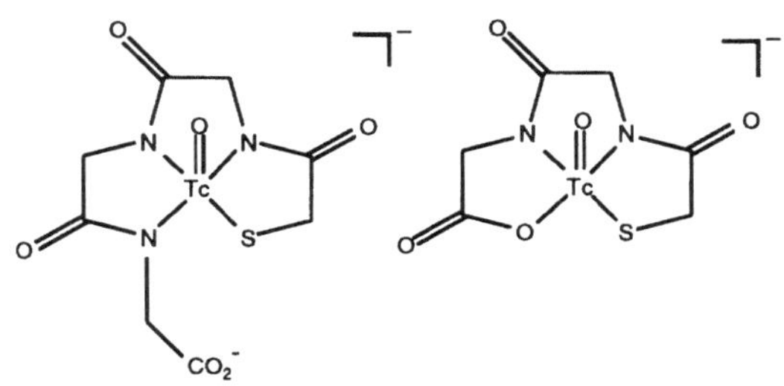

Figure 10A Figure 10B

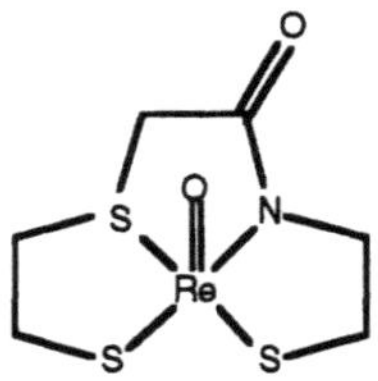

Figure 11

The structure of a rhenium complex of a new hydrophilic tetradentate ligand based on the NS_3 donor set is shown in Figure 11. The overall geometry surrounding the central rhenium atom is closest to being trigonal bipyramidal. This is unusual as all the oxo complexes of the tetradentate N_2S_2/N_3S ligands generally display square based pyramidal geometries [34]. Synthesis of the Re(V) complex can be achieved directly from $[ReO_4]^-$. Reaction of the NS_3 complex with phosphines results in cleavage of the ligand at the thioether sulphur to yield complexes of the type $[ReO(NS_2)(PR_3)]$ containing an unusual tridentate trianionic NS_2 ligand [34].

PHOSPHINE LIGANDS

Phosphorus appears to have a strong stabilising effect on technetium and rhenium complexes, and a number of hybrid donor ligands containing tertiary phosphine groups have been investigated. Technetium and rhenium complexes of the tetradentate mixed amine/phosphine ligand N,N'-bis[2-(diphenylphosphino)phenyl]propane-1,3-diamine, Figure 12, have been synthesised, $[MO(N_2P_2)X]$ where M=Tc or Re and X=Cl, OH, OMe and OEt [35]. The synthesis is successful from $[MO_4]^-$, however, in the case of the rhenium complex significantly higher yields were achieved when starting from the Re(V) precursor $[ReOCl_4]^{--}$. The crystal structures of both the technetium and rhenium complexes show the complexes attain a distorted octahedral configuration with the N_2P_2 donor set occupying the equatorial plane orthogonal to the M=O linkage. A mononegative unidentate nucleophile, such as Cl^-, completes the octahedral geometry. This is a common feature of tetradentate ligands with a maximum dianionic charge of two.

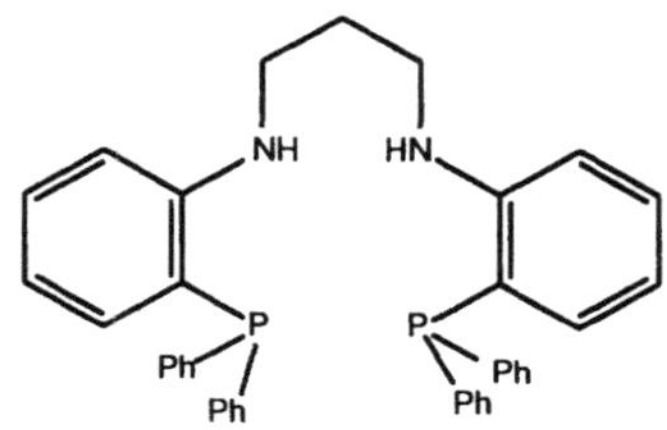

Figure 12

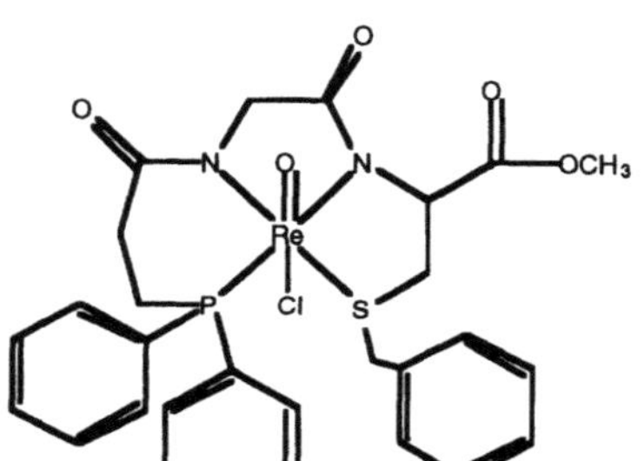

Figure 13

Incorporation of phosphine donors into a peptide backbone has been investigated in an attempt to increase the stability of peptide based complexes of technetium and rhenium. 3-diphenylphosphinopropionylglycyl-L-(S-benzyl)cysteinyl methyl ester (LH_2) is the first example of a phosphine derivatised peptide ligand. In this ligand the phosphine functional group has been coupled to a dipeptide derivative generating a tetradentate ligand, which contains the PN_2S donor atom set. The likely structure of the complex is shown in Figure 13 [36].

Rhenium (V) and technetium(V) complexes of tridentate dibasic phosphine ligand bis(*o*-hydroxyphenyl)phenylphosphine (PO_2H_2) and of the bidentate (*o*-hydroxyphenyl)diphenylphosphine (POH) ligands can be synthesised directly from $[MO_4]^-$ [37]. The complexes have the general formula $[MO(PO_2)(PO_2H)]$ and $[MOCl(PO)_2]$, where M=Tc and Re. Figure 14 shows the proposed octahedral structure of $[TcOCl(PO)_2]$, where one phosphine ligand lies in the equatorial plane and the second ligand spans the equatorial and axial sites.

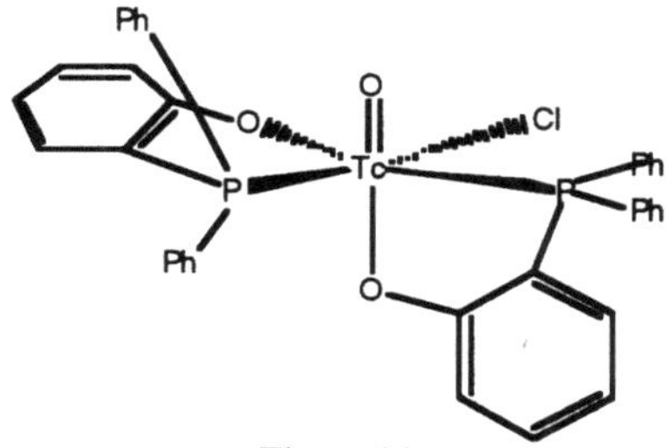

Figure 14

THIOLATE LIGANDS

Complexes containing the potentially tetradentate SSNS ligand such as $[TcO(SCH_2CH_2)_2N(CH_2CH_2R)X]$ where X=Cl or 4-methoxythiophenol and $R=(C_2H_5)_2N$ or C_2H_5S have been synthesised from the reaction of the ligand with $[TcOCl_4]^-$ and Tc(V)-gluconate respectively [38]. The amine Et_2N or EtS groups were found not to have coordinated leaving a tridentate SNS ligand. This type of mixed tridentate/monodentate ligand complex allows for the fine tuning of the biodistribution via manipulation of the monodentate ligand. The structures prove that the complexes attain a trigonal bipyramidal geometry with the basal plane defined by the thiol donors of the tridentate ligand and the oxo group. Biodistribution of the analogous ^{99m}Tc complexes show that there was significant uptake in the brain. Derivatisation of the SNS ligand backbone has been undertaken to produce a series of analogous complexes [39]. It is interesting that contrary to expectations the monodentate SR ligand is stable *in vivo*.

The "3+1" concept of using a mixed tridentate/monodentate ligand set has also been investigated using the tridentate dithiolate ligand $HS\text{-}CH_2CH_2\text{-}X\text{-}CH_2CH_2SH$, where X=O,S or NR. Complexes with the general formula [MO(SXS)(SR)], where M=Tc and Re, were synthesised directly from $[MO_4]^-$ where M=Tc and Re [40]. A representation of the geometry of these complexes is shown in Figure 15. The ligands adopt an overall square pyramidal geometry around the central metal atom with the tridentate/monodentate donors lying in the equatorial plane and the oxo ligand at the apical site.

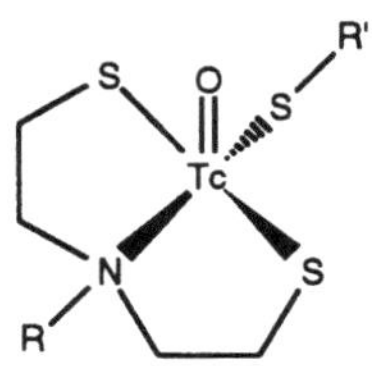

Figure 15

Reaction of $[ReOCl_4]^-$ with the tridentate ligand $HS(CH_2)_2S(CH_2)_2SH$ in the presence of a monodentate thiol such as ethanethiol yields the mixed species [ReO(SSS)(SEt)]. Complexes with highly variable substituents can be synthesised using the mixed tridentate/monodentate ligand approach. In the absence of the monodentate thiol the rhenium (V) species can be isolated [ReO(SSS)Cl]. The crystal structure of this complex shows the geometry surrounding the central rhenium atom to be a distorted square pyramid with the oxo ligand occupying the axial position [41]. Amine/thiolate complexes, [$ReOL_1L_2$] where L_1= $C_2H_5SCH_2CH_2N(CH_2CH_2S)_2$ and L_2=Cl or $SC_6H_4OCH_3$, were synthesised via the rhenium (V) precursors, Re(V)-citrate or [ReO(ethyleneglycol)$_2$] [42]. The structure of the monodentate thiolate complex showed the complex to have a trigonal bipyramidal geometry around the central rhenium atom with the S atom of the monodentate thiol and the N atom of the tridentate ligand occupying the apical positions and the equatorial positions filled by the oxo group and the S atoms of the tetradentate thiol.

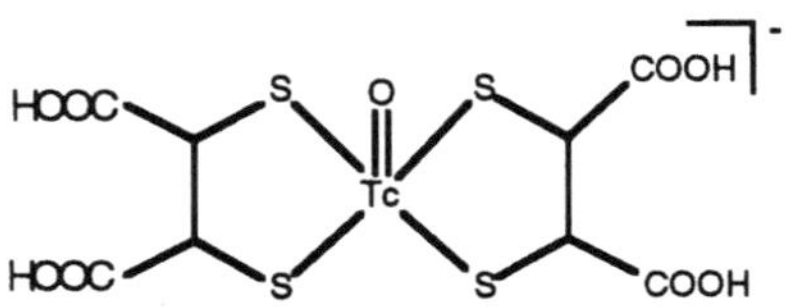

Figure 16

The technetium oxo complex of dimercaptosuccinic acid (DMSA), [$TcO(DMSA)_2$]$^-$ Figure 16, is a commercially available kidney imaging agent [44]. The *meso*-DMSA can adopt three isomer conformations of the carboxylic acid with respect to the Tc=O core. The possibilities are syn-endo, anti or syn-exo orientation. The crystal structure of the ^{99}Tc complex has not been determined to date to confirm which of these isomers is predominant.

HIGHER DENTICITY LIGANDS

^{99m}Tc-pentetate (DTPA) is a renal imaging agent based on the potentially octadentate ligand diethylenetriaminepentaacetic acid. The actual structure of the complex is unclear; there are two possibilities where the oxidation state of the technetium is postulated to be either +4 or +5. The Tc(IV) possibility, Figure 17, contains no oxo-group and two uncoordinating COOH groups. The proposed Tc(V) complex attains an octahedral geometry with a carboxylate group trans to an oxo group and three carboxylates remain uncoordinated [44].

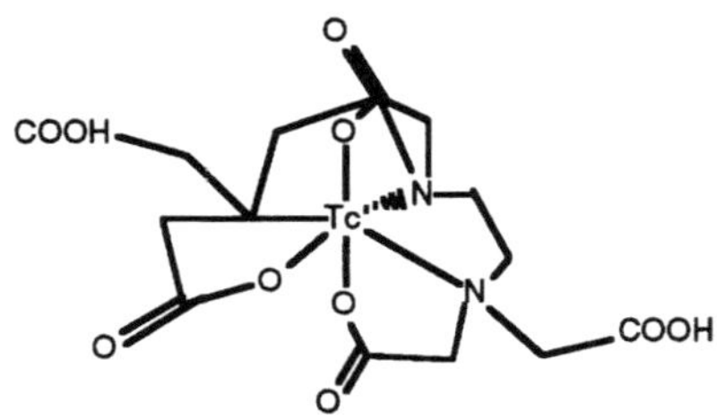

Figure 17

A rhenium-186 complex of (1-hydroxyethylidene) diphosphonate (HEDP) is currently under investigation for use in bone pain palliation [45]. Methylenediphosphonate (MDP) and ethane-1-hydroxy-1,1-diphosphonate complexes of ^{186}Re were synthesised via Sn reduction of perrhenate. Technetium complexes of MDP have been used to image bone.

OTHER LIGANDS

Rhenium complexes of the potentially tridentate diimine ligands di-(2-pyridyl)ketone (DPK) and 2,3-bis(2-pyridyl)benzoquinoxaline (BBQ). $[ReOCl_2(DPK.OH)]$ were synthesised from $[ReOCl_3(PPh_3)_2]$ and the complexes $[MOCl_2(BBQ.OH)]$ were synthesised from $[MOCl_4]^-$, where M= Tc or Re. In both types of complex the overall geometry surrounding the central metal atom was found to be distorted octahedral with the halide ligands and the nitrogen donors occupying the equatorial plane and the oxygen donors occupying the remaining trans positions [46].

The rhenium(VII) complex $[ReO_3\{B(pz)_4\}]$ is easily reduced by PPh_3 to yield a very reactive complex formulated as "$[ReO(-O)\{B(pz)_4\}]_2$". This complex is a suitable precursor for investigation into the chemistry of Re(V). A wide variety of derivatives have been synthesised including $[ReOCl_2\{B(pz)_4\}]$, $[ReO(SPh)\{B(pz)_4\}]$ and $[ReO(C_6H_4O_2)\{B(pz)_4\}]$ [47]. $[TcO(glucoheptonate)_2]^-$ is a kidney imaging agent [44]. The complex is believed to be Tc(V) although the structure has not been determined. Figure 18 shows the proposed structure of the complex, where the glucoheptonate ligands are in the equatorial plane with the oxo ligand at the apex to complete the square pyramidal geometry. The Tc-glucoheptonate complex, like Tc-citrate, is often used as a route into Tc(V) chemistry via ligand exchange.

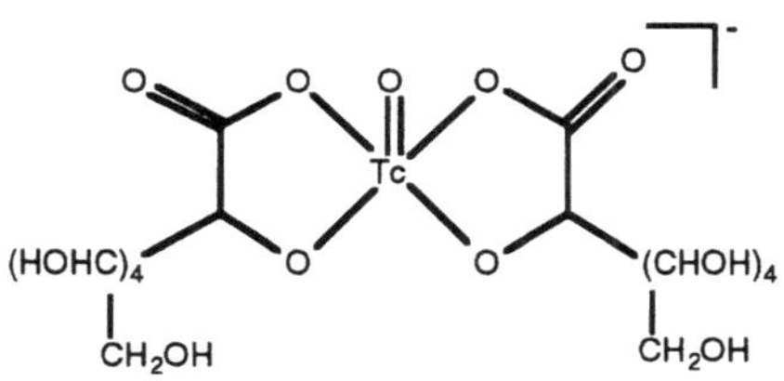

Figure 18

The Dioxo Core

The TcO_2^+ core is thought to be prevalent in no-carrier added concentrations. Neutral nitrogen donor ligands are the most common ligand for the dioxo core. These complexes are generally available directly from $[TcO_4]^-$ with reducing ligands such as diphosphine the pH must be maintained slightly alkaline. One oxo group can be protonated in strong acid to give the $[TcO(OH)]^{2+}$ core. $[TcCl_3(MeCN)(PPh_3)_2]$ has been shown to be a useful precursor into dioxo technetium chemistry [48]. The dioxo complexes can be easily identified by the strong absorbance in the infra-red at ca. 850cm^{-1} which is due to $\nu(M{=}O)$.

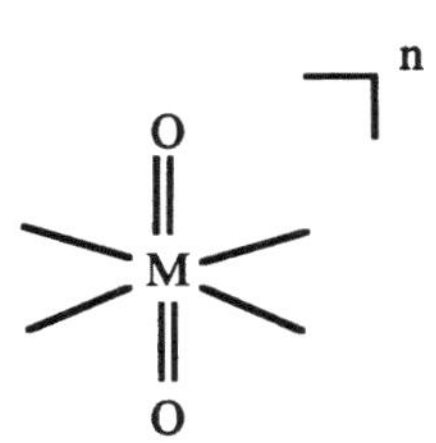

n=0,+1

M(V) M=Tc or Re

The cationic tetraamine dioxo ^{99m}Tc complex in Figure 19 is another example of a preformed chelate complex in which the biologically active molecule, T, is attached for specific targeting. In this case the site of attachment is on the propylene backbone, the incorporation of the chelate is generally carried out during synthesis of the biomolecule. The technetium coordination environment consists of a planar tetraamine ligand with the *trans* dioxo- core [49,50].

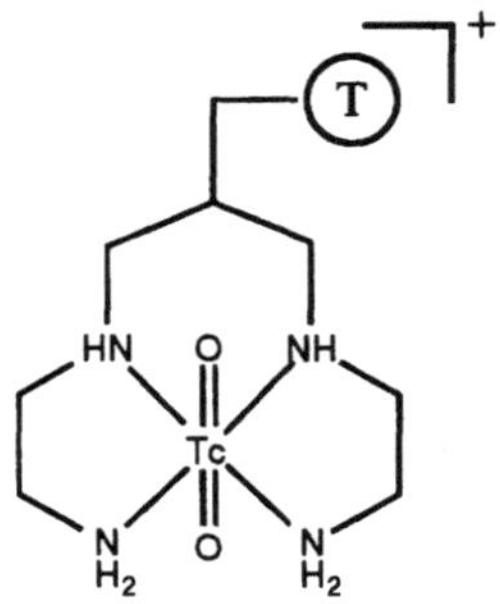

Figure 19

Another nitrogen donor ligand known to stabilise the trans dioxo core is pyridine, $[TcO_2(Py)_4]^+$ is synthesised from the reaction of $[TcOCl_4]^-$ with pyridine and is a widely used precursor for technetium chemistry [51].

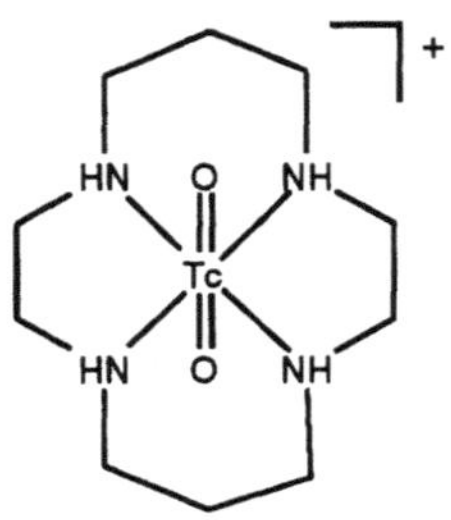

Figure 20

Tetrafosmin, $[TcO_2L_2]^+$, where L is the phosphine 1,2-bis(bis(ethoxyethyl)phosphino)ethane $(EtOCH_2CH_2)_2P(CH_2)_2P(CH_2CH_2OEt)_2$ has been approved as a myocardial perfusion imaging agent [52]. Other co-ligands for Tc=O core include cyclam derivatives (cyclam=1,4,8,11-tetraazacyclotetradecane), Figure 20, which play an important role in diagnostic nuclear medicine as substrates for labelling large proteins and peptides [53, 54].

Dioxo complexes of rhenium cannot be synthesised directly from $[ReO_4]^-$. Complexes of the type $[ReO_2(amine)_2]I$ have been synthesised from the Re(V) precursor $[ReIO_2(PPh_3)_2]$ and amines such as ethylenediamine (en), 1,3-diaminopropane (pn), diethylenetriamine (dien) and triethylenetetramine (trien) [55]. These have the same structures as the Tc analogues discussed above. There are no reports of the synthesis of such complexes directly from $[ReO_4]^-$. The behaviour of the complexes as a function of pH was investigated. $[ReO_2(en)_2]I$ and the 1,3-diaminopropane analogue showed the existence of the protonated species $[Re(OH)_2(amine)_2]^{3+}$ and $[Re(OH)(amine)_2]^{2+}$. In these complexes the site of protonation was found to be the oxo ligand. In contrast the site of protonation for the dien and trien complexes is believed to be the free amine groups on the amine ligand. $[ReO_2(en)_2]I$ and $[ReO_2(pn)_2]I$ are very stable in aqueous solutions whilst $[ReO_2(dien)_2]I$ and $[ReO_2(trien)_2]I$ were found to be rather unstable.

Nitrido-complexes

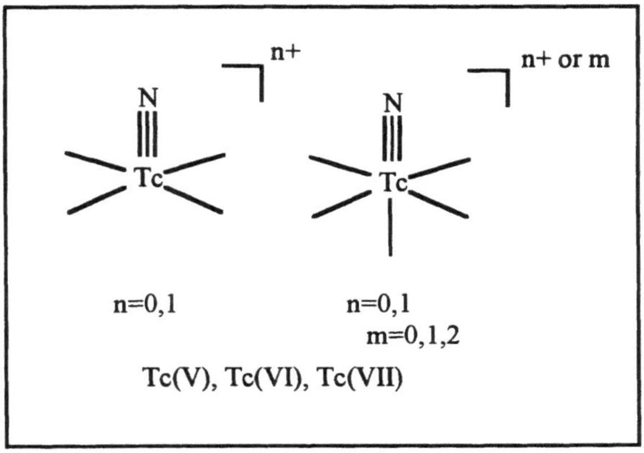

The ability of the Group 7 transition metals to form nitride (M≡N) complexes was first established by Chatt et al in 1964 with the characterisation of $[ReCl_2N(PPh_3)_2]$ [56]. The synthesis of the Tc analogue using a directly analogous route from $[TcO_4]^-$ and hydrazine in the presence of the phosphine did not however follow until 1981[57]. The chemistry of the Tc nitrido-core was initially developed largely by Baldas and co-workers, and early in an extensive series of papers they reported an alternative route to the key precursor $[TcNCl_4]^-$ using the reaction of azide with pertechnetate in acid solution [58]. This nitride formally contains Tc(VI) and is paramagnetic. They also reported the synthesis and structure (Figure 21) of the dithiocarbamato-complex $[TcN(S_2CNEt_2)_2]$ [59]. It transpires that five coordinate square pyramidal geometry is relatively common for nitrido-complexes and reflects the orbital requirements of the strongly π-donating nitride ligand and its very high *trans* effect which labilises any ligand in a *trans* coordination site.

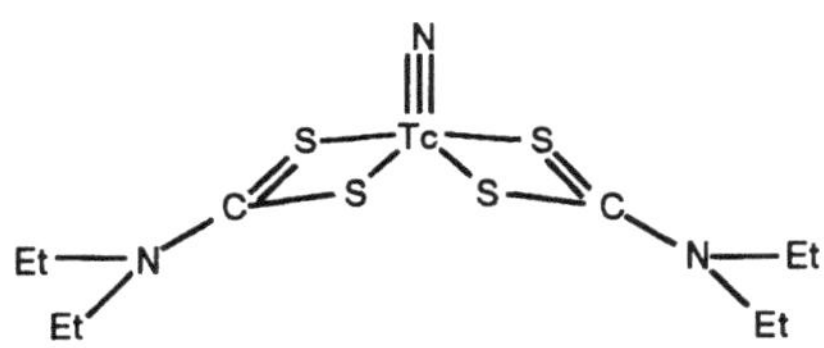

Figure 21

The analogous dithiocarbamato nitride with N-ethyl-N-ethoxy substituents (TcNOET) shows considerable promise as a myocardial imaging agent [60]. It differs from other heart imaging agents in not having a positive charge, and the details of the mechanism by which it is accumulated in the heart remain to be determined. An essential feature of the viability of the complex for pharmaceutical use has been the development of a high yield synthesis from N-methyl-S-methyldithiocarbazate and $[TcO_4]^-$ (^{99}Tc or ^{99m}Tc) in the presence of a tertiary phosphine as reducing agent [61]. This generates an intermediate of uncertain structure containing the nitride ligand which however can be readily derivatised with a wide range of polydentate ligands to give nitride complexes in high yields. The lower overall charge on the $[Tc{\equiv}N]^{2+}$ core as compared with $[Tc{=}O]^{3+}$ means that in complexes with comparable ligands the nitrides will generally be more negatively charged. Some recent comparisons of the biological behaviour of oxo and nitrido-complexes of DADS and MAG_3 support this view [62].

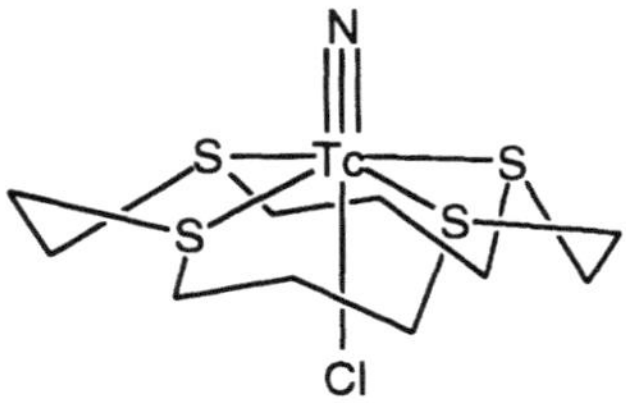

Figure 22

The substitution chemistry of $[TcNCl_4]^-$ has been studied in detail, and recent examples include cationic complexes of the type [TcNCl(TCE)] where TCE = a macrocyclic thiacrown ether [63] (see Figure 22). Other co-ligands for the Tc≡N core include EDTA, EDDA and DTPA [64], SNO donor tridentate ligands [65], an amido-sugar Schiff base ligand (from $[TcNCl_2(PPh_3)_2]$) [66] and a tetradentate bis(thiosemicarbazone) ligand [67]. The substitution chemistry of $[TcNCl_2(PMe_2Ph)_3]$ with a wide range of bidentate and monodentate ligands has also been studied in detail [68]. Much of the substitution chemistry described in this paragraph has thus far been mostly restricted to technetium-99 and it remains to be seen if it can be universally successfully extrapolated to the technetium-99m level.

Although as indicated above rhenium nitrides can be generated from $[ReO_4]^-$, there are as yet no reported examples of rhenium nitrides with the ^{186}Re and ^{188}Re isotopes.

Imido-complexes

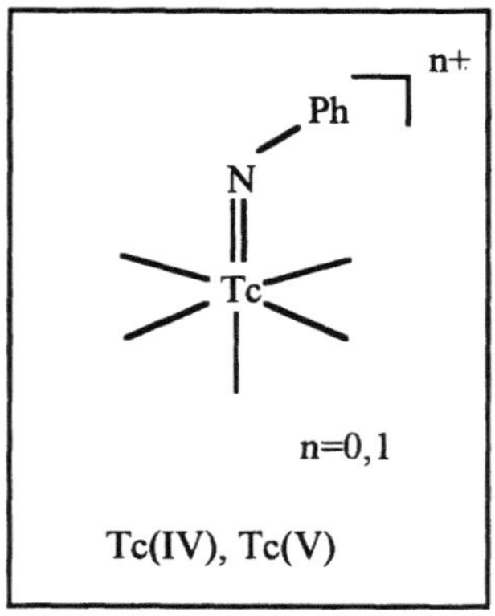

The imido-ligand M=NR (R=alkyl or aryl) is formally isoelectronic with the oxo-ligand and also functions as dianionic ligand. An important distinction from the oxo-ligand is that imide rarely acts as a bridging ligand and the much reduced *trans* effect means that five coordination with a vacant site trans to imide is not found. In the majority of its complexes the lone pair of electrons on nitrogen is involved in the metal nitrogen multiple bond and formally six electrons are donated to the metal[1]. Rhenium(V) imido-complexes such as $[ReCl_3(NPh)(PPh_3)_2]$ were first reported in the 1960's and 70's from reaction of oxo-complex precursors with aromatic amines [56], phosphinimines [69], or hydrazines of the type ArNHNHCOR [69]. Much later it was shown that the technetium analogue $[TcCl_3(NPh)(PPh_3)_2]$ can also be prepared from aromatic amines and $[TcOCl_4]^-$ [70] and the complex has the structure (for Ar = 4-tolyl) shown in Figure 23.

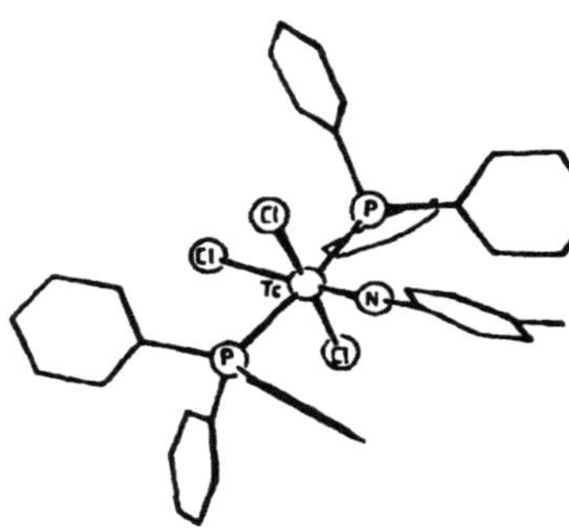

Figure 23

[1] If imide is regarded as dianionic, the convention for electron counting for the metal is that it donates 6 electrons

The Tc-N distance of 1.78Å is consistent with a strong Tc-N multiple bond. A key development of this imide chemistry in a radiopharmaceutical context was the demonstration that the imido-core can be generated from $[TcO_4]^-$ by reaction with the hydrazines $ArNHNHCOCH_3$ in the presence of triphenylphosphine [71].In order for imides to be viable as radiopharmaceuticals it is also necessary to replace the PPh_3 by smaller more hydrophilic ligands, and there have been extensive studies on the substitution chemistry of $[TcCl_3(NPh)(PPh_3)_2]$. Reaction with neutral ligands such as phosphines generally produces cationic complexes such as $[TcCl_2(NPh)(PMe_2Ph)_3]^+$ [72] or with diphosphines the paramagnetic Tc(IV) complexes $[TcCl(NPh)(P\text{-}P)_2]^+$ (P-P = bidentate diphosphine) [69]. However with anionic ligands there is generally replacement of the imide ligand by an oxo-group, presumably due to hydrolysis to the aromatic amine [69,73]. This can be prevented by the use of bulky ligands such as 2,6-disubstituted aromatic thiols and stable complexes of the type $[Tc(NPh)(SAr)_4]^-$ have been isolated and structurally characterised. [73]. In view of the requirement for small, neutral and hydrophilic complexes this comparative instability of the imide core does not augur well for its use in actual imaging agents, although astute selection of the co-ligand may yet produce appropriate compounds. There are also no reports to date of the imide chemistry being successfully extended to the technetium-99m isotope. Also although there is an extensive reported chemistry of rhenium imido-complexes, this has not been extrapolated to the radioactive Re isotopes.

Finally mention should be made of the remarkable complexes $[TcX(NAr)_3]$ (X=I, CH_3 etc, Ar= 1.2,6-$Pr^i{}_2C_6H_3$) which are prepared from pertechnetate by reaction with Me_3SiNAr in aprotic solvents [74].These strikingly demonstrate the predilection for Tc to form M-N multiple bonds. The complexes are stable to aerial oxidation and reduction, but their behaviour in protic media has not been reported.

Hydrazido (2-) complexes

The hydrazido (2-) ligand is analogous to both oxo- and imido- and acts formally as a dianionic ligand and shares with imide a reluctance to act in a bridging mode, a relatively small *trans* influence and the formal donation of six electrons when regarded as dianionic.

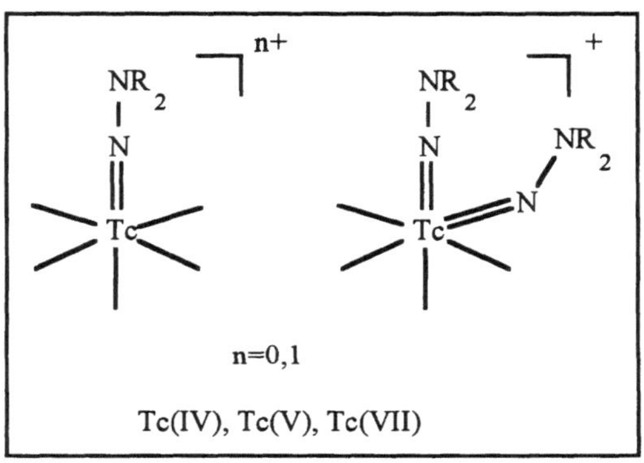

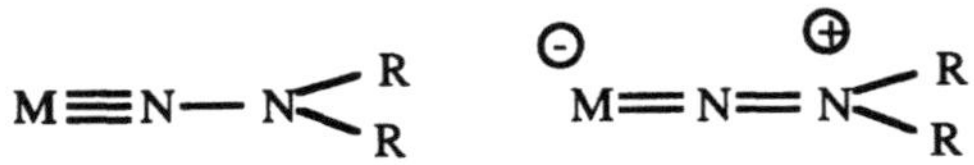

A B

Figure 24

However a significant difference from imide (and oxo-) is the possibility of the involvement of canonical form B in which the hydrazide ligand has an overall neutral charge (see figure 24). An accumulating body of evidence suggests that in many hydrazido complexes form B plays a significant part and the formal overall charge on the NNR_2 ligand is less than 2.

The technetium(V) hydrazide complexes $[TcCl_3(NNR_2)(PPh_3)_2]$ (R_2 = Me_2 ,MePh, Ph_2) were first prepared from simple reaction of $[TcOCl_4]^-$ with one equivalent of the appropriate hydrazine in methanol [75].The X-ray crystal structure is shown in Figure 25. The short Tc-N distance of 1.734(5)Å confirms a strong Tc-N multiple bond, and the N-N distance of 1.285(7)Å indicates a degree of N-N multiple bonding consistent with a contribution from resonance form B above (an N-N single bond is ca 1.41Å). It was subsequently shown that hydrazides could be generated directly from pertechnetate by reaction with the hydrazine hydrochloride. The reducing power of the hydrazines ensures that no additional reducing agent is required. The nature of the intermediate so produced is not clear (as with the nitride synthesis discussed above), but addition of a ligand such as dithiocarbamate (dtc) gives the cationic, formally Tc(VII) complexes $[Tc(NNR_2)_2(dtc)_2]^+$ in high yield. In contrast to the well known dioxo-complexes of Tc(V) the hydrazide ligands are *cis* rather than *trans*. Reaction of the intermediate with bidentate phosphines gives the Tc(IV) complexes $[TcCl(NNR_2)(P\text{-}P)_2]^+$ which were shown by X-ray crystallography to have the structure shown schematically in Figure 26.

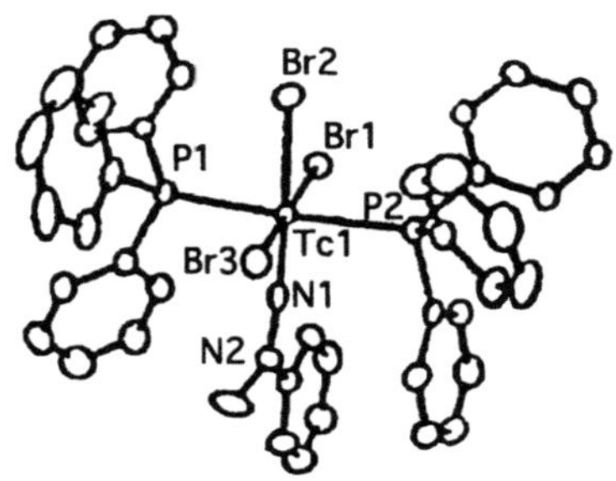

Figure 25

A promising feature of the chemistry of these ligands in radiopharmaceutical terms is that they appear to be far more robust towards hydrolysis than the corresponding imides [76]. In common with imido and diazenido- (see below) complexes they share the possibility of optimising biodistribution by altering the hydrazide substituents and using these as the site of attachment of biological targeting molecules.

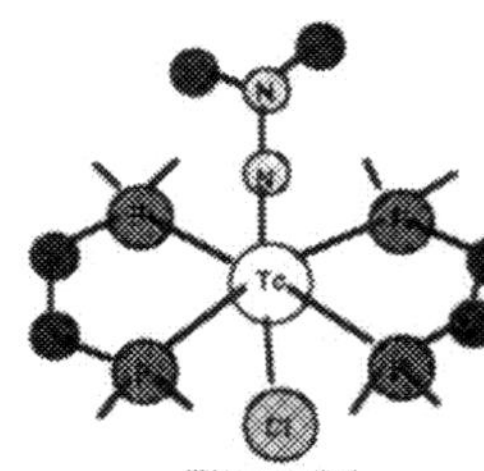

Figure 26

Much of this hydrazide chemistry is available for Re using $[ReO_4]^-$ as precursor, and work is currently in progress to extend it to the radioactive isotopes of Tc and Re.

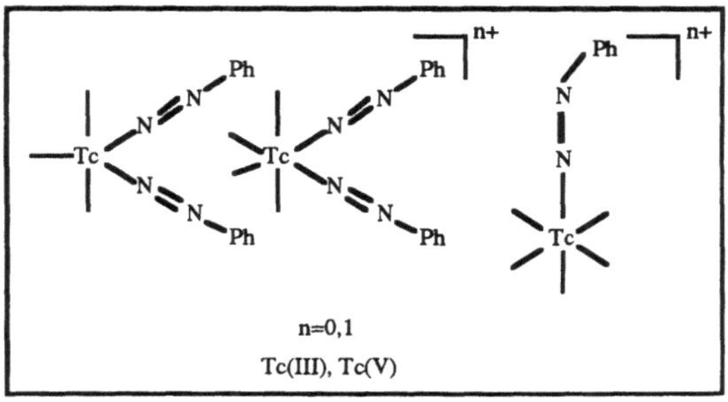

Diazenido-complexes

The diazenide ligand (M-N=N-R) is formally analogous to nitrosyl and can donate four or two electrons to the metal depending on whether the lone pair of electrons on the nitrogen adjacent to the metal is involved in the M-N bond (see Figure 27) and is generally regarded as being monoanionic. R can in principle be alkyl or aryl, but to date there are no reported examples of technetium alkyl diazenide complexes.

Aryldiazenide complexes can be prepared for other metals from the corresponding diazonium salts, but the most commonly used route involves the reaction of a suitable metal precursor with an aryl hydrazine. This latter route was used independently by two research groups [77,78,79] to prepare $[TcCl(NNAr)_2(PPh_3)_2]$, the first reported technetium diazenide complex, from $[TcOCl_4]^-$ in the presence of PPh_3.

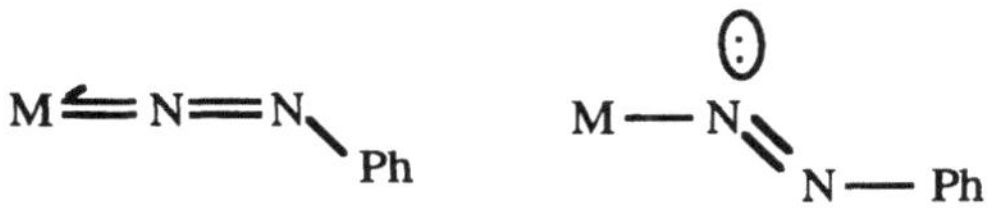

Figure 27

The X-ray structure of this complex with Ar = C_6H_4Cl-4 showed as expected the same trigonal bipyramidal geometry found (Figure 28) for the Re analogue prepared some years earlier [80]. The two diazenide ligands lie in the equatorial plane, and the linear M-N-N systems indicate that the ligands are formally donating four electrons each to the metal. The substitution chemistry of this species has been investigated in some detail [81], and complexes such as $[Tc(NNPh)(salen)(PPh_3)]^+$ (salen = N,N-bis(2-hydroxybenzylidene)-1,4-diazabutane) and $[TcCl(NNPh)(P\text{-}P)_2]^+$ where P-P is a bidentate tertiary diphosphine. The X-ray crystal structure of the former is shown in Figure 29 .

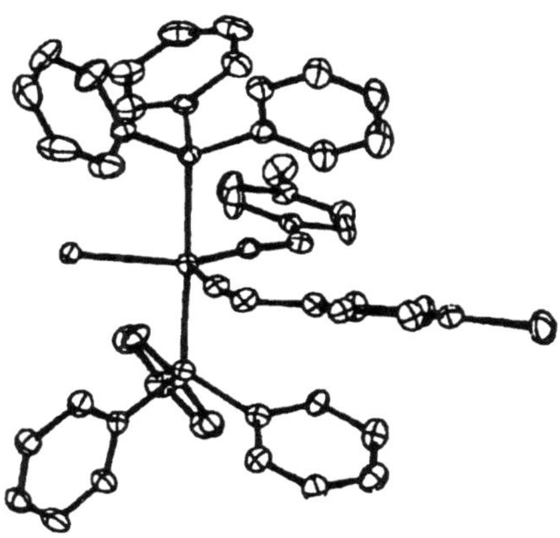
Figure 28

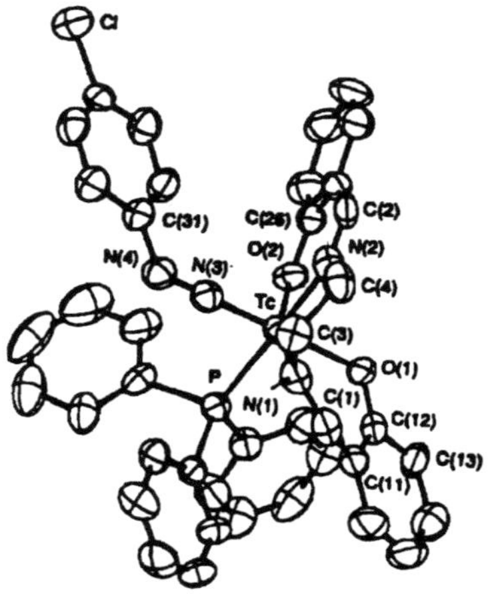

Figure 29

One of the diazenide ligands is lost in these reactions and although its fate is not certain, the free hydrazine is probably formed. The single diazenide ligand has a linear M-N-N system, consistent with the formal donation of four electrons. It has also been shown that these diazenido-complexes can be prepared directly from pertechnetate by reaction with an arylhydrazine hydrochloride in combination with an appropriate co-ligand [81]. The vast majority of the Tc diazenide complexes reported to date have phosphine co-ligands and the only other type of complex reported is $[Tc(NNAr)_2(dtc)_2]^+$ (dtc = dithiocarbamate). Much remains to be done to understand fully the coordination chemistry of the Tc diazenide core.

As mentioned above, an attractive possibility for the hydrazido and diazenido cores is to use the core substituents to control the biodistribution. This principle has been elegantly exploited by the use of a 2-hydrazinopyridine with a succinimidyl activated ester group in the 4-position (HYNIC, see Figure 30) [82]. This is first coupled to the biologically active molecule and the conjugated system so formed is then reacted with pertechnetate to give species with Tc bound to the protein, presumably via diazenide or hydrazide type ligation. However these have as yet not been characterised at the 99-Tc level. The related aryldiazenides $[TcCl(NNC_6H_4COOsuc\text{-}4)(P\text{-}P)_2]^+$ have been totally characterised with 99-Tc [83], but work on the extension to 99m-Tc is still in progress.

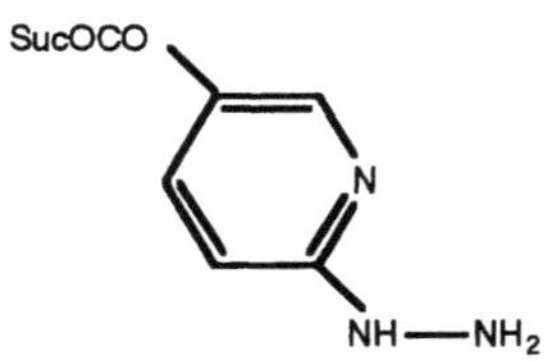

Figure 30

In a recent paper [84] the HYNIC system has been used to label a protein that is an antagonist for the IIb/IIIa receptors on platelets. Efficient labelling of the protein was achieved, but with tricine as co-ligand HPLC showed that several Tc-containing species were obtained. In an attempt to simplify the coordination chemistry at technetium the more powerful tetradentate chelating ligand EDDA (ethylenediaminediaacetic acid) was used. However even in this case, although higher stability was achieved, there is still evidence for slow conversion to other species. It was suggested that the principal species present is a hydrazido complex (ie a diazenide protonated at the pyridine substituted nitrogen) such as shown in Figure 31 where X is probably chloride.Such a complex could subsequently rearrange to any of several different isomers with different relative orientations of the donor groups (eg diazenide *cis* to X).

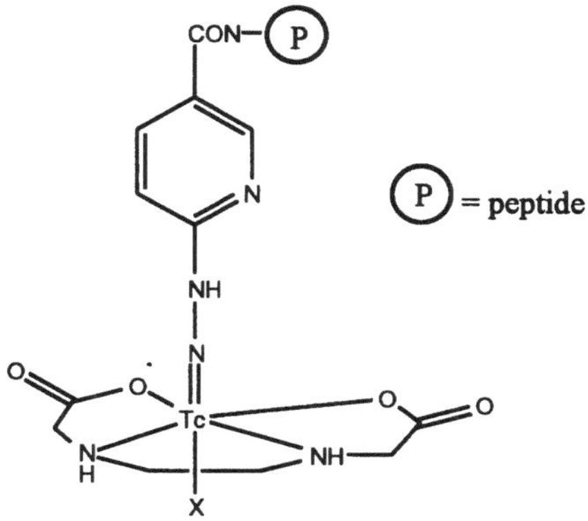

Figure 31

It will be of considerable interest to see if these proposals can be supported by structural studies at the technetium-99 level, and the problems encountered emphasise the need for greater understanding of the fundamental coordination chemistry of diazenido and hydrazido cores.

Lower oxidation state complexes

In the absence of multiply bonded core ligands the oxidation state of the technetium is inevitably lower, and in this section the formal oxidation states span I to IV. The dominant geometry is octahedral for radiopharmaceutically relevant ligand systems.

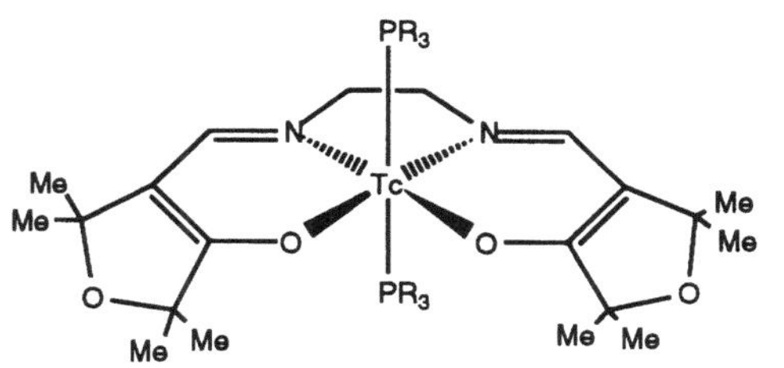

Figure 32

For the Tc(III) state a common synthetic route can be regarded as oxygen abstraction from Tc(V) oxo-complexes with a tertiary phosphine and is exemplified by the synthesis of complexes of the type $[TcL(PR_3)_2]$ (where L = tetradentate dianionic Schiff base ligand) [85,86]. The synthesis can be carried out directly from pertechnetate and the species Q12 (Figure 32) is being evaluated as a myocardial perfusion agent. The well established Cardiotec™ agent is also Tc(III) and comprises a boron-capped tris-dioxime ligand system [87]. A number of other new Tc(III) complexes have been fully characterised including complexes of phosphinothiols such as $[Tc(Ph_2PC_6H_4S\text{-}2)_3]$ [88,89] and $[Tc(SCH_2CH_2PPh_2)_2(SCH_2CH_2Ph_2PO\text{-}S)]$ [89], $[Tc(S_4)(SPh)_2]^-$ (where S_4=$[S(CH_2)_2SCH_2\text{-}]_2$ [90]. The former complex is unusual in having five coordination with one of the phosphinothiolate ligands only bound via the thiolate sulphur.

The Tc(I) oxidation level is surprisingly easily accessible from pertechnetate with even quite modestly reducing ligands. The hexakis(isocyanide) Tc cation is now well established as the basis of the Cardiolite™ heart imaging agent and it has recently been shown that Tc(I) carbonyl complexes of the type $[TcX_3(CO)_3]^{2-}$ can be prepared in high yield from pertechnetate in THF/diglyme using BH_3.THF as reductant [91]. The BH_3 reductant is not necessary if reducing ligands such as tertiary phosphines are present and complexes such as $[TcCl(CO)_3(PPh_3)_2]$ can be obtained in good yield [92]. The carbonyl anions are particularly reactive towards substitution, and a range of $[Tc(CO)_3L_3]^+$ (L=neutral donor) complexes are accessible, some of the reactions proceeding in methanol or even in water. Comparable chemistry can also be carried out for Re, starting from $[ReO_4]^-$. There are no reports of this chemistry for the 99m-Tc isotope, but the stability of some of the complexes in aqueous media is promising in this respect.

At first thought traditional organometallic chemistry might appear inappropriate for radiopharmaceutical applications. However, the development of the synthesis of complexes of the type $[Tc(arene)_2]^+$ directly from $[^{99m}TcO_4]^-$ [93] showed that such complexes are sufficiently stable *in vivo* to show myocardial uptake. An elegant recent development has been the synthesis of estradiol derivatives joined to a $[(\eta^5-C_5H_5)Re(CO)_3]$ fragment via an acetylenic linker [94] (Figure 33). Remarkably the 11-CH_2Cl derivative shows a significantly higher binding at 25°C to estradiol receptors than the free steroid. This was attributed to the ability of the acetylene linked Re unit to locate under the steroid ring system, minimising steric constraints for the binding of the 17-OH group to suitable receptor sites. It remains to be shown if this synthetically demanding chemistry can be carried out from radioactive $[ReO_4]^-$.

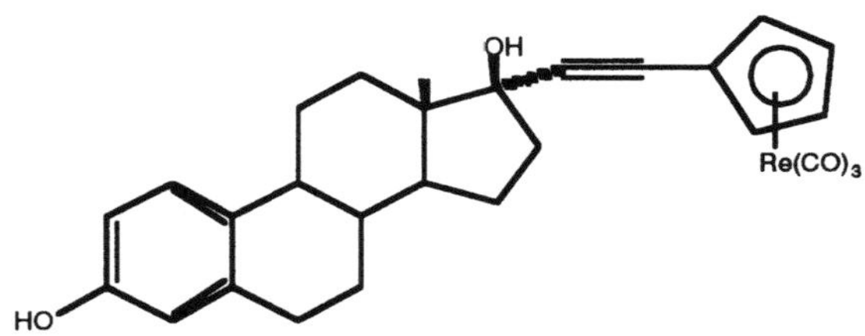

Figure 33

Table 1. Structures of polydentate ligand/TcO species

Donor Set.	Ligand type.	Example.	Acronym.	^{99}Tc/^{99m}Tc	Ref
Cl, Br, I	Halides	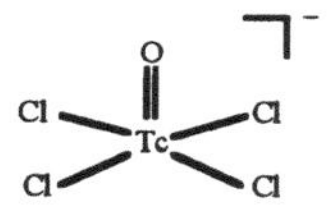	-	^{99}Tc	95
O_2	Diolates, glycolates	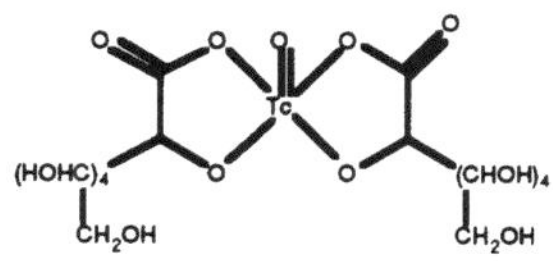	Gluco-heptonate	^{99}Tc/^{99m}Tc	44
S, S_2	Thiolates, dithiolates, dioxalates	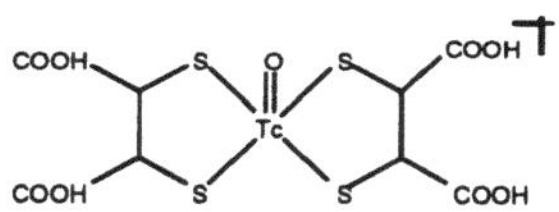	DMSA	^{99}Tc/^{99m}Tc	44
SOS, SNS	Tridentate dithiolates plus monodentate thiolate	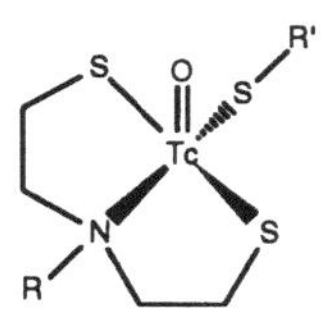	-	^{99}Tc/^{99m}Tc	38, 40
ONO, ONS, ONN	Tridentate Schiff bases	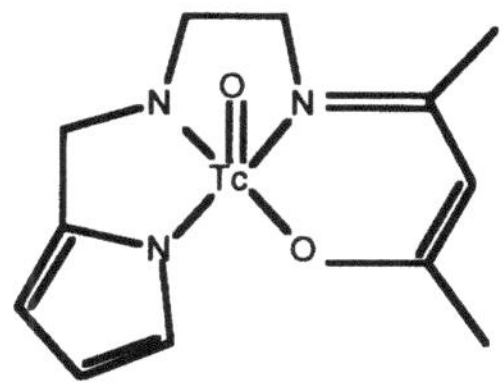	-	^{99}Tc/^{99m}Tc	24
SNNS	Diamine-dithiolates	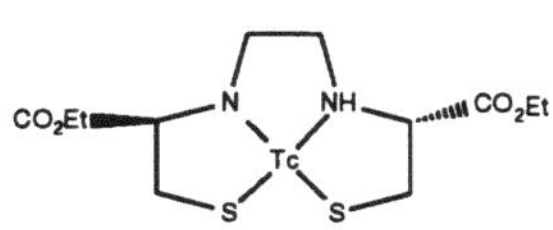	**ECD**, BAT, DADT	^{99}Tc/^{99m}Tc	1,2, 5,9 11, 96, 97
ONNO	Tetradentate Schiff bases	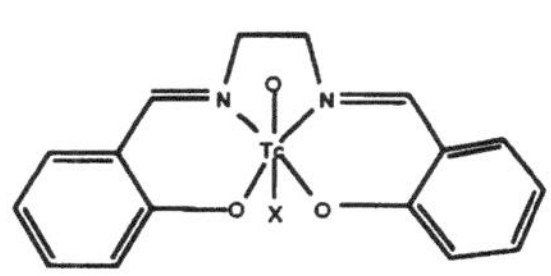	Salen	^{99}Tc/^{99m}Tc	25

Table 1 (cont.). Structures of polydentate ligand/TcO species

SNNN	Mercapto-acetyl triglycine	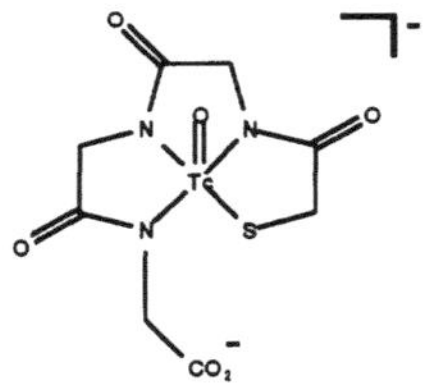	MAG_3	$^{99}Tc/^{99m}Tc$	16
NNNN	Aminoamine oximes	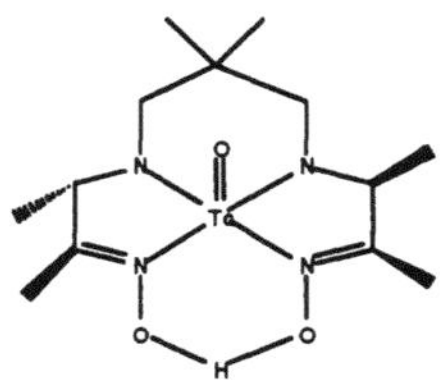	**HMPAO**, PnAO	$^{99}Tc/^{99m}Tc$	28, 98
SNNO	Mercaptoacetyl diglycine	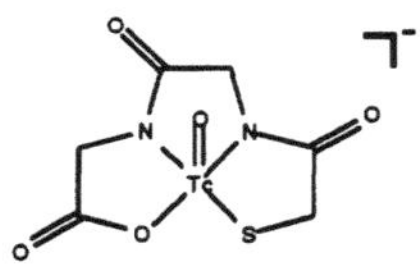	MAG_2	$^{99}Tc/^{99m}Tc$	33
NPPN	Diamine-phosphines	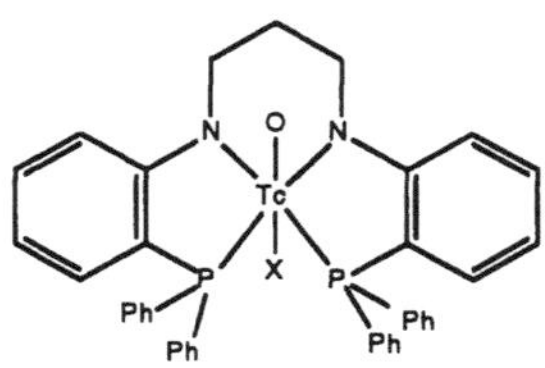	-	^{99}Tc	35
PO	Hydroxy-phosphines	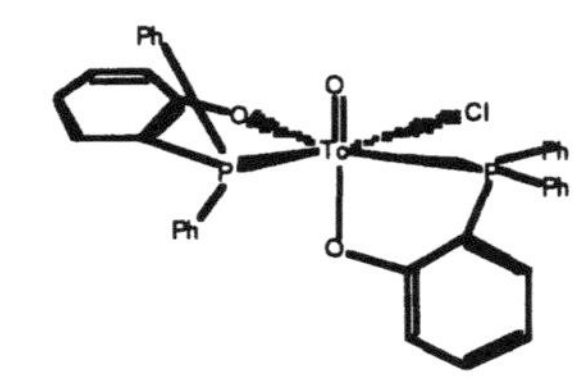	-	^{99}Tc	37

References

1. (a) Deutsch, E.: Perspectives on the history, present and possible future of technetium and rhenium in nuclear medicine. In technetium and rhenium in chemistry and nuclear medicine 4, Ed. Nicolini, M., Bandoli, G., Mazzi, U., SG Editoriali, Padova, 1995, pXXV.
(b) Tisato, F., Refosco, F., Bandoli, G.: Structural survey of technetium complexes, Coord. Chem. Rev.; 1994, 135, 325.
2. (a) Walovitch, RC., Makuch, J., Knapik G., Watson, AD., Williams, SJ., Picard, M., Franceschi, M., Zimmerman, RE., Holman, BL.: Metabolism of Tc99m-ECD in normal volunteers. J. Nucl. Med.; 1988, **29**, 747.
(b) Cheesman, EH., Blanchette, MA., Ganey, MV., Maheu, LJ., Miller, SJ., Watson A. D.: Technetium-99m ECD: ester derivatised diaminedithiol technetium complexes for imaging brain perfusion. J. Nucl. Med.; 1988, **29**, 788.
3. Scheffel, U., Goldfarb, HW., Lever, SZ., Gungon, RL., Burns, HD., Wagner HD.: Comparison of technetium-99m aminoalkyl diaminodithiol (DADT) analogs as potential brain blood flow imaging agents. J. Nucl. Med.; **1988**, **29**, 73.
4. Mahmood, A., Halpin, WA., Baidoo, KE., Sweigart, DA., Lever, SZ.: Acta Crystallog. C: Cryst Struct. Commun. Structure of a neutral N-alkylated diamine dithiol (DADT) Tc-99(V) complex. *syn*[TcO(NET-TMDADT)]; 1991, **47**, 254.
5. (a) Jones, A., Davison, A. DePamphilis, B.: Preparation and crystal structure of tetraphenylarsonium bis(2- mercaptoethanolato) oxotechnetate. Inorg. Chem.; 1981, **20**, 1617.
(b) Kasina, S., Fritzberg, AR., Johnson, DL., Eshima, D.: Tissue distribution properties of technetium-99m diamide-dimercaptide complexes and potential use as renal radiopharmaceuticals. J. Med. Chem.; 1986, **29**, 1933.
6. Rao, TN., Adhikesavalu, D., Camerman, A. and Fritzberg, AR.: Technetium(V) and rhenium(V) complexes of 2,3- bis(mercaptoacetamido)propanoate. Chelate ring stereochemistry and influence on chemical and biological properties. J. Am. Chem. Soc.; 1990, **112**, 5798.
7. Lui, S. and Edwards, DS.: New N_2S_2 diamidedithiol and N_3S triamidethiols as bifunctional chelating agents for labelling small peptides with technetium-99m. In technetium and rhenium in chemistry and nuclear medicine **4**. Ed. Nicolini, N., Bandoli G., Mazzi, U., SG Editorali, Padova; 1995, 383.
8. Guhlke, S., Diekmann, D., Zamora, PO., Knapp, FF., and Biersack H.J.: MAG_3 p-nitrophenyl ester for ^{99m}Tc and ^{188}Re labelling of amines and peptides. In technetium and rhenium in chemistry and nuclear medicine **4**. Ed. Nicolini, N., Bandoli G., Mazzi, U., SG Editorali, Padova; 1995, 363.
9. Shultze, LM., Todaro, L J., Baldwin, RM., Byrne, EF. and McBride, BJ.: Synthesis, characterisation and crystal structure of neutral rhenium(V) complexes with S-substituted N_2S_2 ligands. Inorg. Chem.; 1994, **33**, 5579.
10. Mahmood , A., Wolff, JA , Davison A. and Jones AG.: Technetium and rhenium complexes of amine amide dithiol ligands: ligand synthesis and metal complexes. In technetium and rhenium in chemistry and nuclear medicine **4** Ed. Nicolini, N , Bandoli G., Mazzi, U., SG Editorali, Padova; 1995, 211.
11. Francesconi, LC., Yang, YY., Kung, M-P., Zhang, XX., Billings, JP., Guo, Y-Z. and Kung H. F.: Technetium-99m *N,N'*- Bis(2-mercapto-2-methylprpoyl)-2-aminobenzylamine: Technetium-99m complexes of a novel Bis(aminoethanethiol) ligand. J. Med. Chem.; 1994, 37, 3282.
12. Vassian, EG. and Murmann, RK.: Aromatization of an aliphatic amine oxime Nickel(II) complex by molecular oxygen. Inorg. Chem.; 1967, **6**, 2043.
13. Rhodes, BA.: Direct labelling of proteins with^{99m}Tc. Nucl. Med. Biol., 1991, **18**, 667.
14. Thakur, ML., Marcus, CS., Hennemann, P., Butler, J , Sinow, R., Liu, H., et al.: Imaging inflamatory diseases with neutrophil (PMN) specific technetium-99m monoclonal antibody (MAB). J. Nucl. Med., 1991, **32**, 1836.
15. Chianelli, M., Signore, A., Sobnack, R., Fritzberg, AR , Britton, KE. and Mather, SJ.: 99m-Tc-Interleukin-2: A new radiopharmaceutical for the *in vivo* detection of lymphocytic infiltration. In technetium and rhenium in chemistry and nuclear medicine **4**. Ed. Nicolini, N., Bandoli G., Mazzi, U., SG Editorali, Padova; 1995, 551.

16. Grummon, G., Rajagopalan, R., Palenik, GJ., Koziol, AE. and Nosco, DL.: Synthesis and characterisation and crystal structures of technetium(V)-oxo complexes useful in nuclear medicine. 1. Complexes of Mercaptoacetylglycylglycylglycine (MAG_3) and its methyl ester derivative (MAG_3OMe). Inorg. Chem.; 1995, **34**, 1764.
17. DiZio, JP., Anderson, CJ., Davison, A., Erhardt, GJ., Carlson, KE., Welch, MJ. and Katzenellenbogen J. A.: Technetium- and rhenium-labeled progestins: Synthesis, receptor binding and in vivo distribution of an 11β-substituted progestin labeled with technetium-99 and rhenium-186.J. Nucl. Med.; 1992, **33**, 558.
18. Archer, CM., Canning, LR., Duncanson, P., Gill, HK., Griffiths, DV., Hughes , JM., Kelly, JD., Pitman, MA., Storey, AE. and Tran, AM.: New hydrophilic ligands for ^{99m}Tc-based radiopharmaceuticals. In technetium and rhenium in chemistry and nuclear medicine **4**. Ed. Nicolini, N., Bandoli G., Mazzi, U., SG Editorali, Padova; 1995, 177.
19. Lister-James, J., McBride, WJ., Buttram, S., Civitello, ER., Martel, LJ., Pearson, DA., Wilson, DM. and Dean, RR.: In technetium and rhenium in chemistry and nuclear medicine **4**. Ed. Nicolini, N., Bandoli G., Mazzi, U., SG Editorali, Padova; 1995, 269.
20. Chi, DY., O'Neil, JP., Anderson, CJ., Welch, MJ. and Katzenellenboggen, JA.: Homodimeric and heterodimeric Bis(amino thiol) oxometal complexes with rhenium(V) and technetium(V). Control of heterodimeric complex formation and an approach to metal complexes that mimic steroid hormones. J. Med. Chem.; 1994, **37**, 928.
21. Chi, DY., Wilson, SR. and Katzenellenbogen, JA.: Crystal structure of a Bis(amido)bis(thiolato)oxorhenium(V) complex that forms a methanol-solvated salt with calcium extracted from silica gel. Inorg. Chem.; 1995, **34**, 1624.
22. Hansen, L., Lipowska, M., Taylor Jr, A. and Marzilli, LG.: A new and unexpected arrangement for a $Re^{V}=O(N_2S_2)$ complex. The donor set in the basal plane is NOS_2. Inorg. Chem.; 1995, **34**, 3579.
23. Breitz, H., Weiden, P., Vanderheyden, J-L., Appelaum, J., Bjorn, M., Fer, M., Wolf, S., Ratliff, B., Seiler, C., Foise, D., Fisher, D., Schroff, R., Fritzberg, A. and Abrams, P.: Clinical experience with Rhenium-186 labeled monoclonal antibodies for radioimmunotherapy: Results of phase I trials. J. Nucl Med.; 1992, **33**, 1099.
24. Morgan, G., Deblaton, M., Hussein, W., Thornback, J., Evard, G., Durant, M., Stach, J., Abram, U. and Abram, S.: Rhenium(V) and technetium(V) complexes with N-[2(1*H*-pyroylmethyl)]-N'-(4-pentene-3-one-2)ethane-1,2-diaminale ($C_{12}H_{16}N_3O$, MRP20). X-ray crystal structures of H_3MRP 20 and TcO(MRP 20). Inorg. Chim. Acta; 1991, **190**, 257.
25. Jurrison, DS., Dancey, K., McPartlin, M., Tasker, PA. and Deutsch, E.: Synthesis and characterisation, and electrochemical properties of technetium complexes containing both tetradentate Schiff Base and monodentate tertiary phosphine ligands: Single-Crystal Structure of *trans*-(*N*, *N*'-Ethylenebis(acetylacetone iminato))bis(triphenylphosphine)technetium(III) hexafluorophosphate. Inorg. Chem.; 1984, **23**, 4743.
26. Leonard JP., Nowotnik DP. and Neirinckx RD. J.: Technetium-99m D,L HMPAO a new radiopharmaceutical for imaging regional brain perfusion using Spect - a comparison with I-123 HIPDM. Nucl. Med.; 1986, **27**, 1819.
27. Solanki, KK., Mather, SJ., Al-Janabi, M. and Britton, KE.: A rapid method for the preparation of Tc-99m hexametazime labelled leucocytes. Nucl. Med. Commun.; 1988, **9**, 713.
28. Fair, CK., Troutner, D.E., Schlemper, EO., Murrmann, RK. and Hoppe, M. L.: Oxo[3,3'-(1,3-propane-diyliimino)-bis(3- methyl-2-butanone oximato)(3-)-N,N',NN'',N''']technetium (V), $[TcO(C_{13}H_{25}N_4O_2]$. Acta Cryst.; 1984, **C40**, 1544.
29. Neirinckx, RD., Burke, JF., Harrison, RC., Forster, AM., Andersen, AR. and Lassen, NA.: The retention mechanism of technetium-99m-HM-PAO: intracellular reaction with glutathione. J. Cereb. Blood Flow Metab.; 1988, **8**, S4.
30. Linder, K., Chan, YW., Cyr, JE., Malley, MF., Nowotnik, DP. and Nunn, AD.: TcO(PnAO-1-(2-nitroimidazole)) [BMS- 181321], a new technetium-containing nitroimidazole complex for imaging hypoxia: Synthesis, characterisation, and xanthine oxidase-catalyzed reduction. J. Med. Chem.; 1994, **37**, 9.

31. Archer, CM., Edwards, B., Kelly, JD., King, AC., Burke, JF. and Riley, A. L. M.: Technetium labelled agents for imaging tissue hypoxia *in vivo*. In technetium and rhenium in chemistry and nuclear medicine **4**. Ed. Nicolini, N., Bandoli G., Mazzi, U., SG Editorali, Padova; 1995, 535.
32. Verbruggen, AM.: A new renal imaging agent based on mercaptoacetyl triglycine (MAG_3). Eur. J. Nucl. Med.; 1990, **7**, 346.
33. Johannsen, B., Noll, B., Leibnitz, P., Reck, G., Noll, S. and Spies, H.: Technetium and rhenium complexes of mercapto- containing peptides 1. Tc(V) and Re(V) complexes with mercaptoacetyl diglycine (MAG_2) and X-ray structure of $AsPh_4[TcO(MAG_2)].C_2H_5OH$. Inorganica Chimica Acta; 1993, **210**, 209.
34. Dilworth, JR. and Al-Jebori M. Unpublished Results.
35. Tisato, F., Refosco, F., Meresco, A., Bandoli, G., Dolmella, A. and Bolzati, C.: Synthesis and structural characterisations of six-coordinate oxo-M(V) complexes (M=Tc, Re) containing a tetradentate P_2N_2-phosphino-amido ligand. Inorg. Chem.; 1995, **34**, 1779.
36. Santimaria, M., Maina, T., Mazzi, U. and Nicolini, M.: *Trans*-Oxochloro[3-Diphenylphosphinopropionylglycinato-L-(S-Benzyl)CysteinatoMethylEster-P,N,N',S]Rhenium(V): Synthesis, characterisation and HPLC analysis. In technetium and rhenium in chemistry and nuclear medicine **4**. Ed. Nicolini, N., Bandoli G., Mazzi, U., SG Editorali, Padova; 1995, 149.
37. Luo, H., Setyawati, I., Rettig, SJ. and Orvig, C.: Rhenium(V) and techentium(V) complexes of Bis(*o*- hydroxyphenyl)phenylphosphine (PO_2^{2-}) and (*o*-Hydroxyphenyl)diphenylphosphine (PO^-) ligands. Inorg. Chem.; 1995, **34**, 2287.
38. Mastrostamatis, SG., Papdopoulos, MS., Pirmettis, IC., Paschali, E., Varvarigou, AD., Stassinopoulou, CI, Raptopoulou, CP., Terzis, A. and Chiotellis, E.: Tridentate ligands containing the SNS donor atom set as a novel backbone for the development of technetium brain-imaging agents. J. Med. Chem.; 1994, **37**, 3212.
39. Spyriounis, DM., Pelecanou, M., Stassinopoulou, CI., Raptopoulou, CP., Terzis, A. and Chiotellis, E.: Synthesis and characterisation of oxotechnetium(V) complexes with aza-subsituted 2,6-Dimethyl-4-azaheptane-2,6-dithiol ligands and benzyl mercaptan as coligand. Inorg. Chem.; 1995, **34**, 1077.
40. Spies, H., Fietz, T., Glaser, M., Pietzsch, HJ. and Johannsen, B.: The "n+1" concept in the synthesis strategy of novel technetium and rhenium tracers. In technetium and rhenium in chemistry and nuclear medicine **4**. Ed. Nicolini, N., Bandoli G., Mazzi, U., SG Editorali, Padova; 1995, 243.
41. Fietz, T., Spies, H., Pietzsch, HJ. and Leibnitz, P.: Synthesis and molecular structure of chloro(3-thiapentane 1,5- dithiolato)oxorhenium(V). Inorganica Chimica Acta; 1995, **231**, 233.
42. Papadopoulos, M., Primettis, I., Raptopoulou, CP., Terzis, A. and Chiotellis, E.: Synthesis and characterisation of oxorhenium(V) complexes of tripodal NS_3 containing a monodentate ligand as coligand. In technetium and rhenium in chemistry and nuclear medicine **4**. Ed. Nicolini, N., Bandoli G., Mazzi, U., SG Editorali, Padova; 1995, 223.
43. Pietzsch, H., Spies, H., Leibnitz, P., Reck, G. and Johannsen, B.: Technetium and rhenium complexes with multidentate thioether ligands. In technetium and rhenium in chemistry and nuclear medicine **4**. Ed. Nicolini, N., Bandoli G., Mazzi, U., SG Editorali, Padova; 1995, 231.
44. Ponto, JA., Chilton, HM. and Watson, NE.: Pharmaceuticals in medical imaging, Swanson, DP., Chilton, HM., Thrall, JH., Eds., Macmillan Publishing Co., New York; 1990, 501.
45. Maxon, HR., Schroder, LE., Thomas, SR., Hertzberg, VS., Deutsch, EA., Scher, HI., Samarantunga, RC., Libson, KF., Williams, CC., Moulton, JS. and Schneider, HJ.: Re186(Sn)HEDP for treatment of painful osseous metastases: Initial clinical experience in 20 patients with hormone-resistant prostate cancer. Radiology; 1990, **176**, 155.
46. Gerber, TIA., Adendorff, H., Jacobs, R., du Preez, JGH. and Bandoli G.: Angular strain as driving force for nucleophilic attack on diimines in complexes of rhenium(V) and technetium(V). In technetium and rhenium in chemistry and nuclear medicine **4**. Ed. Nicolini, N., Bandoli G., Mazzi, U., SG Editorali, Padova; 1995, 189.
47. Paulo, A., Domingos, A., Marcalo, J., Pires de Matos, A. and Santos, I.: Reactivity of a tetra(pyrazolyl)borate oxorhenium complex. Inorg. Chem.; 1995, **34**, 2113.

48. Riche, F. , Vidal, M., Bolzati, C., Uccelli, L. and Duatti, A.: $Tc(IV)Cl_4(PPh_3)_2$ and $Tc(III)Cl_3(CH_3CN)(PPh_3)_2$ as precursor into *Trans* dioxo technetium(V) complexes with chelating amine and tetraazamacrocycles. Inorg. Chem.; 1995, **231**, 147.
49. Maina, T., Stolz, B., Albert, R., Nock, B., Bruns, C. and Macke, H.: Synthesis, radiochemical and biological evaluation of $^{99m}Tc[N4\text{-}(D)PHE^1]$-Octreotide. In technetium and rhenium in chemistry and nuclear medicine **4**. Ed. Nicolini, N., Bandoli G., Mazzi, U., SG Editorali, Padova; 1995, 395.
50. Nock, B., Koch, P., Evard, F., Paganelli, G. and Macke, H.: $^{99m}TcN_4$-Lys-Biotin, a new biotin derivative useful for pretargeted avidin-biotin immunoscintigraphy: Synthesis, evaluation and comparison with other ^{99m}Tc-biotin conjugates. In technetium and rhenium in chemistry and nuclear medicine **4**. Ed. Nicolini, N., Bandoli G., Mazzi, U., SG Editorali, Padova; 1995, 429.
51. Kastner, E., Fackler, PH., Clarke, MJ. and Deutsch, E.: Synthesis and structure of *trans*-$[O_2(TBP)_4Tc]^+$ (TBP=4-*tert*-Butylpyridine) and related complexes. Inorg. Chem.; 1984, **23**, 4683.
52. Lahiri, A., Higley, B., Smith, T., Crawley, J., Edwards, B., Archer, C., Chiu, W., Latham, I. and Kelly, D.: Myocardial perfusion imaging in man using new ^{99m}Tc-labelled diphosphine complexes. Nucl. Med. Communications; 1989, **10**, 245.
53. Delmon-Moingeon, LI., Mahmood, A., Davison, A., and Jones, A.: J. Nucl. Biol. Med.; 1991, **35**, 47.
54. Simon, J., Troutner, DE., Volkert, WA. Radiochemical characterisation of Tc-cyclam. J.: Radiochem. Radioanal. Lett.; 1981, **47**, 111.
55. Kremer, C., Dominguez, S., Chinea, E., Mederos, A. and Kremer, E.: Synthesis, characterisation and potentiometric studies of rhenium(V) dioxo complexes with acyclic polyamine ligands. In technetium and rhenium in chemistry and nuclear medicine **4**. Ed. Nicolini, N., Bandoli G., Mazzi, U., SG Editorali, Padova; 1995, 197.
56. Chatt, J., Garforth, JD., Johnson, NP., Rowe, GA.: Nitrido and arylimido complexes of rhenium, J. Chem. Soc.; 1964; 1012.
57. Kaden, K., Lorenz, B., Schmidt, K., Sprinz, H., Wahren, M.: Nitridokomplexe des technetium(V) Isotopenpraxis; 1981, 17, 174.
58. Baldas, J., Bonnyman, J., Williams, GA.: Studies of technetium complexes 9. Use of tetrachloronitridotechnetate(VI) anion for the preparation of nitrido complexes of technetium. Crystal structure of bis(8-quinolinethiolato)nitridotechnetium(V): Inorg. Chem.; 1986; 25; 150.
59. Baldas, J., Bonnyman, J., Pojer, PM., Williams, GA., Mackay, MF.: Synthesis and structure of bis(diethyldithiocarbamato)nitridotechnetium(V); J. Chem. Soc. Dalton Trans.; 1981; 1798.
60. Pasqualini, R., Duatti, A.: Synthesis and characterisation of the new neutral myocardial imaging agent $[^{99m}TcN(noet)_2]$ (noet = N-ethyl-N-ethoxydithiocarbamato): J. Chem. Soc. Chem. Commun.; 1992; 1354.
61. Pasqualini, R., Duatti, A., Bellande, E. et al: Bis(dithiocarbamato)nitrido technetium-99m radiopharmaceuticals: a class of neutral imaging agents; J. Nucl. Med.; 1994; 35, 334.
62. Mang'era, KO., Bellande, E., Vanbilloen, H., Boonen, C., Pasqualini, R., Verbruggen, AM.; Comparative evaluation of the biological behaviour of ^{99m}Tc-nitrido and ^{99m}Tc-oxo complexes of LJL-EC and L,L-ECD, In the Technetium and rhenium in chemistry and nuclear medicine 4, Ed. Nicolini, M., Bandoli, G., Mazzi, U., SG Editorali, Padova, 1995, p405.
63. Pietzsch, H-J, Spies, H., Liebritz, P., Reck, G., Johannsen, B.: Technetium and rhenium complexes with multidentate thioether ligands, In technetium and rhenium in chemistry and nuclear medicine 4, Ed. Nicolini, M., Bandoli, G., Mazzi, U., SG Editorali, Padova, 1995, p231.
64. Takayama, T., Kane, Y., Sekine, T., Yoshihara, K., Kudo, H.: Synthesis and characterisation of nitridotechnetium complexes of EDTA, EPDA and DPTA. In technetium and rhenium in chemistry and nuclear medicine 4, Ed. Nicolini, M., Bandoli, G., Mazzi, U., SG Editorali, Padova, 1995, p33.
65. Cros, G., Coulais, Y., Tahor, HB., Gleizes, A., Guirand, R.: Synthesis and chacterisation of oxo- and nitrido-complexes and 99m-technetium(V) and rhenium(V) with new SNO and SN_2O ligands. Biodistribution studies of the related 99m-Tc complexes. In technetium and rhenium in chemistry

and nuclear medicine 4, Ed. Nicolini, M., Bandoli, G., Mazzi, U., SG Editorali, Padova, 1995, p85.

66. Vicelli, L., Bolzati, C., Zucchini, GL., Marinelli, M., Duatti, A.: Synthesis of a nitrido technetium complxes containing an amido-sugar-Schiff base ligand. In technetium and rhenium in chemistry and nuclear medicine 4, Ed. Nicolini, M., Bandoli, G., Mazzi, U., SG Editorali, Padova, 1995, p165.
67. Bellande, E., Laine, J., Comazzi, V. et al. Preparation and biodistribution of bis(thiosemicarbazone)nitrido technetium(V) complexes. Evaluation as potential blood flow tracers. In technetium and rhenium chemistry and nuclear medicine 4. Ed. Nicolini, M., Bandoli, G., Mazzi, U., S.G. Editoriali, Padova, 1995, p333.
68. Abram, U., Ritter, S., Hubener, R.: Mixed ligand technetium and rhenium complexes with metal nitrogen multiple bonds. In technetium and rhenium in chemistry and nuclear medicine 4, Ed. Nicolini, M., Bandoli, G., Mazzi, U., SG Editorali, Padova, 1995, p45.
69. Chatt, J., Dilworth, JR.: Novel routes to organoimido-complexes of molybdenum, rhenium and osmium: Chem. Commun.: 1972, 519.
70. Dilworth, JR., Thompson, RM., Archer, CM., Kelly, JD., Povey, DC. New technetium cores with metal nitrogen multiple bonds. The synthesis and characterisation of Tc(V) and Tc(IV) imido-complexes. In Technetium and Rhenium in Chemistry and Nuclear Medicine 3. Ed. Nicolini, M., Bandoli, G., Mazzi, U., New York Raven Press, 1990, 109.
71. Nicholson T, Davison A, Jones AG; The synthesis of technetium imido-complexes from pertechnetate. Inorg. Chim. Acta: 1991, 187, 51.
72. Nicholson, T., Davison, A., Jones, AG, Zubieta JA, Chen Q.: The synthesis and characterisation of a cationic phenylimido complex. The X-ray crystal structure of $[TcCl_2(NPh)(PMe_2Ph)_3][BPh_4]$. Inorg. Chim. Acta; 1995, 230, 205.
73. Nicolson, T., Cook, J., Davison, A., Jones, AG.: Reactions of the technetium(V) phenylimido complex $[TcCl_3(NPh)(PPh_3)_2]$ with aromatic thiolate ligands (where X=Cl,Br). Inorg. Chim. Acta: 1994, 218, 97.
74. Burrell, A., Clark, D., Gordon, P., Sattelburger, A., Bryan, J.: Synthesis and molecular and electronic structures of tris(arylimido)technetium(V) and tris(arylimido)technetium(VI) complexes derived from successive one electron reductions of tris(arylimido)-iodotechnetium(VII). J. Amer. Chem. Soc.: 1994, 116, 3873.
75. Archer, CM., Kelly, JD., Dilworth, JR., Povey DC, Smith, GW.: The synthesis of technetium hydrazide complexes. In Technetium and Rhenium in Chemistry and Nuclear Medicine 3. Ed. Nicolini, M., Bandoli, G., Mazzi, U. New York Raven Press, 1990, p159.
76. Coutinho, B., Dilworth, JR., Thompson, RM., Archer, CM., Kelly, JD.: Imido complexes of technetium and rhenium. In Technetium and Rhenium in Chemistry and Nuclear Medicine 4, Ed. Nicolini, M., Bandoli, G., Mazzi, U. SG Editorali, Padova, 1995,p 81.
77. Archer, CM., Dilworth, JR., Jobanputra, P., Thompson, RM., McPartlin, M., Hiller, W.: Technetium diazenido complexes I. The synthesis and structures of $[TcCl(NNC_6H_4Cl\text{-}4)_2(PPh_3)_2]$ and $[TcCl(NNPh)(Ph_2PCH_2CH_2PPh_2)_2][PF_6]$. J. Chem. Soc. Dalton Trans., 1993, 897.
78. Archer, CM., Dilworth, JR., Jobanputra, P., McPartlin, M. and Hiller, W.: Development of new technetium cores containing metal-nitrogen multiple bonds. Synthesis and characterisation of some diazenido hydrazido and imido complexes of technetium. Polyhedron; 1990; 9, 1497.
79. Nicholson T, de Vries N, Davison A, Jones AG; Synthesis and chracterisation of aryldiazenido complexes of technetium and their protonation reactions. The X-ray structure of $[TcCl(NNC_6H_4Br\text{-}4)_2(PPh_3)_2]$. In technetium and rhenium in chemistry and nuclear medicine 3. Ed. Nicolini M, Bandoli g, Mazzi U; New York Raven Press, 1990, p95
80. Dilworth, JR., Harrison, SA. Walton, DRM. and Schweda, E.: The preparation and protonation of $[ReBr(N_2Ph)_2(PPh_3)_2]$. The structure of $[ReBr_2(N_2Ph)(NNHPh(PPh_3)_2]$, a complex with hydrazido(2-) ligand with a large angular distortion. Inorg. Chem.: 1985; 24, 2594.
81. Dilworth, JR., Jobanputra, P., Thompson, RM., Povey, D.C., Archer, CM., Kelly, JD.: Technetium diazenido-complexes II. The preparation of $[TcCl(NNC_6H_4\text{-}Cl)_2(PPh_3)_2]$ from $[TcO_4]$ and its substitution chemistry. The crystal and molecular structure of cis-$[Tc(salen)(NNC_6H_4Cl\text{-}4)(PPh_3)_2]$. J. Chem. Soc. Dalton Trans.; 1994, 1251.

82. Schwartz, DA., Abrams, MJ., Mauser, MM. et al: Preparation of hydrazido-modified proteins and their use for the synthesis of ^{99m}Tc-protein conjugate. Bioconjugate Chem.; 1991; 2, 334.
83. Continho, B., Dawson, D., Dilworth, JR. et al.: Towards new radiopharmaceutical agents based on technetium and rhenium complexes with metal-nitrogen multiple bonds. In technetium and rhenium in chemistry and nuclear medicine 4. Ed. Nicolini, M., Bandoli, G., Mazzi, U., SG Editoriali, Padova, 1995, p3.
84. Liu, S., Edwards, S., Looby, RJ. et al.: Labelling a hydrazino-nicotinamide-modified cyclic IIb/IIIa receptor antagonist with ^{99m}Tc using aminocarboxylates as co-ligands. Bioconjugate Chem.; 1996, 7, 63.
85. Marmion, M., DeRosch, M., Bushman, M. et al.: Radiopharmaceutical development of Technescan Q12. In technetium and rhenium in chemistry and nuclear medicine 4. Ed. Nicolini, N., Bandoli, G., Mazzi, U., SG Editorali, Padova, 1995, p253.
86. Jurrisson, S., Dancey, K., McPartlin, M., Tasker, P., Deutsch, E.: Synthesis and characterisation and electrochemical properties of technetium complexes containing both tetradentate Schiff base ligands and monodentate tertiary phosphine ligands; single crystal X-ray structure of trans(N,N'-ethylene bis(acetylacetano iminato)bis(triphenylphosphine) technetium(III) hexafluorophosphate. Inorg. Chem., 1984, 23, 4743.
87. Treler, EN., Francesconi, LC., Gougontas JZ., Malley, MF., Nunn, AD.: Mono-capped tris(dioxane) complexes of technetium(III). Synthesis and structural characterisation of [TcX(dioxime)$_3$Br]. Inorg. Chem.; 1989, 28, 3411.
88. Dilworth, JR., Hutson, AJ., Morton, S. et al.: The preparation and electrochemistry of technetium and rhenium complexes of 2-diphenylphosphinobenzenethiol. The crystal and molecular structures of [M(Ph$_2$PC$_6$H$_4$S-2)$_3$] (M=Tc,Re). Polyhedron; 1992; 11, 2151.
89. Tisato, F., Refosco, F., Bandoli, G. et al.: Synthesis and characterisation of neutral technetium(III) complexes with S,P-bidentate phosphinethiolate ligands. Crystal structure of [Tc(SCH$_2$CH$_2$PPh$_2$)$_2$(SCH$_2$CH$_2$Ph$_2$PO)]. J. Chem. Soc. Dalton Trans.; 1994, 1453.
90. Pietzsch, H-J., Spies, H., Lubritz, P., Reck, G., Johannsen, B.: Technetium and rhenium complexes with multidentate thioether ligands. In technetium and rhenium in chemistry and nuclear medicine 4. Ed. Nicolini, M., Bandoli, G., Mazzi, U., SG Editorali, Padova, 1995, p231.
91. Alberto, R., Schlibi, R., Schubiger, PA., Abram, U., Kadem, TA.: Reactions with the technetium and rhenium complexes [NEt$_4$]$_2$[TcX$_3$(CO)$_3$]. Synthesis and structure of [Tc(CNBu^t)$_3$(CO)$_3$]NO$_3$ and [Et$_4$N] [Tc$_2$(mSCH$_2$CH$_2$OH)$_3$(CO)$_6$]. Polyhedron; 1996; 15, 1079.
92. Alberto, R., Schebli, R., Egli, A. et al.: Low pressure synthesis of [Et$_4$N]$_2$[MX$_3$(CO)$_3$] (M=Tc, Re, X=Cl, Br) and its substitution behaviour in water and organic solvents. In technetium and rhenium in chemistry and nuclear medicine 4. Ed. Nicolini, M., Bandoli, G., Mazzi, U., SG Editorali, Padova, 1995, p7.
93. Nosco DL, Tofe AJ, Dunn TJ et al; New developments in radiophrmaceuticals at Mallinkrodt. In technetium and rhenium in chemisry and nuclear medicine, 3. Ed Nicolini M, Bandoli G, Mazzi U, New York Raven Press, 1990, p 381.
94. Top S, Elhafa H, Vessieres A et al; Rhenium carbonyl complexes of beta estradiol derivatives with high affinity for the estradiol receptor - an approach to selective organometallic radiopharmaceuticals; J. Amer. Chem. Soc.; 1995, 117, 8372.
95. Cotton, FA., Davison, A., Day, VM., Gage, LG. and Trop, HS.: Preparation and structural characterisation of salts of oxotetrachlorotechnetium(V). Inorg. Chem.; 1979, **18**, 3024.
96. Edwards, D., Cheesman, E.,Watson, M., Maheu, L., Nguyen, S., Dimitre, L., Nason, T., Watson, A. and Walovitch, R. C.: Synthesis and characterisation of technetium and rhenium complexes of N,N'-1,2-Ethylenedilylbis-L-cysteine. Neurolite and its metabolities. In technetium and rhenium in chemistry and nuclear medicine **3**. Ed. Nicolini, N., Bandoli G., Mazzi, U., SG Editoriali, New York; 1989, 433.
97. Lever, SZ., Baidoo, KE. and Mahmood, A.: Structure proof of syn/anti isomerism in N-alkylated (DADT) complexes of technetium. Inorg. Chim. Acta.; 1990, **176**, 183.

98. Jurrison, S., Aston, K., Kay Fair, C., Schlemper, E., Sharp, P. and Troutner, D.: Effect of ring size on properties of technetium amine oxime complexes. X-ray structures of $TcO_2Pent(AO)_2$, which contains an unusual eight-membered chelate ring, and of $TcOEn(AO)_2$. Inorg. Chem.; 1987, **26**, 3576.

BIFUNCTIONAL CHELATORS FOR TECHNETIUM-99m

Alfons M. Verbruggen

Introduction

Technetium-99m has nearly optimal characteristics as a radionuclide for diagnostic radiopharmaceuticals: (1) a low radiation dose to the patients due to the absence of α- and ß-radiation and the short physical half-life (6.02 h), (2) the excellent quality of its scintigraphic images as a result of the favourable energy of its gamma radiation (140.5 keV) which is efficiently detected by the NaI(Tl) crystals of conventional gamma cameras and on the other hand has a good tissue penetration and (3) its continuous availability as pertechnetate from a ^{99m}Mo- ^{99m}Tc generator. However, an inconvenience associated with technetium is the fact that it cannot simply replace a hydrogen atom as it is the case with halogens like ^{123}I and ^{18}F, nor can be a substitute for one of the other common atoms in biologically interesting compounds, i.e. carbon, nitrogen or oxygen.

Labelling of bioactive compounds with technetium-99m therefore requires their conjugation to a bifunctional chelating agent (BCA). Such BCA is characterised by the fact that it contains in its structure (1) a functional group through which it can be covalently bound to a bioactive compound. The bond can be of varying nature, e.g. amide, thiourea, ester, alkylated amine, or even a carbon-carbon bond; (2) a set of donor atoms arranged in such a way that a stable complex with Tc can be formed. The bifunctional chelate approach is in use already since many years as a strategy to label proteins and antibodies with a radionuclide and the different techniques have been described in a number of review articles [1-6].

In recent years, bifunctional chelators have also been used for the labelling of non-protein compounds such as peptides, receptor binding agents and other drugs with ^{99m}Tc. New BCA's and interesting modifications have been introduced and they will be discussed together with the earlier techniques in this chapter.

Generally, two basic approaches to the labelling of biologically interesting compounds with ^{99m}Tc can be distinguished, i.e. the preformed chelate approach and the postconjugation direct or exchange labelling.

S. J. Mather (ed.), Current Directions in Radiopharmaceutical Research and Development, 31–46.

The preformed chelate approach

The earliest attempts to label antibodies with ^{99m}Tc via a BCA used diethylenetriaminepentaacetate (DTPA), coupled to the protein using DTPA cyclic anhydride, DTPA-N-hydroxysuccinimide ester or a p-isothiocyanatobenzyl derivative of DTPA [7-11]. Alternative BCA's in the same period were derivatives of bis-N-methylthiol semicarbazone, derivatised with a phenylpronionic acid side chain for coupling to the ε-amino groups of lysine residues of the proteins [12-14]. In both cases, however, problems were observed such as adventitious binding of the metal to the protein, formation and binding of colloids to the antibody and low yields of specifically bound ^{99m}Tc. To overcome these inconveniences, Fritzberg and co-workers designed the so-called preformed chelate technique (Figure 1).

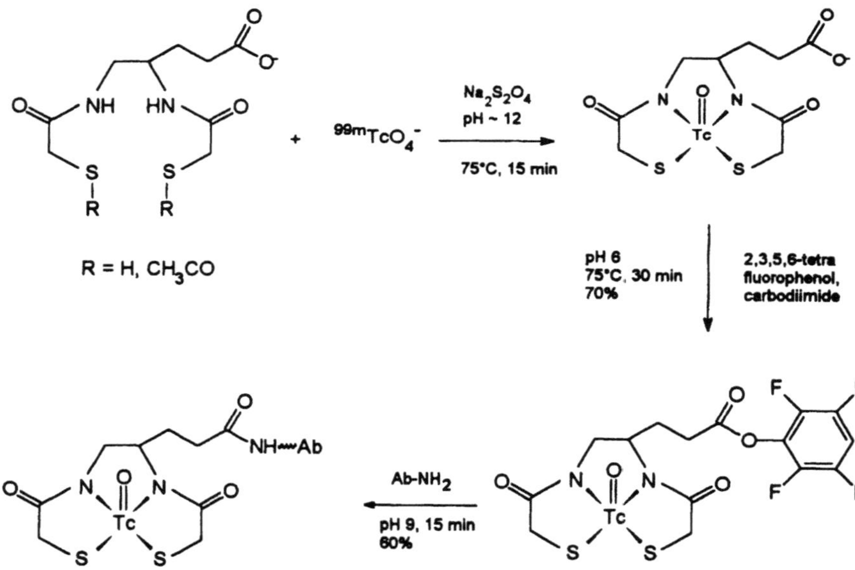

Figure 1. Schematic representation of the preformed chelate approach using a diamide dithiolate chelating agent and activation of the carboxylic group via ester formation with tetrafluorophenol [15]

A carboxyl derivatised diamide dithiolate tetraligand (a derivative of carboxy DADS with extended side chain) is first reacted with ^{99m}Tc-pertechnetate at elevated temperature to form a highly stable tetradentate complex with ^{99m}Tc at the +5 oxidation level, after which the carboxylate is converted to the reactive tetrafluorophenyl ester in the presence of a carbodiimide. The ^{99m}Tc labelled active ester is finally conjugated to the antibody [2,15]. This three-step procedure is rather lengthy (2-3h) and requires purification of the intermediates and final ^{99m}Tc-labelled conjugate, which is obtained in overall yields of 35-50%. However, it provides ^{99m}Tc-N_2S_2-bound antibodies and fragments with high stability and reasonably well retained immunoreactivity.

A number of modifications to this preformed ^{99m}Tc-chelate approach have been proposed by different authors :

- replacement of the diamide dithiolate chelating agent by mercaptoacetyltriglycine and labelling with ^{186}Re [16] or ^{99m}Tc [17];
- preparation of the activated ester with tetrafluorothiophenol [17, 18] or with 4-nitrophenol and enhancement of the conjugation yield with an acylation catalyst [19];
- the use of structurally modified diamide dithiolates and triamidemonothiolates, in which the carboxylic group is well separated from the technetium atom by a rigid aromatic benzene ring, an alicyclic ring or an extended aliphatic chain [20].

The preformed chelate technique has, independently, also been proposed by another group [21]. These authors used derivatives of cyclam such as aminopropyl methyl cyclam which after labelling with ^{99m}Tc at alkaline pH was reacted with 2-iminothiolane to introduce a sulphydryl group. The ^{99m}Tc labelled SH-derivatised cyclam was then reacted with a m-maleimidobenzoyl derivatised antibody at neutral pH to obtain the labelled protein in a low yield, but without non-specific binding of ^{99m}Tc to the macromolecule.

The advantages of the preformed ^{99m}Tc-chelate approach are obvious : application of a well defined chemistry without non-specific binding of ^{99m}Tc to the bioactive compound; moreover, this compound is not exposed to the sometimes harsh labelling conditions (high temperature, alkaline pH, presence of reducing substances). This is particularly important for the preservation of the tertiary structure and immunoreactivity of proteins and antibodies. On the other hand, however, the technique is complex and lengthy and the yields are low. Therefore, it is rather unlikely that it can be adapted for use by the common hospital nuclear medicine laboratory. Without doubt, it is of great value to research laboratories as it permits to prepare and evaluate quite rapidly new ^{99m}Tc-labelled bioactive compounds. Moreover, it can become of interest for use in well equipped and well staffed regional radiopharmacies.

Postconjugation labelling

In view of the difficulties and inconveniences associated with the preformed chelate technique, most efforts in the field of BCA's for ^{99m}Tc-labelling have during the last years been devoted to agents that allow a postconjugation labelling. Such BCA's can first be coupled efficiently with the bioactive compound, after which the conjugate is labelled by the simple addition of ^{99m}Tc-pertechnetate or a weak ^{99m}Tc-complex such as ^{99m}Tc-gluconate. To assure the formation of a really stable final ^{99m}Tc-complex, the majority of approaches has made use of a tetradentate ligand system with sulphur and nitrogen donor atoms, but also other tetradentate besides monodentate and bidentate ligands have been proposed.

TRIAMIDEMONOTHIOLATES

Ram and Buchsbaum [22] prepared a derivative of S-acetyl MAG3-ethyl ester, containing a p-isothiocyanatobenzyl substituent. This precursor was conjugated with the formation of a thiourea bond to a monoclonal antibody at room temperature and slightly alkaline pH. Without isolation or purification of the conjugate, the reaction mixture was incubated with ^{99m}Tc-gluconate for 1.5-2 h to finally yield 9-18% of the ^{99m}Tc-MAG3-antibody conjugate (Figure 2).

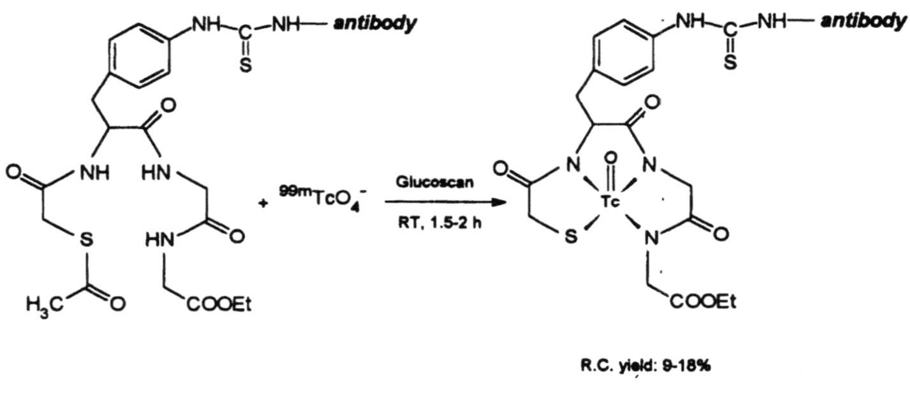

Figure 2. Postconjugation labelling of an S-acetyl MAG3-ethyl ester benzylthiourea-antibody conjugate [22]

The relatively low yield can probably be attributed to the fact that the binding of Tc to the triamidemonothiolate requires deprotonation of the MAG3 amide functions, which normally proceeds efficiently only at elevated temperature or at high pH, but not at neutral pH and room temperature. The proposed procedure might therefore be more successful for labelling of peptides or other bioactive compounds that are stable in the more appropriate labelling conditions.

DIAMINODITHIOLATES

Diaminodithiols (DADT), also named bis-aminoethanethiols (BAT), do easily form very stable complexes with ^{99m}Tc at room temperature in the presence or absence of a weak chelating agent [23, 24]. Examples of radiopharmaceuticals containing this tetradentate donor atom set are the brain perfusion agent ^{99m}Tc-ethylcysteinate dimer (^{99m}Tc-ECD) [25] and the renal function agent ^{99m}Tc-ethylene dicysteine [26]. Lever and co-workers designed a diaminedithiol thiolactone (Figure 3) as a reactive precursor for conjugation of a DADT-chelator to a protein or to other bioactive compounds [27-29].

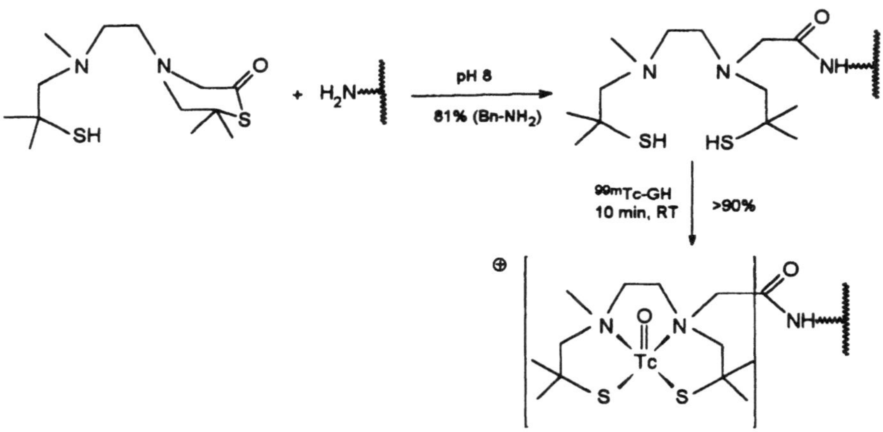

Figure 3. Diaminodithiol thiolactone bifunctional chelating agent which forms a cationic ^{99m}Tc-complex core [27-29]

In this thiolactone precursor both amine nitrogen atoms are substituted with an alkyl substituent and thus tertiary and this prevents inter- and intramolecular reaction with the thiolactone. The free thiol is relatively stable due to the presence of the gem-dimethyl substituent on the a-carbon atom. In this way, the reactive precursor is sufficiently stabilised to allow storage for several months at low temperature. The thiolactone is, in fact, an activated form of a carboxylic acid and it reacts efficiently with primary amino groups of proteins and other compounds to form an amide bond, with the simultaneous release of the strong Tc-chelating diaminodithiol moiety. Incorporation of ^{99m}Tc can easily and efficiently be done by incubation of the conjugate with ^{99m}Tc-glucoheptonate. The technique has been successfully applied for ^{99m}Tc-labelling of simple amines such as benzylamine, proteins such as serum albumin and chemotactic peptides [28, 30].

As this BCA results in the formation of a positively charged Tc complex core, it is inappropriate for preparing radiopharmaceuticals intended for use in the uninjured brain. For this reason, the same group of investigators designed a related BCA (Figure 4) that forms a neutral Tc complex, as the +3 charge on the TcO core is compensated by the deprotonation of two thiols and one amine upon binding of Tc. In this precursor one of the amines is secondary but it is prevented from reaction with the thiolactone by the presence of a gem-dimethyl substituent on the α-carbon atom. This thiolactone BCA has been used to prepare a neutral ^{99m}Tc-labelled conjugate with benzovesamicol as a potential marker for cholinergic neurons in the brain [33]. Although the lipophilicity was similar to that of 5-iodobenzovesamicol, the brain uptake of the ^{99m}Tc-benzovesamicol complex in mice was very low and no regional selectivity was observed in the radioactivity distribution in the brain.

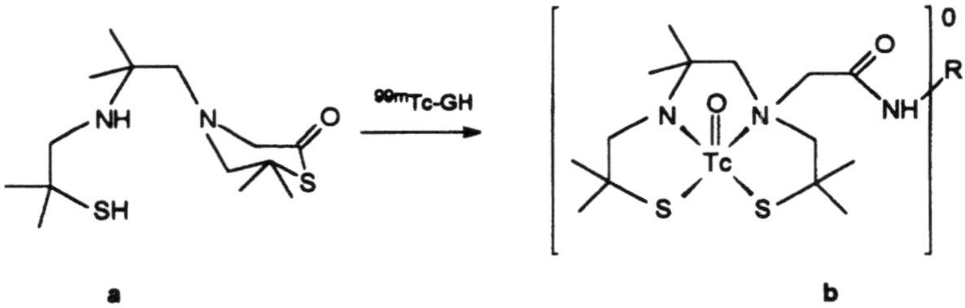

Figure 4. Bifunctional diaminodithiol thiolactone precursor (a) which forms a neutral complex core with ^{99m}Tc (b) [31-32]

In a slightly different synthetic approach, Lever and co-workers prepared a similar ^{99m}Tc-DADT conjugate with part of quinuclidinyl benzilate (QNB) [34, 35]. It was hypothesised that the Tc-DADT chelate could replace the iodobenzhydrol portion of I-QNB and the overall three-dimensional size of the resulting complexes would be similar. This is a first example of the 'partial structure concept' in which a ^{99m}Tc-chelate replaces part of the bioactive compound. In *in vivo* studies in mice, the formed ^{99m}Tc-QNB complexes crossed the blood-brain barrier and showed some limited affinity for the muscarinic cholinergic receptor.

A different approach to a diaminodithiol precursor that can be easily and efficiently coupled to proteins prior to labelling with ^{99m}Tc has been elaborated by Eisenhut and co-workers [36-38]. They developed the N-hydroxysuccinimide (NHS) ester of a diaminodithiol which is derivatised with 4-n-butoxybenzoic acid (Figure 5). This activated ester contains in its structure two secondary amines and two thiols, but is stable for several months at -18 °C if stored in the form of the dihydrochloride.

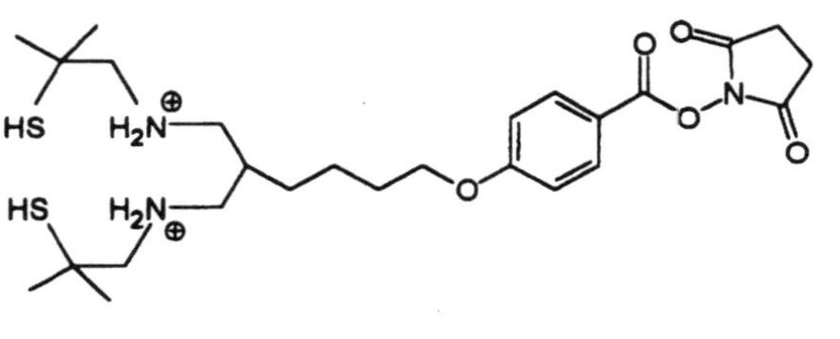

Figure 5. Bifunctional N-hydroxysuccinimide ester of bis(aminoethanethiol) for antibody conjugation and stable ^{99m}Tc labelling [38]

As in the higher discussed thiolactone precursors, the thiols of this NHS-ester are stabilised against oxidation by the presence of gem-dimethyl substituents on the a-carbon atoms. The so-called NHS-BAT ester is coupled with antibodies in a precursor/antibody ratio of 10:1 and the DADT-antibody conjugate is then efficiently (80-85%) labelled with ^{99m}Tc by incubation for 5 min at room temperature with generator eluate and 5 μmol $SnCl_2$ in 0.1M tartaric acid. Any unreacted ^{99m}Tc can simply be removed by ultrafiltration. The antibodies labelled in this way are reported to retain 90-95% of their immunoreactivity.

Different groups have used a diaminodithiol as part of structurally modified receptor binding agents for facile labelling with ^{99m}Tc. In these cases the DADT-moiety was not coupled to the bioactive drug via an amide bond, but incorporated in the global structure via alkylation of one of the DADT amines or through a C-C bond. Samnick and co-workers [39] investigated the ^{99m}Tc labelling and biodistribution in rats of two DADT-derivatives of spiperone, in which the ^{99m}Tc-DADT moiety replaces part of the spiperone structure (Figure 6).

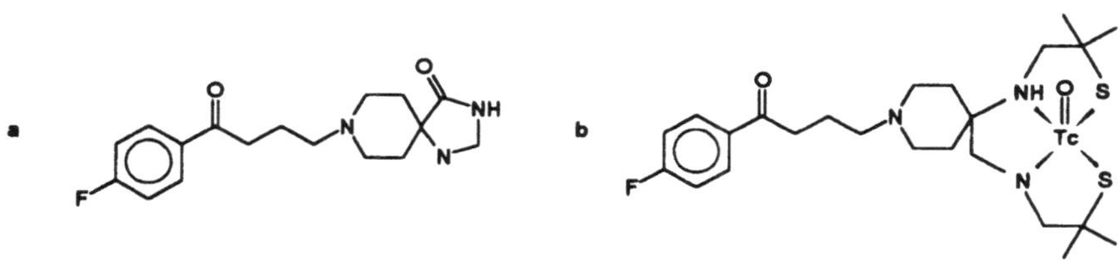

Figure 6. Structure of spiperone (a) and of a ^{99m}TcO-DADT-spiperone derivative (b) [39]

Both compounds could be labelled with ^{99m}Tc in high yield (92-98%) by simple addition of generator eluate and stannous ions at pH 11-12, but the brain uptake of the highly lipophilic ^{99m}Tc-labelled derivatives in rats was negligible.

DiZio and co-workers prepared three technetium and rhenium labelled DADT-progestin derivatives to study the possibility of developing diagnostic imaging agents for steroid-receptor positive tumours [40, 41]. The progestins were linked to the N_2S_2 metal chelate system by alkylation of one of the secondary amines of the diaminodithiol using the triflate or mesylate of hydroxyalkyl derivatised progestins (Figure 7a). As could be expected for N-substituted diaminodithiols, labelling with ^{99m}Tc (via ^{99m}Tc-gluconate) resulted in the formation of diastereomers and they showed different but in all cases clearly reduced affinities for the progesterone receptor. To reduce the high lipophilicity of the ^{99m}Tc-DADT-progestin complexes (about 100 times higher than for the parent steroid) the DADT chelate system was replaced in further studies by a monoamine monoamide dithiol (MAMA) ligand (Figure 7b). However, the in vivo behaviour of the new derivatives was similar to that of the DADT-linked progestins [42-43].

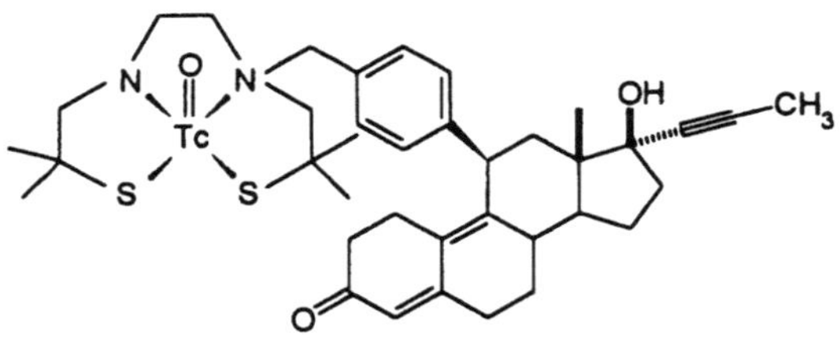

a

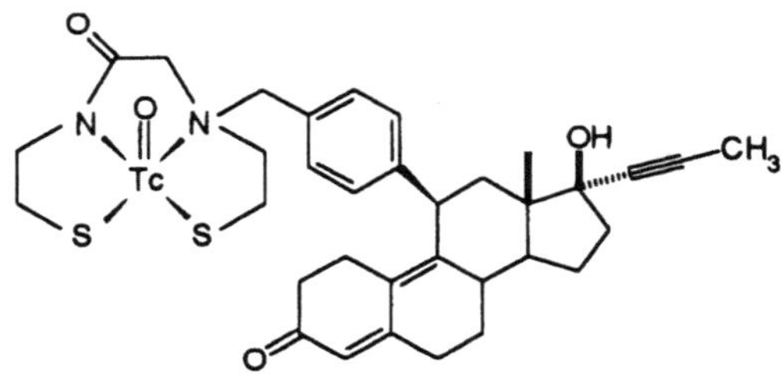

b

Figure 7. ^{99m}Tc-labelled progestins linked to a diaminodithiol (a) or a monoamine-monoamide dithiol (b) [40,43]

Several authors have reported the synthesis and evaluation of different diaminodithiols substituted with a short or long alkanoic acid side chain on one of the amines or on the central alkylene bridge between the two amines [44-47]. These ligands were designed as bifunctional chelating agents for labelling of small molecules or proteins with ^{99m}Tc or as analogs of fatty acids that can be labelled with ^{99m}Tc.

Peptide sequences as bifunctional chelators for ^{99m}Tc

During the last years there has been a growing interest in developing ^{99m}Tc-labelled peptides as target specific imaging agents [48,49], e.g. for diagnosis of infection and inflammation, deep vein thrombosis, pulmonary embolism, atherosclerosis and certain types of tumours. Specific peptides have been designed with high binding affinity for receptors which are over-expressed in the case of these pathologies. One of the approaches to permit efficient labelling of such peptides with ^{99m}Tc is to incorporate in the peptide a sequence that contains a donor atom set that allows stable complexation of technetium. Such sequences are (1) cysteinyl-glycyl-cysteinyl, (2) acylglycyl-glycyl-cysteinyl and (3) glycyl-glycyl-cysteinyl (Figure 8).

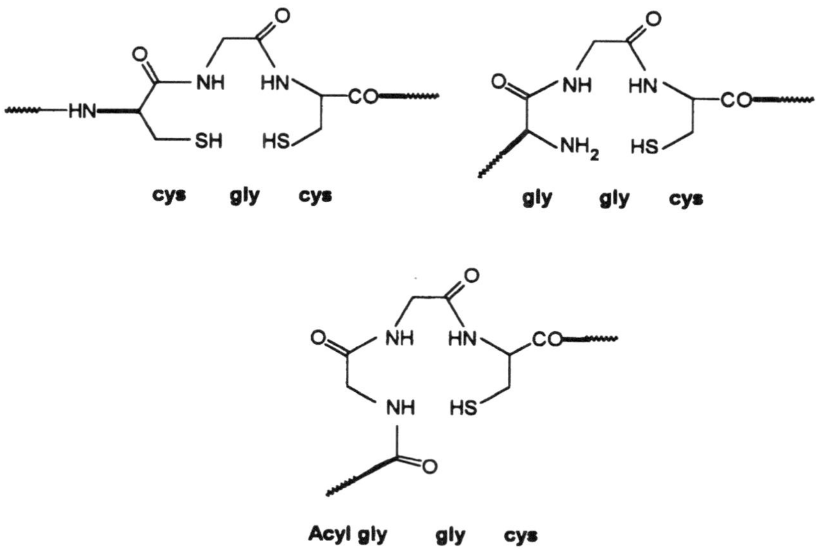

Figure 8. Peptide sequences as bifunctional chelators for ^{99m}Tc [50-52]

These peptide sequences are, in fact, respectively a diamide dithiolate, a triamide monothiolate and a diamide monoamino monothiolate and have been designed by Lister-James and co-workers at Diatide Inc. in the development of their ^{99m}Tc-labelled peptides, called "Techtides" [50-51].

The cys-gly-cys sequence is being used in peptide 280 with the thiols of the two cysteine moieties protected with an acetamidomethyl group. P280 requires therefore heating at 100°C for 15 minutes for complete labelling by ligand exchange with ^{99m}Tc-glucoheptonate. ^{99m}Tc-P280 has given excellent images of deep vein thrombosis in initial clinical studies. In a second generation derivative of P280 a diaminodithiol chelator has been incorporated in the structure and the resulting P357 peptide can be labelled with ^{99m}Tc at room temperature. ^{99m}Tc-P357 showed higher thrombus uptake and thrombus:background ratios than ^{99m}Tc-P280 in animal studies and has given excellent clinical images of deep vein thrombosis and of pulmonary embolism.

The acyl-gly-gly-cys sequence (triamide thiol) was incorporated in peptide P587, which was designed to have a high affinity for somatostatin receptors (SSTR). It requires heating for 5 min at 100°C in the presence of ^{99m}Tc-glucoheptonate for complete labelling. Replacement of one of the amides of the Tc-binding sequence by an amine resulted in derivative P829 and this amine-amide-amide-thiol sequence allows to perform the labelling reaction by incubation for 15-30 min at room temperature. ^{99m}Tc-P829 is presently being tested in clinical studies.

Other tetradentate ligands as bifunctional chelators for ^{99m}Tc

To a limited extent, propylene diaminedioxime (PnAO) tetraligands covalently bound to a bioactive compound have been used to allow labelling of these molecules of biological interest with ^{99m}Tc (Figure 9). PnAO tetraligands can easily be labelled in high yield with ^{99m}Tc at room temperature with or without a transfer ligand. Coupling of the PnAO backbone with other substances has been done either by a global synthesis or by derivatisation of the propylene bridge between the two amines with a reactive thiocyanatobenzyl group that allows thiourea formation with a primary amine of the bioactive compound.

Linder and co-workers at Bristol-Myers Squibb Pharmaceutical Research Institute prepared ^{99m}TcO- (PnAO)-1-(-2-nitroimidazole) via global synthesis of the PnAO-nitroimidazole conjugate as a tracer agent for imaging hypoxia [53]. Mäcke and co-workers designed a complex synthesis for a thiocyanatobenzyl substituted PnAO chelator and coupled it to biotin and to (D)Phe[1]-octreotide [54,55]. The ^{99m}Tc labelled biotin conjugate was used for visualisation of tumours in a pre-targeting approach in combination with avidin and monoclonal antibodies. The ^{99m}Tc-labelled somatostatin analogue was evaluated in tumour-bearing animals and specifically interacted with somatostatin binding sites on the tumour. However, because of its pronounced hepatobiliary clearance, it was found inappropriate for the in vivo visualisation of somatostatin receptor positive tumours and/or their metastases in the abdomen. To reduce the lipophilicity of the ^{99m}Tc-labelled PnAO conjugates, the authors substituted later the PnAO chelator by a bifunctional tetraamine (N_4) chelating group (Figure 10), which on binding of ^{99m}Tc leads to a monocationic, hydrophilic ^{99m}Tc(V) dioxo complex [56,57].

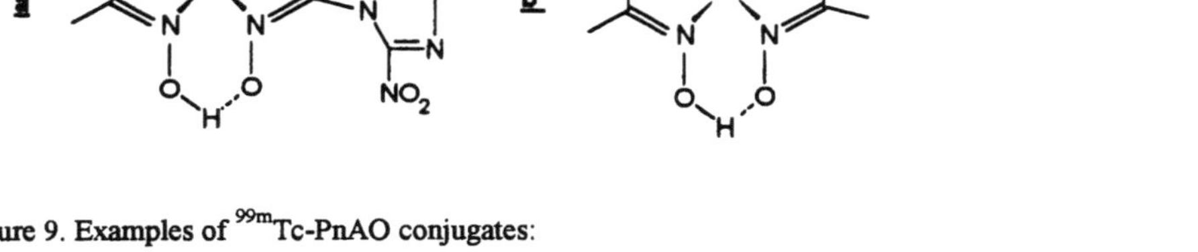

Figure 9. Examples of ^{99m}Tc-PnAO conjugates:

a: ^{99m}TcO-(PnAO)-1-(2-nitroimidazole) [53]

b: ^{99m}Tc(PnAO)-5-benzylthiourea octreotide [55]

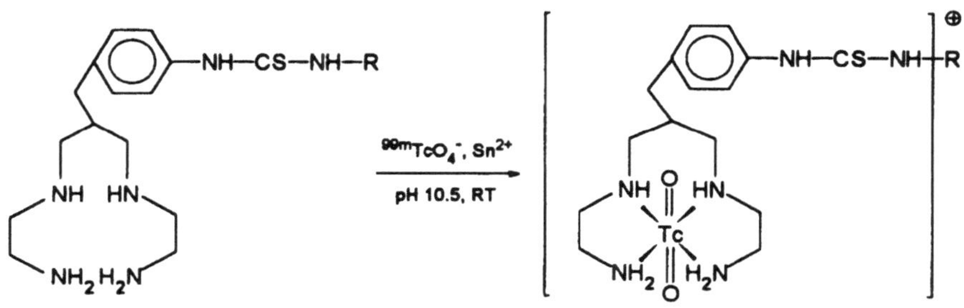

Figure 10. Tetra-amine (N_4) bifunctional chelator which forms a hydrophilic cationic $^{99m}Tc(O_2)$-complex [56,57]

The labelling can be performed at low ligand amounts (2.8 x 10^{-8} mol) in aqueous alkaline conditions (pH 10.5) and results in ≥97% yields of ^{99m}Tc complexes with high specific activity (1.6 Ci/μmol). Both the ^{99m}Tc-N_4-lysin-biotin and the $^{99m}Tc[N_4$-(D)Phe[1]]-octreotide are cleared mainly through the kidneys with minimal liver uptake and thus show a more favourable biodistribution than the PnAO conjugates.

Mono- and diligands as bifunctional ^{99m}Tc chelating agents

N-hydroxysuccinimidyl hydrazinonicotinate (S-Hynic) has been shown to be a valuable bifunctional chelating agent that can be coupled easily, mostly via a linker, to free amino groups of proteins and peptides. Labelling of the Hynic-conjugates with ^{99m}Tc proceeds at room temperature in high yields if a co-ligand such as tricine is present. The usefulness of Hynic was first demonstrated by Schwartz and co-workers for stable labelling of proteins with ^{99m}Tc [58,59], a finding recently confirmed by Verbeke [17]. Later it was used extensively to prepare ^{99m}Tc-labelled chemotactic peptides [48,49,60]. The exact nature of the ^{99m}Tc-Hynic complex remained unclear for several years [4]. Recently, Liu and co-workers at the DuPont Merck Pharmaceutical Company studied Hynic conjugates of peptides in a research program toward developing thrombus imaging agents based on cyclic IIb/IIIa receptor antagonists [61]. The radiolabelling of the Hynic conjugated cyclic peptide (Hynictide) was carried out by reaction with pertechnetate in the presence of excess tricine and $SnCl_2$ at pH 4-5 and room temperature. From their studies the authors concluded that the complex, which was formed in high yields and with high specific activity (≥20 Ci/μmol) has a $^{99m}Tc(Hynictide)(tricine)_2$ structure (Figure 11). However, HPLC analysis indicated that the complex exists as multiple species, some of which inter-convert, depending on the temperature, reaction time and pH of the mixture. The presence of these multiple species is most likely due to different bonding modalities of either the hydrazine moiety of the Hynictide or the two tricine co-ligands. Replacement of tricine by other co-ligands such as ethylenediamine-N,N-diacetic produced complexes with higher stability and fewer coordination isomers. These results indicate that hydrazinonicotinamide acts as a monodentate ligand, requiring the presence of a co-ligand to form a stable complex with ^{99m}Tc.

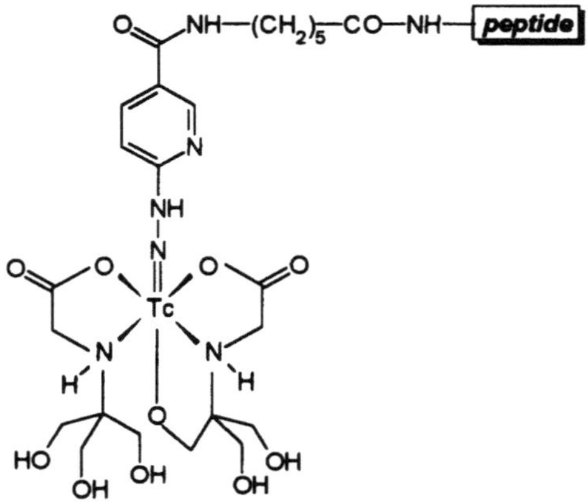

Figure 11. One of the proposed structures of a ^{99m}Tc-(tricine)$_2$ hydrazinonicotinamide (Hynic) peptide for thrombus imaging [61]

Other monodentate bifunctional chelators have been used to improve the ^{99m}Tc-binding characteristics of proteins. These are the thiolating agents iminothiolane and N-acetylhomocysteine (Figure 12). Coupling of immunoglobulins with iminothiolane to introduce a number of 1-amidino-4-mercaptobutyl side chains was proposed nearly simultaneously by two groups [62,63]. This method is now employed by Mallinckrodt Medical Holland in their HIG labelling kit. ^{99m}Tc-human immunoglobulin is in clinical use for detection of inflammatory foci. Mahmood and co-workers reported recently a new method for labelling blood cells with ^{99m}Tc via hydrophilic, polycationic poly-D-lysine modified by coupling of N-acetyl homocysteine [64]. The modified polylysine is labelled with ^{99m}Tc in >95% yield by transchelation via ^{99m}Tc-glucoheptonate during 45-60 min at room temperature. ^{99m}Tc is probably bound to one or more of the released thiols, but also amino groups from poly-lysine and glucoheptonate may be involved in the binding of Tc.

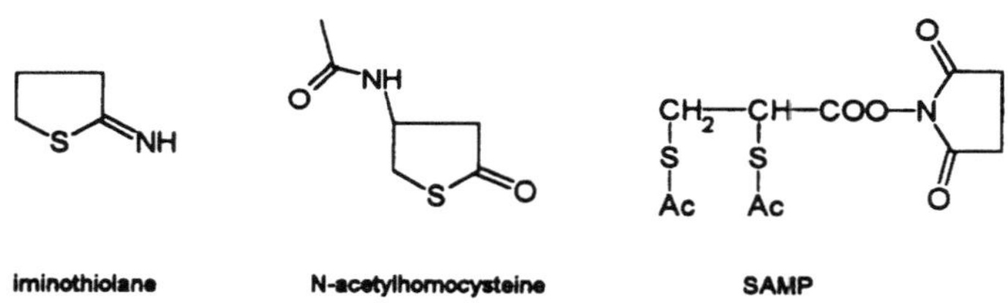

Figure 12. Bifunctional thiolating agents used to improve the ^{99m}Tc-binding strength of proteins [61,62]

A bidentate bifunctional thiolating agent for coupling to proteins and enhancement of their ^{99m}Tc binding strength has been developed by Verbeke and co-workers [65,66], i.e. 2,3-di-acetylmercaptopropionic acid N-hydroxysuccinimide ester (SAMP) (Figure 12). The authors coupled SAMP to human serum albumin and the resulting dimercaptopropionyl albumin (DMP-HSA) forms very easily stable complexes with ^{99m}Tc by addition of pertechnetate and stannous ions and incubation for a few minutes at room temperature. After promising results in a volunteer, ^{99m}Tc-DMP-HSA is now being evaluated in clinical studies as a potential practical substitute for in vitro labelled ^{99m}Tc-labelled erythrocytes for radionuclide ventriculography.

Acknowledgement is made to M.J. Vangoetsenhoven and B.J.Cleynhens for the typing of the manuscript and the professional drawing of the figures.

References

1. Sunberg MW, Meares CF, Goodwin DA, Diamanti CI. Chelating agents for the binding of metal ions to macromolecules. Nature 1974;250:587-8.
2. Fritzberg A. Advances in ^{99m}Tc-labeling of antibodies. Nucl-Med 1987;26:7-12.
3. Hansen HJ, Jones AL, Grebenau R, Kunz A, Goldenberg DM. Labeling of anti-tumor antibodies and antibody fragments with Tc-99m. Cancer treatment research 1990;51:233-44.
4. Delmon-Moingeon LI, Mahmood A, Davison A, Jones AG. Strategies for labeling monoclonal antibodies and antibody-like molecules with technetium-99m. J Nucl Biol Med 1991;35:47-59.
5. Griffiths GL, Goldenberg DM, Jones AL, Hansen AJ. Radiolabeling of monoclonal antibodies and fragments with technetium and rhenium. Bioconjug Chem 1992;3:91-9.
6. Jurisson S, Berning D, Jia W, Ma D. Coordination compounds in nuclear medicine. Chem Rev 1993;93:1137-56.
7. Khaw BA, Strauss HW, Carvalho A, Locke E, Gold HK, Haber E. ^{99m}Tc labeling of antibodies to cardiac myosin Fab and to human fibrinogen. J Nucl Med 1982;23:1011-9.
8. Paik CH, Murphy PR, Eckelman WC, Volkert WA, Reba RC. Optimization of the DTPA mixed-anhydride reaction with antibodies at low concentration. J Nucl Med 1983;24:932-6.
9. Lanteigne D, Hnatowich DJ. The labeling of DTPA-coupled proteins with ^{99m}Tc. Int J Appl Radiat Isot 1984;35:617-21.
10. Childs RL, Hnatowich DJ. Optimum conditions for labeling of DTPA-coupled antibodies with technetium-99m. J Nucl Med 1985;26:293-9.
11. Paik CH, Ebbert MA, Murphy PR et al. Factors influencing DTPA conjugation with antibodies by cyclic DTPA anhydride. J Nucl Med 1983;24:1158-63.
12. Arano Y, Yokoyama A, Magata Y, Horiuchi K, Saji H, Torizuka K. In the procurement of stable ^{99m}Tc labeled protein using bifunctional chelating agent. Appl Radiat Isot 1986;37:587-92.
13. Arano Y, Yokoyama A, Magata Y, Saji H, Horiuchi K, Torizuka K. Synthesis and evaluation of a new bifunctional chelating agent for ^{99m}Tc labeling of proteins: p-carboxyethylphenylglyoxal-di-(N-methylthiosemicarbazone). Nucl Med Biol 1986;12:425-30.
14. Arano Y, Yokoyama A, Furukawa T et al. Technetium-99m-labeled monoclonal antibody with preserved immunoreactivity and high in vivo stability. J Nucl Med 1987;28:1027-33.
15. Fritzberg AR, Abrams PG, Beaumier PL et al. Specific and stable labeling of antibodies with technetium-99m with a diamide dithiolate chelating agent. Proc Natl Acad Sci USA 1988;85:4025-9.
16. Visser GWM, Gerretsen M, Herscheid JDM et al. Labelling of monoclonal antibodies with rhenium-186 using MAG3 chelate for radioimmunotherapy of cancer. A technical protocol. J Nucl Med 1993;34:1953-63.

17. Verbeke K, Hjelstuen O, Debrock E, Cleynhens B, De Roo M, Verbruggen A. Comparative evaluation of $^{99}Tc^{m}$-Hynic-HSA and $^{99}Tc^{m}$-MAG3-HSA as possible blood pool agents. Nucl Med Commun 1995;16:942-57.
18. Fritzberg AR. personal communication.
19. Guhlke S, Diekmann D, Zamora PO, Knapp FF, Biersack HJ. MAG3 p-nitrophenyl ester for ^{99m}Tc and ^{188}Re labelling of amines and peptides. In: Nicolini M, Bandoli G, Mazzi U, editors. Technetium and rhenium in chemistry and nuclear medicine 4. Padova: SGEditoriale,1995:363-6.
20. Liu S, Edwards DS. New N_2S_2 diamidethiol and N_3S triamidethiols as bifunctional chelating agents for labelling small peptides with technetium-99m. In: Nicolini M, Bandoli G, Mazzi U, editors. Technetium and rhenium in chemistry and nuclear medicine 4. Padova: SGEditoriale,1995:383-93.
21. Franz J, Volkert WA, Barefield EK, Holmes RA. The production of ^{99m}Tc-labeled conjugated antibodies using a cyclam-based bifunctional chelating agent. Nucl Med Biol 1987;14:569-72.
22. Ram S, Buchsbaum D. A peptide-based bifunctional chelating agent for ^{99m}Tc- and ^{186}Re-labeling of monoclonal antibodies. Cancer Res 1994;3:769-73.
23. Liang FH, Virzi F, Hnatowich DJ. Serum stability and non-specific binding of technetium-99m labeled diaminodithiol for protein labeling. Nucl Med Biol 1987;14:555-61.
24. Efange SMN, Kung HF, Billings JJ, Blau M. Synthesis and biodistribution of ^{99m}Tc-labeled piperidinyl bis(aminoethanethiol) complexes: Potential brain perfusion imaging agents for single photon emission computed tomography. J Med Chem 1988;31:1043-7.
25. Walovitch RC, Hill TC, Garrity ST et al. Characterization of technetium-99m-L,L-ECD for brain perfusion imaging, Part 1: Pharmacology of technetium-99m ECD in nonhuman primates. J Nucl Med 1989;30:1892-901.
26. Verbruggen AM, Nosco DL, Van Nerom CG, Bormans GM, Adriaens PJ, De Roo MJ. Technetium-99m-L,L-ethylenedicysteine: a renal imaging agent. I. Labeling and evaluation in animals. J Nucl Med 1992;33:551-7.
27. Lever SZ, Baidoo KE, Kramer AV, Burns HD. Synthesis of a novel bifunctional chelate designed for labeling proteins with technetium-99m. Tetrahedron Lett 1988;29:3219-22.
28. Baidoo KE, Scheffel U, Lever SZ. ^{99m}Tc labeling of proteins: initial evaluation of a novel diaminedithiol bifunctional chelating agent. Cancer Research (Suppl) 1990;50:799s-803s.
29. Baidoo KE, Lever SZ. Synthesis of a diaminedithiol bifunctional chelating agent for incorporation of technetium-99m into biomolecules. Bioconjug Chem 1990;1:132-7.
30. Baidoo KE, Stathis M, Scheffel U, Lever SZ, Wagner HN. High affinity Tc-labeled chemotactic peptides. J Nucl Med 1993;34:18P (abstract).
31. Baidoo KE, Lever SZ. Design and synthesis of a versatile precursor to neutral technetium and rhenium complexes. Tetrahedron Lett 1990;31:5701-4.
32. Baidoo KE, Lever SZ, Scheffel U. Bifunctional chelator for facile preparation of neutral technetium complexes. Bioconjug Chem 1994;5:114-8.
33. Del Rosario RB, Jung Y-W, Baidoo KE, Lever SZ, Wieland DM. Synthesis and in vivo evaluation of a $^{99m/99}Tc$-DADT-benzovesamicol: a potential marker for cholinergic neurons. Nucl Med Biol 1994;21:197-203.
34. Lever SZ, Baidoo KE, Mahmood AM, Matsumura K, Schefel U, Wagner HN. Novel technetium ligands with affinity for the muscarinic cholinergic receptor. Nucl Med Biol 1994;21:157-64.
35. Lever SZ, Wagner HN. The status and future of technetium-99m radiopharmaceuticals. In: Nicolini M, Bandoli G, Mazzi U, editors. Technetium and rhenium in chemistry and nuclear medicine 4. Padova: SGEditoriale,1995:649-59.
36. Eisenhut M, Brandau W, Missfeldt M. Synthesis and in vivo testing of a bromobutyl substituted 1,2,5,9-diazocycloundecane: a versatile precursor for new ^{99m}Tc-bis(aminoethanethiol) complexes. Nucl Med Biol 1989;8:805-11.
37. Eisenhut M, Missfeldt M, Lehmann WD, Karas M. Synthesis of a bis(aminoethanethiol) ligand with an activated ester group for protein conjugation and ^{99m}Tc labeling. J Labelled Compd Radiopharm 1991;29:1283-91.
38. Eisenhut M, Lehmann WD, Becker W et al. Bifunctional NHS-BAT ester for antibody conjugation and stable technetium-99m labeling: conjugation chemistry, immunoreactivity and kit formulation. J Nucl Med 1996;37:362-70.

39. Samnick S, Brandau W, Sciuk J, Steinsträsser A, Schober O. Synthesis, characterization and biodistribution of neutral and lipid-soluble ^{99m}Tc-bisaminoethanethiol spiperone derivatives: possible ligands for receptor imaging with SPECT. Nucl Med Biol 1995;22:573-83.
40. DiZio JP, Fiaschi R, Davison A, Jones AG, Katzenellenbogen JA. Progestin-rhenium complexes. metal-labeled steroids with high receptor binding affinity, potential receptor-directed agents for diagnostic imaging or therapy. Bioconjug Chem 1991;2:353-66.
41. DiZio JP, Anderson CJ, Davison A et al. Technetium- and rhenium-labeled progestins: synthesis, receptor binding and in vivo biodistribution of an 11ß-substituted progestin labeled with technetium-99 and rhenium-186. J Nucl Med 1992;33:558-69.
42. O'Neil JP, Wilson SR, Katzenellenbogen JA. Preparation and structural characterization of monoamine-monoamide bis(thiol) oxo complexes of technetium(V) and rhenium(V). Inorg Chem 1994;33:319-23.
43. O'Neil JP, Carlson KE, Anderson CJ, Welch MJ, Katzenellenbogen JA. Progestin radiopharmaceuticals labeled with technetium and rhenium: synthesis, binding affinity, and in vivo distribution of a new progestin N_2S_2-metal conjugate. Bioconjug Chem 1994;5:182-93.
44. Liang FH, Virzi F, Hnatowich DJ. The use of diaminodithiol for labellling small molecules with technetium-99m. Nucl Med Biol 1987;14:63-7.
45. Liang FH, Virzi F, Hnatowich DJ. Serum stability and non-specific binding of technetium-99m labeled diaminodithiol for protein labeling. Nucl Med Biol 1987;14:555-61.
46. Misra HK, Virzi F, Hnatowich DJ, Wright G. Synthesis of a novel diaminodithiol for labelling proteins and small molecules with technetium-99m. Tetrahedron Lett 1989;30:1885-8.
47. Mach RH, Kung HF, Jungwiwattanaporn P, Guo Y-Z. A new synthesis of bis-aminoethanethiol (BAT) chelating agents containing a gamma carboxylate. Tetrahedron Lett 1989;30:4069-72.
48. Fischman AJ, Babich JW, Strauss HW, A ticket to ride: peptide radiopharmaceuticals. J Nucl Med 1993;34:2253-63.
49. Fischman AJ, Babich JW, Rubin HR. Infection imaging with technetium-99m-labeled chemotactic peptide analogs. Semin Nucl Med 1993;24:154-68.
50. Lister-James J, McBride WJ, Buttram S et al. Technetium-99m chelate-containing receptor-binding peptides. In: Nicolini M, Bandoli G, Mazzi U, editors. Technetium and rhenium in chemistry and nuclear medicine 4. Padova: SGEditoriale,1995:269-74.
51. Pearson DA, Lister-James J, McBride WJ et al. Somatostatin receptor-binding peptides labeled with technetium-99m: chemistry and initial biological studies. J Med Chem 1996;39:1361-71.
52. Pearson DA, Lister-James J, McBride WJ et al. Thrombus imaging using technetium-99m-labeled high-potency GPIIb/IIIa receptor antagonists. Chemistry and initial biological studies. J Med Chem 1996;39:1372-82.
53. Linder KE, Chan Y-W, Cyr JE, Malley MF, Nowotnik DP, Nunn AD. TcO(PnAO-1-(2-nitromidazole)) [BMS-181321], a new technetium-containing nitroimidazole complex for imaging hypoxia: synthesis, characterization, and xanthine oxidase-catalyzed reduction. J Med Chem 1994;37:9-17.
54. Koch P, Mäcke HR. ^{99m}Tc labeled biotin conjugate in a tumor "pretargeting" approach with monoclonal anitibodies. Angew Chem Int Ed Engl 1992;31:1507-9.
55. Maina T, Stolz B, Albert R, Bruns C, Koch P, Mäcke H. Synthesis, radiochemistry and biological evaluation of a new somatostatin analogue (SDZ 219-387) labelled with technetium-99m. Eur J Nucl Med 1994;21:437-44.
56. Maina T, Stolz B, Albert R, Nock B, Bruns C, Mäcke H. Synthesis, radiochemical and biological evaluation of ^{99m}Tc[N_4-(D)Phe^1]-octreotide, a new octreotide derivative with high affinity for somatostatin receptors. In: Nicolini M, Bandoli G, Mazzi U, editors. Technetium and rhenium in chemistry and nuclear medicine 4. Padova: SGEditoriale,1995:395-400.
57. Nock B, Koch P, Evard F, Paganelli G, Mäcke H. ^{99m}TcN_4-lys-biotin, a new biotin derivative useful for pretargeted avidin-biotin immunoscintigraphy: synthesis, evaluation and comparison with other ^{99m}Tc-biotin conjugates. In: Nicolini M, Bandoli G, Mazzi U, editors. Technetium and rhenium in chemistry and nuclear medicine 4. Padova: SGEditoriale,1995:429-36.
58. Schwartz DA, Abrams MJ, Hauser MM et al. Preparation of hydrazino-modified proteins and their use for synthesis of ^{99m}Tc-protein conjugates. Bioconjug Chem 1991;2.333-6.

59. Abrams MJ, Juweid M, tenKate CI et al. Technetium-99m-human polyclonal IgG radiolabeled via the hydrazino nicotinamide derivative for imaging focal sites of infection in rats. J Nucl Med 1990;31:2022-8.
60. Babich JW, Solomon H, Pike MC et al. Technetium-99m-labeled hydrazino nicotinamide derivatized chemotactic peptide analogs for imaging focal sites of bacterial infection. J Nucl Med 1993;34:1967-74.
61. Liu S, Edwards DS, Looby RJ et al. Labeling a hydrazino nicotinamide-modified cyclic IIb/IIIa receptor antagonist with ^{99m}Tc using aminocarboxylates as coligands. Bioconjug Chem 1996;7:63-71.
62. Goedemans WT, Panek KJ, Ensink GJ, de Jong MTM. A new, simple method for labelling of proteins with ^{99m}Tc by derivatization with 1-imino-4-mercaptobutyl groups. In: Nicolini M, Bandoli G, Mazzi U, editors. Technetium and rhenium in chemistry and nuclear medicine 3: Verona: Cortina International and New York: Raven Press, 1990:595-604.
63. Joiris E, Bastin B, Thornback JR. A new method for labelling of monoclonal antibodies, their fragments and other proteins with technetium-99m. In: Nicolini M, Bandoli G, Mazzi U, editors. Technetium and rhenium in chemistry and nuclear medicine 3: Verona: Cortina International and New York, Raven Press: 1990:609-14.
64. Mahmood A, Delmon-Moingeon LI, Limpa-Amara N, Davison A, Jones AG. A new approach to labeling cells with technetium-99m, part 1. Preparation of modified polylysine and in vitro cell labeling. Nucl Med Biol 1996;23:79-85.
65. Verbeke KA, Vanbilloen HP, De Roo MJ, Verbruggen A. Technetium-99m mercaptoalbumin as a potential substitute for technetium-99m labelled red blood cells. Eur J Nucl Med 1993;20:473-82.
66. Verbeke KA, Vanhecke WB, Mortelmans LA, Verbruggen AM. First evaluation of technetium-99m dimercaptopropionyl albumin as possible tracer agent for ventriculography in a volunteer. Eur J Nucl Med 1994;21:906-12.

MEDIUM HALF-LIFE INORGANIC RADIONUCLIDES FOR PET IMAGING

Jamal Zweit

Introduction

In vivo radiotracer imaging continues to grow in importance and consideration is constantly given to the relative merits of the different techniques of radionuclide imaging and how they complement each other. The aim of this review is to highlight the role of inorganic medium-lived radionuclides within the field of Positron Emission Tomography (PET). PET has evolved around the use of short-lived radioactive tracers of natural organic elements such as ^{11}C (20 min.), ^{13}N (10 min.) and ^{15}O (2 min). Although fluorine is not a commonly natural constituent of organic molecules, ^{18}F (110 min.), as a hydrogen analogue, is the radionuclide most commonly used and ^{18}F-FDG is currently the most widely used PET radiotracer. This is due at least in part to the longer half-life of ^{18}F which offers both practical and technical advantages to study prolonged biochemical interactions that are not possible even with the longest half-life organic radionuclide (^{11}C, 20 min.). This review therefore focuses on exploiting the use of medium half-life radionuclides in PET imaging. This expansion could aid in realising the true potential of PET by combining the sensitivity and quantitative accuracy of the technique with a large number of specific tracers developed for single photon imaging using for example, ^{99m}Tc, $^{123,\ 131}I$, ^{111}In, ^{67}Ga and ^{67}Cu radionuclides. Here, the positron-emitters ^{94m}Tc, $^{120,124}I$, ^{110}In, $^{66,68}Ga$ and $^{61,64}Cu$ could be used as the PET imaging analogues. The abundance of inorganic positron-emitting radionuclides span a wide range of half-lives (~ 1-100 hours) and spectrum of chemical properties ranging from the alkali metals to transition elements to lanthanides and the halogens (although not strictly 'inorganic' elements, the halogens are included for completion). This diversity of physical, chemical and biochemical properties justifies further exploration into this area of inorganic PET in order to take advantage of the opportunities offered by such radionuclides in PET research. In addition to the practical benefits of medium half-life radiotracers, certain applications particularly in oncology, require tracer kinetics to be followed for periods exceeding the limits of conventional short-lived PET radionuclides. This is often necessary for pharmacokinetic studies of radiolabelled anti-cancer drugs and other molecules such as monoclonal antibodies (MAbs), where

S. J. Mather (ed.), Current Directions in Radiopharmaceutical Research and Development, 47–61.

tissue uptake kinetics far exceeding the 20 min. half-life of ^{11}C are not uncommon. This is further supported by our experience using the tamoxifen analogue, idoxifen [1], where peak levels of uptake into experimental tumours were not found until 24 hours post i.v. administration. This implies that ^{124}I with its 100 h half-life is a suitable PET radiolabel to study the pharmacokinetics of this anti-estrogen drug in breast cancer patients.

From a logistic point of view such a review is currently appropriate as PET facilities continue to expand, and concern has been raised with respect to the cost effectiveness of the technique. To this end, the use of inorganic tracers based on medium half-life and generator-produced radionuclides enables PET to be carried out at centres remote from a cyclotron. The longer half-life of such radionuclides allows regional distribution of a number of radiotracers to be a viable option and the goal of significantly reducing the cost of PET can finally be achieved.

The choice of inorganic radionuclides described here is based on realistic forecast in terms of their production, radiolabelling and imaging feasibility. These and other aspects pertinent to the radionuclides will be discussed in this chapter.

Decay Properties of Inorganic PET Radionuclides

Unlike the conventional short-lived PET radionuclides, the vast majority of inorganic positron-emitting radionuclides combine both electron capture (EC) and positron (β^+) decays as means to achieve stability. The emission of non-annihilation gamma-rays following EC decay results in an increase in the signal due to single events with a reduction in the 511 keV photon flux leading therefore to reduced sensitivity. This however does not negate their use as positron-emitting tracers thanks in part to the high detection efficiency of the coincident event compared to single photon imaging. The EC decay, however has implications on both image performance and radiation dosimetry. Table 1 lists the decay properties of the radionuclides that are related to PET imaging. The radionuclides included are those with half-lives > 1 hour and a positron emission rate of ≥ 19. Decay data are from Lederer & Shirley [2] and Sowby [3]

Radionuclide Production

RADIOPHYSICAL ASPECTS

Compared to conventional PET radionuclides (Z = 6-9), the higher atomic number (Z ~ 21-70) of medium-lived radionuclides implies that higher energy particles are needed for their production. This is essential in order to overcome the higher coulomb barrier, a repulsive force between the incident particle and the target nucleus. Radionuclide yields however, are also modulated by the available phase space, spin changes and other spectroscopic factors [4]. The production of some of these radionuclides is therefore feasible through (p,n) and (p,α) reactions for which low energy cyclotrons (10-15 MeV) are adequate for large scale production particularly for the lighter nuclei [5-8]. All the radionuclides listed in table 1, except for ^{52}Fe, ^{57}Ni and ^{83}Sr, can be produced through (p,n) or (p,α) reactions using a small cyclotron. Where a medium or a high energy cyclotron is available, alternative production reactions are possible and a choice is therefore available especially when consideration is given to cost of enriched materials and power dissipation and target cooling problems.

Table 1 Decay properties of medium-half life (1-100 h) PET radionuclides

Nuclide	$T_{1/2}$ hours	β^+ decay [a] %	$E_{\beta+}$ [b] MeV	Δ_{np} g-rad/μCi-h	Δ_p g-rad/μCi-h
^{52}Fe	8.2	57	0.804	0.41	1.58
^{55}Co	18	77	1.51	0.91	4.24
^{57}Ni	36	40	0.850	0.31	4.07
^{61}Cu	3.3	62	1.21	0.66	1.75
^{64}Cu	12.7	19	0.575	0.26	0.41
^{66}Ga	9.5	57	4.15	2.06	5.21
^{68}Ga	1.1	89	1.90	1.57	2.02
^{75}Br	1.6	76	1.74	1.11	2.56
^{76}Br	16	57	3.98	1.47	5.50
^{83}Sr	33	24	1.23	0.32	1.66
^{86}Y	15	34	3.15	0.48	7.46
^{89}Zr	78	22	0.900	0.22	2.47
^{94m}Tc	0.9	72	2.47	1.60	3.94
^{94g}Tc	4.9	11	0.816	0.10	5.69
^{120}I	1.4	46 -81 [c]	4.59	3.03	5.75
^{124}I	100	22	2.14	0.41	2.30

[a] Remainder of decay is by electron capture in all listed radionuclides.
[b] maximum positron energy.
[c] Positron emission is quoted as 46% in ref [2] and 81% in ref [3].
Δ_{np} / Δ_p = equilibrium dose constant for non-penetrating / penetrating radiation.

RADIOCHEMICAL ASPECTS

In addition to the radiophysical and targetry aspects of production, the radiochemical aspects for the production of inorganic radionuclides are even more demanding than those encountered in the production of conventional PET tracers. This is due to the need for radiochemical separation of the product from the target material as well as other stable and radioactive elements which are also produced either from competing reactions on the target nucleus or from other isotopic impurities present particularly when using enriched targets. The task therefore of radiochemical separation must account for all possible impurities which in some cases necessitates multi-step purification in order to obtain a product of the highest possible purity.

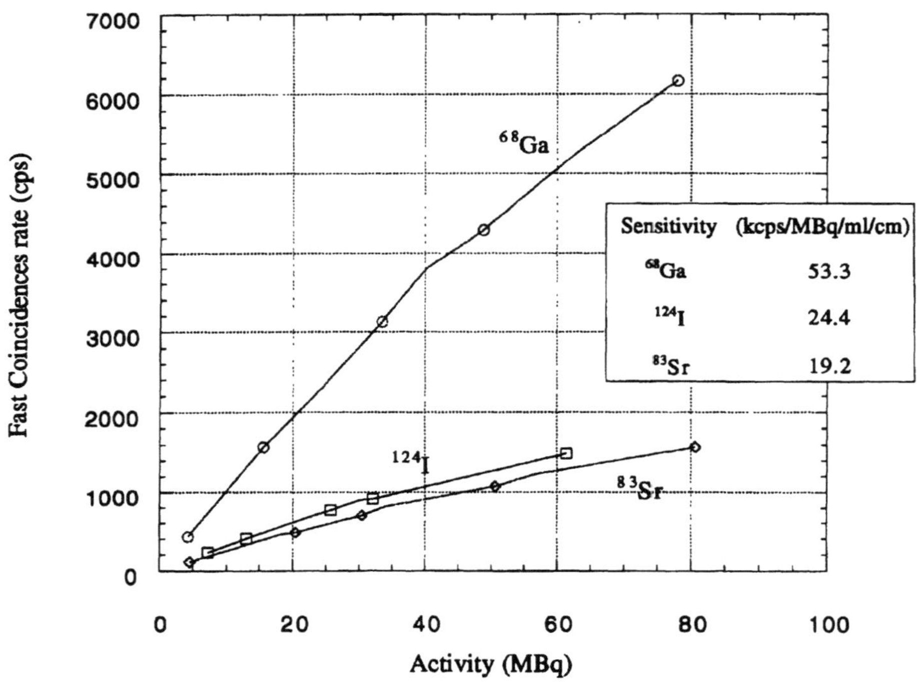

Figure 1. MUP-PET fast coincidences rate as a function of activity in the centre of the field of view for three radionuclides with different positron emmissions and variation in their electron capture decays.

Image Performance

The imaging feasibility and characteristics of such radionuclides must be investigated as part of their pre-clinical evaluation. Due to the complication of EC decay and the emission of high energy positrons from some of these radionuclides, image evaluation of such tracers is more crucial and must be more rigorous than that carried out for conventional PET isotopes. We and others have demonstrated beyond doubt the use of such radionuclides with positron emission rates as low as 19 % for ^{64}Cu [9, 10], 22% for ^{124}I [11-15] and 24% for ^{83}Sr [16, 17]. Although the rate of positron emission is directly related to the sensitivity of detection, it is not the only determinant of image quality. In a study, using the MUP-PET camera [18], we have compared the imaging performance of a number of inorganic positron emitters representing a range of half-lives, positron emission rates and non-annihilation gamma photons. For example, as shown in figure 1, when the data rates of ^{68}Ga (β^+ = 89%), 83Sr (β^+ = 23%) and 124I (β^+ = 22%) were compared the system sensitivity (in kcps/MBq/ml/cm) of ^{83}Sr was similar to that of ^{124}I reflecting the similarities in their positron emission rates. However the signal to noise ratio for ^{83}Sr was superior to that of ^{124}I and slightly worse than that of ^{68}Ga. This is probably due to the stronger γ-emissions, above 511 keV, of ^{124}I (90%) than for ^{83}Sr (38 %) [16]. It should be emphasised that current 3-D PET systems have approximately a 60-fold greater sensitivity than the MUP-PET camera used in this evaluation study. Using therefore a state of the art high sensitivity PET system will even allow the use of low β^+ emitting radionuclides and further improve image quality and quantitation in general. Table 2 shows the sensitivity figures, for a number of radionuclides, measured using the MUP-PET camera and the values extrapolated the most advanced BGO-based PET system (e.g., ECAT-EXACT).

Table 2 Volume sensitivity of MUP-PET and ECAT-EXACT PET scanners for a number of Medium-lived PET radionuclides

Radionuclide	MUP-PET sensitivity [kcps / (MBq/ml)]	ECAT-EXACT sensitivity [kcps / (MBq/ml)]
^{18}F	580	35000
^{62}Cu	490	29400
^{64}Cu	65	3900
^{68}Ga	370	22000
^{83}Sr	190	11000
^{120}I	390	23000
^{124}I	180	10800

Inorganic Radionuclides and Radiopharmaceuticals

The medium half-life radionuclides discussed in this section are those that have been conjugated to molecules and / or their production methods have been developed.

IRON (^{52}Fe, $T_{1/2}$ = 8.2 h, β^+ =57%)

Iron-52 is a useful β^+-emitting radionuclide with attractive physical, chemical and biological properties. ^{52}Fe-citrate (transferrin) is the most suitable radiopharmaceutical for in-vivo monitoring of bone marrow function. Compared to $^{111}InCl_3$ and ^{99m}Tc-sulphur colloid, it can differentiate between haematopoietic and reticuloendothelial activity, a relationship that is not always maintained in pathological conditions . Recent clinical studies conducted in patients with myelofibrosis demonstrated good quality PET imaging using The ECAT-ART scanner and a small amount (5.5 MBq) of ^{52}Fe injected activity [19].

^{52}Fe could also be a useful PET label for peptides such as octreotide through a desferroxamine (DFO) conjugation. It has been established that the biodistribution of ^{68}Ga-DFO-octreotide is similar to that of ^{111}In-DTPA-D-Phe^1-octreotide [20]. The longer half-life of ^{52}Fe (8.3h) could provide superior images to ^{68}Ga (68 min.) since background activity in humans injected with ^{111}In-DTPA-D-Phe^1-octreotide was significantly lower at 24 h compared to 4 h post injection. A serious problem with ^{52}Fe is its availability which is currently confined to a few centres in which the radionuclide is produced by a helium-3 or alpha-particle irradiation of natural chromium targets. This problem can be partially circumvented by using higher yield production methods such as $^{50}Cr(\alpha,2n)^{52}Fe$ on an enriched target [21], $^{55}Mn(p,4n)^{52}Fe$ on natural target [22] or high energy (72 MeV) protons on natural Ni targets [23].

COBALT (^{55}Co, $T_{1/2}$ = 18 h, β^+ = 77%)

The interest in ^{55}Co arose from its potential to replace stable cobalt in bleomycin complexes for use in tumour imaging with PET [24]. The physical properties of ^{55}Co are excellent for PET imaging, possessing a high β^+ emission rate (77%) and a suitable half-life (18h) that is compatible with the biokinetics of many molecules including monoclonal antibodies (Mabs) and peptides.

Another application, which has been explored by the Groningen Group [25], is to use $^{55}Co^{2+}$ (to mimic Ca^{2+}) to identify and quantify damage as a result of the detrimental intracellular influx of Ca^{2+} in the process of cell death. The method reveals even mild changes of the degenerative process, irrespective of the integrity of the blood brain barrier.

Several nuclear reactions can be used for the production of ^{55}Co. These include proton / deuteron irradiation on Fe [24, 26], proton bombardment of Ni [27] and ^3He

bombardment of Mn [28]. These production possibilities allow diversity of cyclotrons, in terms of particles and energies, to be utilised for ^{55}Co production; thereby making the radionuclide available to a wider number of users.

NICKEL (^{57}Ni, $T_{1/2} = 36$ h, $\beta^+ = 40\%$)

The nuclear characteristics of ^{57}Ni combined with amenable chemical properties of nickel make ^{57}Ni-based radiopharmaceuticals potentially attractive agents for PET imaging. The 1.5 d half-life is compatible with the kinetics of small and large molecules including Mabs and peptides. In this context macrocyclic ligands based on 13N4 core, developed as Cu chelates [29, 30] are directly applicable to conjugation of Ni. The use therefore of the ^{57}Ni-13N4 linked to Mabs and peptides in targeting tumours is worth investigating. Once such radioconjugates are evaluated, the ^{57}Ni PET imaging agent can be combined, with the isotopic analogue ^{66}Ni ($T_{1/2}$ = 55 h, E_{β^-} = 0.2 MeV), in a targeted radionuclide therapy approach. The decay of ^{66}Ni to ^{66}Cu ($T_{1/2}$ = 5 min, E_{β^-} = 2.6 MeV) could be advantageous in a cocktail emission of a low and a high range β^--particles to target small and large tumours simultaneously.

The reasonably long half-life of ^{57}Ni allows for wider distribution of the radionuclide from regional cyclotrons. We have already reported on an efficient production method via the $^{59}Co(p,3n)^{57}Ni$ reaction using inexpensive natural target material [31]. Cation-exchange chromatography was used to produce a product with high radionuclide, radiochemical and chemical purity. Using this method a typical run yields about 400 - 500 MBq of ^{57}Ni activity based on 1 hour irradiation and a 25 μA beam current.

COPPER (^{61}Cu, $T_{1/2} = 3.3$ h, $\beta^+ = 62\%$; ^{64}Cu, $T_{1/2} = 12.7$ h, $\beta^+ = 19\%$)

Copper radionuclides undergo beta, electron capture and positron decays leading to particulate (beta and Auger electron) emissions for therapy and gamma rays (following beta, electron capture or positron decay) for tomographic imaging. Indeed ^{64}Cu combines all three types of decay making it a unique radionuclide for use in both PET imaging and targeted therapy. The two PET nuclides of copper with medium half-lives are ^{61}Cu (3.4h) and ^{64}Cu (12.7h) with positron emissions of 62 and 19% respectively. The added attraction is that copper chemistry has the versatility characteristic of the transition elements [32] without the complexities introduced by the wide range of oxidation states exhibited by, say, Tc and Re (oxidation states I-VII). The chemistry of Cu is dominated by two oxidation states, I and II and within each of theses states also, the co-ordination chemistry remains relatively simple compared to earlier transition elements. The chemistry of copper radionuclides and radiopharmaceuticals has been extensively addressed in a recent review [33].

Earlier work on the production of ^{61}Cu has centred on α-particle induced reactions on natural Ni [34]. Using a low energy medical cyclotron, ^{61}Cu can be produced using $^{61}Ni(p,n)$ [35] and $^{61}Ni(d,2n)$ reactions on enriched ^{61}Ni targets. Using the former reaction the ^{61}Cu yield amounted to 573 MBq /μAh for an 88% enriched target. The use of an enriched ^{60}Ni target and the $^{60}Ni(d,n)^{61}Cu$ reaction will reduce the cost by about a factor of 20 due to the much lower cost of ^{60}Ni. Biological or clinical uses of the radionuclide have not yet been reported.

The majority of pre-clinical and clinical research with Cu-radiopharmaceuticals has been carried using ^{64}Cu and to a lesser extent ^{67}Cu. These included Mabs [10, 36, 37] and peptides [38]. This is mainly due to the wider availability of ^{64}Cu (compared to ^{67}Cu) through reactor and cyclotron production. Production methods feasible for nuclear medicine applications have been developed only relatively recently. ^{64}Cu can be either reactor- [39] or cyclotron- [35, 40] produced, thus allowing wider availability. Reactor production can lead to high or low specific activity, depending on whether production is by direct activation (n,γ) or indirectly through (n,p) reaction on a Zn target. The highest specific activity (3.5 - 11.5 GBq / (g) is, however, achieved by cyclotron irradiation of enriched ^{64}Ni target [41].

The proton and deuteron irradiation of Ni targets leads predominantly to the production of Cu radionuclides with trace quantities of Co isotopes. Radiochemical separation from Ni and Co is best achieved using anion-exchange chromatography, which is simple and highly selective. The columns are easily shielded and the method is amenable to automated processing, reducing radiation exposure to personnel. The method is also well suited to the recovery of the expensive enriched ^{64}Ni which, unlike Cu and Co, is not adsorbed on the column [40, 41]. The trace quantity of Co is eliminated with 5M HCl followed by the recovery of the Cu activity using water as eluent. It must be emphasised that the complete elimination of metal impurities is essential as these will compete with radioactive Cu for sites particularly when using, for example, a chelate compound such as a macrocycle ligand with similar metal affinity.

GALLIUM (^{66}Ga, $T_{1/2}$ = 9.5, β^+ = 57%; ^{68}Ga, $T_{1/2}$ = 68 min, β^+ = 89%)

The radiopharmaceutical chemistry of gallium has been extensively reviewed [42] and in this section only more recent reports on preliminary use of Ga radionuclides in PET imaging are briefly described. There are two gallium radioisotopes, ^{66}Ga and ^{68}Ga, that can be used in PET imaging. The 9.5 h half-life of ^{66}Ga allows distribution from a regional cyclotron whilst ^{68}Ga is conveniently available from a long shelf life (~ 1 year) $^{68}Ge/^{68}Ga$ generator system. Despite commercial availability of such system, clinical PET with ^{68}Ga has been limited to well established radiopharmaceuticals such as ^{68}Ga-citrate, an analogue of the non-specific tumour imaging agent ^{67}Ga-citrate used in single photon imaging, and ^{68}Ga-EDTA used for blood brain barrier permeability (BBB) studies [43]. More recently a preclinical study using ^{68}Ga-DFO-octreotide has been reported [20]. This agent has shown, in tumour-bearing rats, a biodistribution pattern similar to that of the commercially available ^{111}In-DTPA-D-Phe-octreotide. Since the background radioactivity in humans injected with ^{111}In-DTPA-D-Phe-octreotide was significantly lower at 24 h compared to 4 h post-injection, 68Ga may not be an ideal radionuclide for labelling octreotide [38]. The longer half-life of ^{66}Ga may be an alternative in this case provided that the radionuclide can be produced economically and in sufficient quantities. Several efficient methods for its production from Cu targets [44, 45] and from Zn targets [46] have been reported but its use is still limited to a very few centres. An important parameter, related to PET imaging with ^{66}Ga that needs to be carefully assessed is the influence of the high energy (4.2 MeV) positrons on image resolution particularly when using state of the art, High resolution PET scanners.

BROMINE (^{75}Br, $T_{1/2}$ = 1.6 h, β^+ = 76%; ^{76}Br, $T_{1/2}$ = 16 h, β^+ = 57%)

Compared to radioiodines, bromine radionuclides have so far enjoyed only a limited use in few research applications despite some attractive nuclear properties for both imaging and therapy. This is entirely due to non-availability and lack of serious efforts in developing economic and efficient production methods that would allow wider use. The production of ^{75}Br and ^{76}Br has been reviewed by Qaim a decade ago [47] and radiohalogenation of proteins, using bromine radionuclides, have been addressed in great detail by Wilbur [48]. Since then interest in the use of ^{76}Br has been revitalised thanks to the efforts of the Orsay group in their development and evaluation of the mIBG analogue, mBBG, labelled with ^{76}Br as a potential PET radiopharmaceutical [49, 50]. ^{76}Br has also been produced by the Uppsala group and used to label Mabs [51]. Many more compounds can potentially be brominated with ^{76}Br including peptides , proliferation markers such as BUdR [52] and even anti-cancer drugs providing thereby a non-invasive, in-vivo method, to quantify radiotracer kinetics in target and non-target tissues.

STRONTIUM (^{83}Sr, $T_{1/2}$ = 33 h, β^+ = 24%)

The bone seeking radionuclide ^{89}Sr has been shown to be effective in the palliation of pain from bone metastases in breast and prostate cancer. Although ^{89}Sr treatment is simple to administer, it is not uniformly effective. A possible explanation for this is the variability in the radiation dose delivered to metastases. The use of ^{83}Sr and PET would accurately quantify the radiotracer distribution in metastases and normal bone and therefore provide more accurate dosimetry and a means to predict radiotoxicity. Despite the low positron emitting rate and the use of a low sensitivity PET camera, we have demonstrated imaging feasibility of this radionuclide in preliminary phantom studies [16]. An efficient and simple production method has been developed based on proton irradiation of a natural RbCl targets and ion-exchange chromatography technique for the radionuclide purification [53]. The production yield using this method results in a thick target yield of 70 MBq / μAh compared to 4.4 MBq / μAh using a more expensive enriched ^{82}Kr target and a helium-3 beam [17]. A clinical dosimetry study using ^{83}Sr and PET in patients receiving ^{89}Sr therapy for palliation of bone metastases secondary to prostatic cancer, is currently underway at our Institution.

YTTRIUM (^{85g}Y, $T_{1/2} = 2.7$ h, $\beta^+ = 55\%$; ^{85m}Y, $T_{1/2} = 5$ h, $\beta^+ = 70\%$; ^{86}Y, $T_{1/2} = 15$ h, $\beta^+ = 34\%$)

The pure beta-emitter ^{90}Y is a useful radionuclide for targeted therapy due to its suitable half-life ($T_{1/2}$ = 64 h) and high energy (2.3 MeV) beta particles. The pharmacokinetics of ^{90}Y-labelled compounds however, can not be adequately and accurately monitored by external imaging due to the lack of gamma-ray emission. The PET radionuclides of yttrium (^{85g}Y, ^{85m}Y, ^{86}Y) particularly ^{86}Y, can be directly applied to ^{90}Y radiopharmaceuticals and PET imaging can be carried of such radiotracers. This will provide quantitative means of tracer kinetics and would provide accurate dosimetry estimates for ^{90}Y agents.

The production of ^{86}Y from enriched $^{86}SrCO_3$ (96.3%) has been reported by the Julich group [54]. A radiochemical separation, that provides a batch yield of about 1.5 GBq of ^{86}Y activity, was also developed. Whole body biodistribution using ^{86}Y-citrate was carried out using PET imaging and the pharmacokinetic data obtained was used to calculate radiation doses from the ^{90}Y-citrate analogue [55].

ZIRCONIUM (^{89}Zr, $T_{1/2} = 78$ h, $\beta^+ = 22\%$)

^{89}Zr is an attractive isotope for protein and peptide labelling due to its suitable half-life of 3.3 days and sufficient (22%) positron emission. In fact the feasibility of PET imaging with ^{89}Zr has been demonstrated by the Seattle group about a decade ago [56]. The same group has reported on a production method using the $^{89}Y(p,n)$ reaction, but using a somewhat complicated and lengthy separation method involving both solvent extraction and ion-exchange chromatography [57]. A similar method, using a small energy (11MeV) cyclotron was also reported [58]. A simplified production method using the $^{89}Y(d,2n)$ reaction and a one step ion-exchange separation procedure was developed by us [59] and adapted by Meijs et al [60]. The high complexation affinity of DFO, as a chelating agent for Zr, has been utilised in the radiolabelling of Mabs with ^{89}Zr [61]. This study has shown the feasibility of labelling without altering the pharmacokinetic behaviour of the antibody.

TECHNETIUM (^{94g}Tc, $T_{1/2}$= 4.9 h; $\beta^+ = 11\%$; ^{94m}Tc, $T_{1/2} = 0.9$ h, β^+= 72%)

The transverse from SPET to PET can be exemplified in the case of Tc-radionuclides and radiopharmaceuticals. Here the positron emitter ^{94m}Tc could be used with a number of compounds developed for ^{99m}Tc in single photon imaging. Both decays of ^{94}Tc lead to excited levels in ^{94}Mo. The ^{94m}Tc isomer has a high positron emission rate (72%) with an end point energy of 2.5MeV, whilst the longer half-life ground state decays predominantly through electron capture resulting in the emission of high energy γ-rays above the 511 keV line. Depending however, on the sensitivity of detection and the specificity of the radiotracer, the 11% positron emission from the ground state could possibly be utilised in later imaging of the cocktail tracer (^{94m}Tc, ^{94g}Tc). The feasibility of such imaging protocol however needs to be validated on a specific radiotracer basis.

The production of ^{94}Tc from a natural Mo target was reported by Nickles et al [62] and the radionuclide was used to label the neutral Tc complex, terboroxime, a potential heart perfusion agent. Production from natural Mo led to a product of low radionuclide purity and a high radiation dose mixture of activity. In order to improve the radionuclide purity, enriched $^{94}MoO_3$ target was used and the quality of the product was found significantly superior to that from natural targets [63]. The higher purity ^{94m}Tc was successfully used in cardiac imaging using PET [62, 64]. Production via different routes was investigated, in detail, by the Julich group [69-71]. The conclusion of this work is that neither the ^{92}Mo(α,2n) ^{94}Ru → ^{94m}Tc and the ^{92}Mo(α,pn)^{94}Tc routes nor the ^{93}Nb(^{3}He,2n)^{94}Tc reaction are suitable alternatives to the reaction of choice, ^{94}Mo(p,n)^{94}Tc, when using a small cyclotron.

IODINE (^{120}I, $T_{1/2}$ = 1.4 h, β^+ = 46-81% ; ^{124}I, $T_{1/2}$ = 100 h, β^+ = 22%)

Here the transfer from SPET and planar imaging to PET is similar to the Tc case as many compounds currently used with ^{123}I and ^{131}I can be equally labelled with the positron emitters ^{120}I and ^{124}I. At our Institution, where no cyclotron is available, the number of studies carried out with ^{124}I PET is only second to those using ^{18}F-FDG. The 4 d half-life allows for target irradiations at regional cyclotrons and in-house radiochemistry to be carried out post irradiation. Using this system, ^{124}I has been regularly produced in support of our PET programme for the last 5 years [15, 43, 67, 68]. Over that period we have developed production methods based on enriched Te targets and dry chemistry separation procedures which enabled immediate re-use of intact targets [69]. Production reactions reported for ^{124}I production have been recently summarised by Scholten et al [70]. These included ^{124}Te(p,n) [70], ^{124}Te(d,2n) [71-73] and ^{126}Te(p,3n) [69]. The advantage of the (p,n) reaction is that a low energy (11 MeV) cyclotron such as the RDS-111/112, can be used.

In applications where a shorter half-life and increased positron emission are of value, ^{120}I could be used as an alternative to ^{124}I. The 1.4 h half-life is compatible with the kinetics of mIBG and some PET radiopharmaceuticals currently labelled with ^{11}C may alternatively be iodinated, thereby extending the observation of radiotracer kinetics. We are currently developing the large scale production of ^{120}I having recently reported on excitation measurements and a production method using the ^{122}Te(p,3n)^{120}I reaction [74]. Image evaluation using the MUP-PET camera has also been carried out along with radiolabelling experiments of no-carrier added mIBG [75]. The uncertainty regarding the positron emission (quoted values are 46% [2] to 81% [3]) of ^{120}I was also investigated. Preliminary results from volume sensitivity measurements using MUP-PET and gamma-spectroscopy indicate a value between 65-80% positron emission. Future work will include production via the ^{120}Te(p,n)^{120}I reaction and image evaluation using a 3D high sensitivity PET system.

Summary and Conclusion

The limited number of clinical studies, using inorganic PET radionuclides, carried out so far have demonstrated the feasibility of such an approach in PET imaging. This trend needs to continue and more effort needs to be devoted in order to take advantage of the opportunities offered. There is a wealth of inorganic medium half-life radionuclides waiting to be explored in PET imaging. Inorganic PET could add another dimension to conventional PET, offering a broad range of radiopharmaceuticals possessing a wider choice of physical, chemical and biochemical properties. This however needs to be accomplished through serious investment in the development of efficient, high performance targetry and production methods capable of large scale production on regional basis. The long term objectives of this strategy is to enable the operation of a cost-effective PET programme in more hospitals and medical institutions.

Acknowledgements

I would like to thank my colleagues at The Institute of Cancer Research, The Royal Marsden and Hammersmith Hospitals for encouragement and helpful discussions. Also thanks to Mrs Jane Sosabowski and Mr Demitrios Visvikis for helping with the manuscript. Finally I would like to thank The Cancer Research Campaign for the funding of our PET radiopharmaceutical development programme.

References

1 Young, Carnochan P, Trivedi M et al. Pharmacokinetics and biodistribution of radiolabelled idoxifene: prospects for the use of PET in the evaluation of a novel antioestrogen for cancer therapy. Nucl Med Biol 1995; 22: 405-411.

2 Lederer C M and Shirley V S. Table of isotopes. 7th ed. New York: John Wiley & Sons, Inc, 1977.

3 Sowby F D. Radionuclide transformations, energy and intensity of emissions. ICRP38. Oxford: Pergamon Press, 1983.

4 Nickles RJ. A shotgun approach to the chart of the nuclides. Acta Radiologica 1991; 376: 69-71.

5 Zweit JH. The production of medium half-life radionuclides for positron emission tomography [dissertation]. Manchester: Univ. of Manchester, 1989.

6 Ruth TJ, Pate BD, Robertson R, Porter JK. Radionuclide production for the biosciences. Nucl Med Biol 1989; 16: 323-336.

7 Qiam S M, Rosch F, Scholten B, Stocklin G, Kovacs Z, Trkanyi F. Nuclear data relevant to the production of medically important positron emitters Br-75, Y-86, Tc-94m and I-124. In: Dickens J K, editor , Proc. Int. Conf. on Nuclear Data for Science and Technology, 1994, Gatlinburg, Tenn.. American Nuclear Society.

8 Nickles RJ, Sunderland JJ. Low-energy cyclotrons: will they meet performance standards? In: Colman J, editor. Mosby Year Book. St Louis , Mosby Pub. Co., 1992: 95-100.

9 Cutler PD, Schwarz SW, Anderson CJ et al. Dosimetry of copper-64-labeled monoclonal antibody 1A3 as determined by PET imaging of the torso. J Nucl Med 1995; 36: 2363-2371.

10 Philpott GW, Schwarz SW, Anderson CJ et al. RadioimmunoPET: detection of colorectal carcinoma with positron-emitting copper-64-labeled monoclonal antibody. J Nucl Med 1995; 36: 1818-1824.

11 Wilson CB, Snook DE, Dhokia B et al. Quantitative measurement of monoclonal antibody distribution and blood flow using positron emission tomography and ^{124}Iodine in patients with breast cancer. Int J Cancer 1991; 47: 344-347.

12 Ott RJ, Tait D, Flower MA, Babich JW and Lambrecht RM. Treatment planning for ^{131}I-mIBG radiotherapy of neural crest tumours using ^{124}I-mIBG positron emission tomography. Br J Radiol 1992; 65: 787-791.

13 Larson SM, Pentlow KS, Volkow ND et al. PET scanning of iodine-124-3F9 as an approach to tumor dosimetry during treatment planning for radioimmunotherapy in a child with neuroblastoma. J Nucl Med 1992; 33: 2020-2023.

14 Daghighian F, Pentlow KS, Larson SM et al. Development of a method to measure kinetics of radiolabelled monoclonal antibody in human tumour with applications to microdosimetry: positron emission tomography studies of iodine-^{124} labelled 3F8 monoclonal antibody in glioma. Eu J Nucl Med 1993; 20:402-409.

15 Flower MA, Al-Saadi A, Harmer CL, McCready VR, Ott RJ. Dose-response study on thyrotoxic patients undergoing positron emission tomography and radioiodine therapy. Eu J Nucl Med 1994; 21: 531-536.

16 Visvikis D, Zweit J, Flower M, Carnochan P, Ott RJ. ^{83}Sr, a positron emitting radionuclide for dose estimation of ^{89}Sr therapy: imaging feasibility using MUP-PET. Nucl Med Comm 1994; 15: 229 (abstract).

17 R^sch F, Blessing G, Linse KH, Herzog H, Qaim SM. Production of the positron emitting strontium isotope Sr-83 and PET phantom measurements preparatory to the evaluation of Sr-89 pharmacokinetics and dosimetry. J Nucl Med 1996; 37:166P (abstract).

18 Marsden PK, Ott RJ, Bateman JE, Cherry SR, Flower MA, Webb S. The performance of a multiwire proportional chamber positron camera for clinical use. Phys Med Biol 1989; 34: 1043-1062.

19 Glass D, Young H, Myers M et al. Comparison of a rotating, partial ring PET scanner (ECAT-ART) with a dual-headed gamma camera for whole-body imaging with Fe-52 transferrin. J Nucl Med 1996; 37: 148P (abstract).

20 Smith-Jones PM, Stolz B, Bruns C et al. Gallium-67/Gallium-68-[DFO]-octreotide - A potential radiopharmaceutical for PET imaging of somatostatin receptor-positive tumors: synthesis and radiolabeling in vitro and preliminary in vivo studies. J Nucl Med 1994; 35: 317-325.

21 Zweit J, Downey S, Sharma H. A method for the production of iron-52 with a very low iron-55 contamination. Appl Radiat Isot 1988; 39: 1197-1201.

22 Suzuki K. Production of Fe-52 using proton bombardment of natural manganese. Radioisotopes (Japan) 1985; 34: 537-542.

23 Smith-Jones P, Schwarzbach R, Weinreich R. The production of Fe-52 by means of a medium engergy proton accelerator. Radiochim Acta 1990; 50: 33-39.

24 Nieweg OE, Beekhuis H, Paans AMJ et al. Detection of lung cancer with ^{55}Co-bleomycin using a positron camera. A comparison with ^{57}Co-bleomycin and ^{55}Co-bleomycin single photon scintigraphy. Eur J Nucl Med 1982; 7: 104-107.

25 Vaalburg W. What is new in European PET Centres? EEC concerted action on PET investigations of cellular regeneration and degeneration newsletter 1994; 19: 3.

26 Sharma H, Zweit J, Smith AM, Downey S. Production of cobalt-55, a short-lived positron emitting radiolabel for bleomycin. Appl Radiat Isot 1986; 37: 105-109.

27 Maziere B, Stulzaft O, Verret JM, Comar D, Syrota A. Co-55 and Cu-64-DTPA: new radiopharmaceuticals for quantitative tomocisternography. Appl Radiat Isot 1983; 34: 595-598.

28 Watanabe M, Nakahar H, Murakami Y. Production of Co-55 from helium-3 bombardment of natural manganese. Appl Radiat Isot 1979; 30: 625-629.

29 Parker D, editor. Macrocycle synthesis. Oxford: Oxford University Press, 1996.

30 Zweit J, Foster C, Carnochan P, Hall A, Parker D. Copper-64-13N4-macrocycle-biotin-conjugate: radiolabelling and radiotracer kinetic studies in rodents. J Nucl Med 1996; 37: 166P (abstract).

31 Zweit J, Carnochan P, Goodall R and Ott RJ. Excitation functions of proton induced reactions on cobalt: production of no-carrier added nickel-57, a positron emitting label for doxorubicin.

32 Cotton FA, Wilkinson G. Advanced inorganic chemistry: a comprehensive text. 3rd ed. New York: John Wiley & Sons, 1972.

33 Blower PJ, Lewis JS, Zweit J. Copper radionuclides and radiopharmaceuticals in nuclear medicine. Nucl Med Biol, in press.

34 Muramatsu H, Shirai E, Nakahara H, Murakami Y. Alpha particle bombardment of natural nickel target for the production of ^{61}Cu. Int J Appl Radiat Isot 1978; 29: 611-614.

35 SzelecsÈnyi F, Blessing G, Qaim SM. Excitation functions of proton induced nuclear reactions on enriched ^{61}Ni and ^{64}Ni: possibility of production of no-carrier-added ^{61}Cu and ^{64}Cu at a small cyclotron. Appl Radiat Isot 1993; 44: 575-580.

36 Anderson CJ, Connett JM, Schwarz SW et al. Copper-64-labeled antibodies for PET imaging. J Nucl Med 1992; 33: 1685-1691.

37 Shen S, DeNardo GL, DeNardo SJ et al. Dosimetric evaluation of copper-64 in copper-67-2IT-BAT-Lym-1 for radioimmunotherapy. J Nucl Med 1996; 37: 146-150.

38 Anderson CJ, Pajeau TS, Edwards B, Sherman ELC, Rogers BE, Welch MJ. In vitro and in vivo evaluation of copper-64-octreotide conjugates. J Nucl Med 1995; 36: 2315-2325.

39 Zinn KR, Chaudhuri TR, Cheng T, Morris SJ, Meyer WA. Producton of no-carrier-added ^{64}Cu from zinc metal irradiated under boron shielding. Cancer 1994; 73: 774-778.

40 Zweit J, Smith AM, Downey S and Sharma HL. Excitation functions for deuteron induced reactions in natural nickel: production of no-carrier-added ^{64}Cu from enriched ^{64}Ni targets for positron emission tomography. Appl Radiat Isot 1991; 42:193-197.

41 McCarthy DW, Shefer RE, Klinkowstein RE et al. The efficient production high specific activity copper-64 using a biomedical cyclotron. J Nucl Med 1996; 37: 61P (abstract).

42 Green MA, Welch MJ. Gallium radiopharmaceutical chemistry. Nucl Med Biol 1989; 16: 435-448.

43 Ott RJ, Brada M, Flower MA, Babich JW, Cherry SR, Deehan BJ. Measurements of blood-brain barrier permeability in patients undergoing radiotherapy and chemotherapy for primary cerebral lymphoma. Eur J Cancer 1991; 27: 1356-1361.

44 Zweit J, Sharma H, Downey S. Production of gallium-66, a short-lived positron emitting radionuclide. Appl Radiat Isot 1987; 38: 499-501.

45 Goethals P, Coene M, Slegers G, Agon P, Deman J, Schelstraete K. Cyclotron production of carrier-free Ga-66 as a positron emitting label of albumin colloids for clinical use. Eur J Nucl Med 1988; 14: 152-154.

46 Tarkanyi F, Szelecsenyi F, Kovacs Z. Excitation functions for proton induced reactions on enriched Zn-66, Zn-67 and Zn-68. Radiochimica Acta 1990; 50: 19-26.

47 Qaim SM. Recent developmnets in the production of F-18, Br-75, 76, 77 and I-123. Appl Radiat Isot 1986; 37: 803-810.

48 Wilbur DS. Radiohalogenation of proteins: An overview of radionuclides, labelling methods and reagents for conjugate labelling. Bioconjugate Chem 1992; 3: 433-470.

49 Locíh CH, Mardon K, Valette H, et al. Preparation and pharmacological preparation of Br-76-metaobromobenzylguanidine (Br-76-MBBG). Nucl Med Biol 1994; 21: 49-55.

50 Clerc J, Mardon K, Galons H et al. Assessing intratumour distribution and uptake with MBBG versus MIBG imaging and targeting xenografted PC12-pheochromocytoma cell line. J Nucl Med 1995; 36: 859-866.

51 Lovqvist A, Sundin A, Ahlstrom H, Carlsson J, Lundqvist H. Br-76-labelled monoclonal anti-CEA antibodies for radioimmuno-positron emission tomography. Nucl Med Biol 1995; 22: 125-131.

52 Lundqvist H, Malmborg P, Langstrom B, Chiengmai SC. Simple production of Br-77- and I-123- in the labelling of Br-77-BrUdR and I-123-IUdR. Appl Radiat Isot 1979; 30: 39-43.

53 Zweit J, Flower MA, Visvikis D, Carnochan P, Ott RJ. Strontium-83, a positron emitting radionuclide for dose estimation of strontium-89 therapy: production, biodistribution and preliminary imaging. Eur J Nucl Med 1993; 20: 862 (abstract).

54 Rosch F, Qaim SM, Stocklin G. Production of the positron emitting radioisotope Y-86 for Nuclear medical application. Appl Radiat Isot 1993; 44: 677-681.

55 Herzog H, Rosch F, Stocklin G, Christoph L, Qaim SM, Feinendegen LE. Measurement of pharmacokinetics of yttrium-86 radiopharmaceuticals with PET and radiation dose calculation of analogous yttrium-90 radiotherapeutics. J Nucl Med 1993; 34: 2222-2226.

56 Lewellen TK, Krohn KA, Link JM, Eary JF. Feasibility Zr-89 as a PET imaging agent. Proc. the 72nd Scientific Assembly and Annual Meeting of the Radiological Society of North America; 1986, 70.(abstract).
57 Link JM, Krohn KA, Eary JF. Zr-89 for antibody labelling and positron emission tomography. J Lab Comp Radiopharm 1986; 23: 1297 (Abstract).
58 Dejesus OT and Nickles RJ. Production and purification of Zr-89, a potential PET antibody label. Appl Radiat Isot 1990; 41: 789-790.
59 Zweit J, Downey S, Sharma H. Production of no-carrier added zirconium-89 for positron emission tomography. Appl Radiat Isot 1991; 42: 199-201.
60 Meijs WE, Hercheid JDM, Haisma HJ et al. Production of highly pure no-carrier added Zr-89 for the labelling of antibodies with a positron emitter. Appl Radiat Isot 1994; 45: 1143-1147.
61 Meijs WE, Haisma HJ, Klok RP et al. Production of Zr-89-labelled antibodies and their biodistribution in tumour-bearing mice. J Lab Comp Radiopharm 1995; 37: 560-562.
62 Nickles RJ, Nunn AD, Stone CK, Cristian BT. Technetium-94m-teboroxime: snthesis, dosimetry and clinical PET imaging studies. J Nucl Med 1993; 34: 1058-1066.
63 Christian BT, Nickles RJ, Stone CK, Mulnix TL, Clark J. Improving the radionuclidic purity of Tc-94m for PET imaging. Appl Radiat Isot 1995; 46: 69-73.
64 Stone CK, Christian BT, Nickles RJ, Perlman SB. Technetium-94m-labelled methoxyisobutyl isonitrile: dosimetry and resting cardiac imaging with positron emission tomography. J Nucl Cardiology 1994; 1: 425-433.
65 Rosch F and Qaim SM. Nuclear data relevant to the production of the positron emitting technetium isotope Tc-94m via the Mo-94(p,n) reaction. Radiochimica Acta 1993; 62: 115-121.
66 Denzler FO, Rosch F, Qaim SM. Excitation functions of alpha induced reactions on highly enriched Mo-92: comparative evealuation of production routes for Tc-94m. Radiochimica Acta 1995; 68: 13-20.
67 OíConnel MEA, Flower MA, Hinton PJ, Harmer CL, McCready VR. Radiation dose assessment in radioiodine therapy. Dose response relationships in differentiated thyroid carcinoma using quantitative scanning and PET. Radiother Oncol 1993; 28: 16-26.
68 Bakir A, Eccles S, Babich J et al. c-erb2 protein overexpression in breast cancer as a target for PET using iodine-124 labelled monoclonal antibodies. J Nucl Med 1992; 33: 2154=-2160.
69 Zweit J, Bakir MA, Ott RJ, Sharma H, Cox M, Goodall R.Excitation functions of proton induced reactions in natural tellurium: production of no-carrier added I-124 for PET applications. Proc. IV Int. Workshop on Targetry and Target Chemistry, 1991; Villigen, Switzerland, 76-78. (Weinreich R, ed.).
70 Scholten B, Kovacs Z, Tarkanyi F, Qaim SM. Excitation functions of Te-124(p,xn) I-123, 124 reactions from 6 to 31 MeV with special reference to the production of I-124 at a small cyclotron. Appl Radiat Isot 1995; 46: 255-259.
71 Sharma H, Zweit J, Downey S, Smith AM, Smith AG. Production of I-124 for positron emission tomography. J Lab Comp Radiopharm 1989; 26: 165-167.
72 Lambrecht RM, Sajjad M, Qureshi MA, Al-Yanbawi SJ. Production of I-124. J Radioanal Nucl Chem Letters 1988; 127: 143-150.
73 Firouzbakht ML, Schlyer DJ, Finn RD, Laguzzi G, Wolf AP. Iodine-124 production: excitation functions for the Te-124(d,2n) and Te-124(d,3n) reactions from 7 to 24 MeV. Nucl Instr Meth 1993; B79: 909.
74 Zweit J, Luthra SK, Brady F, Carnochan P, Ott RJ, Jones T. Iodine-120, a new positron emitting radionuclide for PET radiopharmaceuticals. J Lab Comp Radiopharm 1995; 37: 823-825.
75 Zweit J, Flower MA, Brown A et al. Iodine-120-mIBG: production and NCA labelling of a new PET radiotracer. J Nucl Med 1996: 37: 191p (abstract).

THERAPEUTIC RADIONUCLIDES: MAKING THE RIGHT CHOICE

Suresh C. Srivastava

Introduction

Recently, there has been a resurgence of interest in nuclear medicine therapeutic procedures (1-4). Using unsealed sources for therapy is not a new concept; it has been around since the beginnings of nuclear medicine. Treatment of thyroid disorders with radioiodine is a classic example. The availability of radionuclides with suitable therapeutic properties for specific applications, as well as methods for their selective targeting to diseased tissue have, however, remained the main obstacles for therapy to assume a more widespread role in nuclear medicine (4,5). Nonetheless, a number of new techniques that have recently emerged, (e.g., tumor therapy with radiolabeled monoclonal antibodies, treatment of metastatic bone pain, etc.) appear to have provided a substantial impetus to research on production of new therapeutic radionuclides (4-7).

Table 1. Radiotherapy Using Unsealed Sources

Tumor therapy
Radiolabeled monoclonal antibodies
Non antibody methods
Receptor-binding radiotracers for tumor and other specific therapies
Bioactive peptides
Antibody derived agents
Molecular recognition units
Conventional in-vivo receptors
Bone pain palliation therapy
Radiation synovectomy
Miscellaneous therapies
Microspheres, colloids (for ascites, etc.)
Radioimmunoguided surgery

S. J. Mather (ed.), Current Directions in Radiopharmaceutical Research and Development, 63–79.

Table 1 lists the various categories of therapeutic procedures involving the use of internally administered radionuclides. Although there are a number of new therapeutic approaches requiring specific radionuclides, only selected broad areas will be used as examples in this article.

Selection Criteria

The selection criteria for therapeutic radionuclides have to include the physical and chemical characteristics of the radionuclide, feasibility of large-scale production, and the biological factors governing its in-vivo distribution (4,7). Physical properties that are important to consider include half-life, and the type, energy, branching ratio and abundances of particulate and gamma-ray emissions. Ideally, the physical half-life should be matched with the in-vivo pharmacokinetics of the radiolabeled compound. If the half-life is too short, most decay will have occurred before the compound has reached maximum target/background ratio. Conversely, too long a lifetime would cause unnecessary radiation dose to normal tissues following the processing of the labeled compound. The nature of the particulate emission is also important to maximise therapeutic effectiveness. The potent lethality of high-LET (linear energy transfer) Auger and low-energy conversion electrons is well documented (8). This effect, however, can best be achieved with intranuclear localisation of the labeled compound. Beta particles on the other hand are less densely ionising and thus have a longer range but much lower LET. Their distribution requirements are, therefore, less restrictive for effective radiotherapy. The gamma-ray energies and abundances are also important since the presence of gamma rays allows low dose biodistribution studies by external imaging for determining biodistribution and dosimetry. Biodistribution data combined with the physical properties of the radionuclide, and with assumptions about tumor size, etc., can be used to calculate radiation absorbed dose at the cellular level (7,9-11).

The important chemical criteria for selecting a radionuclide for radiotherapy are the specific activity, radiochemical purity, trace metal contamination, the number of metal atoms that can be attached per molecule of the compound without compromising biological activity, and in-vivo stability of the radionuclide attachment. The specific activity is dictated primarily by the method of production. Trace metal contaminants are a concern as they can compete for binding sites on the compound being labeled.

The various above physical and chemical criteria have then to be matched with the in-vivo pharmacokinetics of the labeled compound. For example, substantial variations in localisation of radiobioconjugates and the kinetics of their uptake and excretion have been reported (3,11). For monoclonal antibodies (MAb), it is generally observed that 0.5-3 days are necessary to reach maximum tumor concentration although optimum tumor to normal tissue contrast may take longer. Despite the numerous available antigen sites on cancer cells, a non-uniform cellular distribution of the MAb results in most cases (12). These facts reduce the general attractiveness of short-ranged Auger and alpha-emitting radionuclides for radioimmunotherapy (RIT) with MAbs except in specific situations such as for treating blood tumours and micrometastases. Also, short-ranged particles are more attractive if the radiobioconjugate gets internalised into tumor cells, and binds to nuclear components, thus making it possible to target nuclear antigens (13). The longer range of beta particles, on the other hand, allows more uniform tumor irradiation despite the heterogeneity of radioactivity distribution within the tumor tissue. Ultimately, it becomes a trade-off as to which radionuclide is best for a particular application.

Alpha, Auger, and Conversion Electron Emitters

As mentioned above, nuclides that emit high-LET radiations can be most effective in tumor cell killing (8,9,13). If the nuclide used is an Auger electron or a low-energy conversion electron emitter it will deposit the maximum dose within the targeted tumor cells. The radionuclide will be most effective, however, if it is transported across the cell membrane, and localises into the nucleus or in close proximity to it. Representative examples of radionuclides (halogens and metals) that emit alpha, Auger, or conversion electrons, and are suitable for therapeutic use with this approach, are shown in Table 2.

Table 2. Nuclear and Physical Characteristics of Some Alpha, Auger, and Conversion Electron Emitting Radionuclides for Targeting Nuclear Antigens.

	Halogens			Metals		
Radionuclide	Bromine-77	Iodine-125	Astatine-211	Tin-117m	Thallium-201	Bismuth-212
Half-life	57.0h	60.1d	7.2h	13.6d	3.04d	61m
Decay mode	EC, β^+	EC	EC,α	IT	EC	α, β^-
Principal						
γ KeV	511	35.5	None	159	167	727
% Abundance	1.5	6.7	—	86	11	6.7
Principal						
α KeV	None	None	5868	None	None	6051
% Abundance	—	—	41	-	-	25
Auger						
Electrons #	15	20	20	5	18	1
Range, KeV	0.1-12	0.7-30	3.2-87	0.6-24	2.7-77	2.7
% per decay	376	479	95	281	253	30
Conversion						
Electrons, #	11	6	Negligible	9	20	3
Range, KeV	149-508	3.7-36	—	127-158	1.6-167	25-40
% per decay	1.5	93	—	114	115	25

Attractive radionuclides with short range Auger and conversion electron emission are ^{67}Ga, ^{77}Br, ^{117m}Sn, ^{123}I, and iodine-125. Alpha particles that have a high LET, effective in cell killing,, and a range of several cell diameters (40-80 μm) are also very attractive. Examples of alpha emitters include ^{212}Bi, ^{211}At, and ^{255}Fm. It has been calculated that the dose advantage for ^{211}At compared to ^{90}Y (a long-range beta emitter) increases from a factor of 9 for a 1-mm-diameter tumor to a factor of 1200 for a single tumor cell (10). However, a high degree of selectivity and uniform intracellular localisation are necessary to achieve maximum therapeutic advantage. It should be noted that a number of nuclides from this category, in particular ^{123}I, ^{125}I, ^{67}Ga, and ^{201}Tl are commercially available and should be tested for effectiveness to target nuclear antigens.

Beta Emitters

There are a number of beta emitters, especially radiometals, that possess various particle ranges and chemical properties and thus offer a much wider choice for specific applications (4,7,11). Candidate beta emitters can be arbitrarily grouped into two classes: 1) those emitting low to intermediate energy beta particles and gamma emission suitable (>10%) for imaging; and 2) those with higher beta energy and little (<10%) or no gamma emission (Table 3). This distinction is only arbitrary since many radionuclides in the second category allow imaging at high dose administrations. Low-dose biodistribution and imaging experiments are possible with radionuclides in the first group before administering a therapeutic dose of the exact same preparation. Because it has been observed that the biodistribution can be influenced by the choice of radionuclide alone, even with the same antibody system (14), this would be a real advantage. Clinically, it is considered highly desirable, even necessary, to image each patient prior to therapy in order to assess biodistribution and antigenic status and to calculate tumor and normal tissue doses.

From among the radionuclides listed in Table 3, ^{47}Sc, ^{67}Cu, ^{117m}Sn, ^{153}Sm, and ^{188}Re appear particularly attractive because of their favourable chemistry and/or ease of production. Copper-67 has given promising results in preliminary studies for the RIT of lymphoma (15). However, scaled-up accelerator production of ^{67}Cu of high specific activity, required for many applications, has turned out to be problematic (16). Scandium-47 is considered a better substitute for ^{67}Cu since it can be reactor-produced in larger quantities and also because its nuclear and chemical properties are favourable for developing radiobioconjugates and other labeled compounds (17). Tin-117m and ^{153}Sm that are being developed for bone pain palliation therapy are discussed in a later section. The current specific activity of reactor-produced ^{117m}Sn, although not a problem with its use for bone pain palliation therapy, is not acceptable for developing radioimmunoconjugates. Rhenium-188 is attractive since it is a generator product from the decay of the 69.4 day tungsten-188 (18). It has shown promise in initial studies as a therapeutic label for MAbs and other vehicles, e.g., somatostatin analogs.

Table 3. Potential Beta-emitters for Radiotherapy

Radionuclide	Half-life (d)	Electron energy (keV average)	Gamma photon keV(%)
Group I. >10% Gamma Emission			
Scandium-47	3.4	162	159 (68)
Copper-67	2.6	141	185 (49)
Rhodium-105	1.5	190	319 (19)
Tin-117m	13.6	127*	159 (86)
		152*	
Iodine-131	8.0	181	364 (81)
Samarium-153	1.93	225	103 (28)
Lutetium-177	6.7	133	208 (11)
Rhenium-188	0.71	764	155 (15)
Iridium-194	0.80	808	328 (13)
Gold-199	3.1	86	158 (37)
		143*	
Group II. <10% Gamma Emission			
Phosphorus-32	14.3	695	—
Arsenic-77	1.6	228	239 (1.6)
Strontium-89	50.5	583	—
Yttrium-90	2.7	935	—
Palladium-109	0.56	360	88 (3.6)
Silver-111	7.5	350	342 (6.7)
Praseodymium-142	0.80	860	158 (3.7)
Promethium-149	2.2	364	286 (3.1)
Gadolinium-159	0.77	311	363 (8.0)
Holmium-166	1.1	666	80 (6.2)
Rhenium-186	3.71	329	137 (9.2)

* Conversion electron

The use of ^{90}Y for various radiotherapeutic procedures has been popular because of its high-energy beta particle, suitable half-life, and availability. Since ^{90}Y is unsuitable for quantitative imaging, ^{111}In biodistribution data are utilised to predict dose from ^{90}Y-labeled immunoconjugates. However, it has been shown that although the intravascular kinetics in patients are often similar for many ^{90}Y and ^{111}In labeled MAbs, there are significant differences in the tumor uptake and tissue biodistribution properties of these radionuclides (19). A similar approach has been taken for the pair ^{99m}Tc and ^{186}Re, the former for imaging, and the latter for therapy. These radionuclides share very similar chemistries for radiolabeling MAbs and other compounds.

Radiobioconjugates for Tumor Therapy

Research on radiobioconjugates (used here in a generic sense to include radiolabeled monoclonal antibodies, peptides, receptor specific and other bioactive molecules) has experienced rapid growth due to the promise of a number of these compounds to serve as selective carriers of radionuclides to tumor-associated and other specific antigens/receptors in vivo (1-4). However, although radiobioconjugate therapy has shown initial promise for certain types of tumours, practical benefits of this approach have not matched the expectations that were raised more than ten years ago (1). Radioimmunotherapy (RIT, used here in a generic sense for all radiobioconjugates) is considered best suited for treating tumours that cannot be easily resected or for treatment of small disseminated lesions and/or secondary micrometastases. From various considerations, especially dosimetry, the choice of the optimum radionuclide is a very important factor for a successful exploitation of this technique. Although ^{131}I is marginally suited for RIT, most therapy trials have so far utilised this isotope due to its commercial availability at low cost, the well understood chemistry of iodine, and the experience from the use of ^{131}I in treating thyroid disorders.

The radionuclides listed in Tables 2-3 are among the most promising for RIT. Those in Table 2 require the labeled molecule to be not only efficiently internalised into the tumor cells but to also preferably bind to nuclear antigens. A number of monoclonal antibodies have been observed to internalise into tumor cells of various types and bind to nuclear components (13). Various other important factors involved in radiobioconjugate development include the convenience, efficiency, and gentleness of different radiolabeling procedures as well as the stability of the radionuclide attachment to the immunoconjugate. These topics are outside of the scope of this article but a very brief discussion at this point is considered appropriate.

RIT requires a stable attachment of the radionuclide to the MAb since free radionuclide may target normal tissues thus increasing normal organ and whole body doses. Radiolabeling techniques range widely from well established protein halogenation schemes, simple direct labelling of ^{186}Re, to the use of general purpose bifunctional chelating agents such as the bicyclic anhydride of DTPA (DTPA-DA) for ^{90}Y, ^{109}Pd, and ^{153}Sm, to the use of more structurally complex in-house synthesised bifunctional chelating agents for ^{186}Re, ^{67}Cu, ^{47}Sc and ^{90}Y (13,14).

Due to the chemical similarity between Tc and Re, strategies for labelling MAbs with ^{186}Re have directly paralleled those for ^{99m}Tc. Direct labelling with ^{188}Re has been demonstrated utilising free sulphydryl groups on the MAb; these groups can be generated either by chemical reduction of MAb disulphide bonds or by the reaction of lysines on the MAb with 2-iminothiolane. A more selective approach involves chelation of ^{186}Re to a N_3S-amide mercaptide ligand (MAG_2-GABA) prior to conjugation to MAbs (20). While less convenient, this approach allows more control over radiolabeling and may have wider applicability with various MAb systems.

Antibodies have been labeled with ^{90}Y using DTPA-DA; however, in clinical trials these preparations showed high bone uptake of ^{90}Y. Substantially reduced bone uptake in mice was shown using p-isothiocyanatobenzyl DTPA (the coordination sites on this ligand are 8 compared to 7 for DTPA-DA); however, it was still higher than what is generally observed with the corresponding ^{111}In labeled MAb (21). In mice the bone uptake of ^{90}Y has been reduced to the levels of ^{111}In using the macrocyclic bifunctional chelating agent p-bromoacetamidobenzyl-DOTA (22). Biodistribution studies in mice of ^{47}Sc labeled MAb prepared using DTPA-DA have shown high levels of radioactivity in the liver. Carrier-free ^{47}Sc has been prepared at BNL and successfully attached to MAbs 17-1A and anti-CEA F(ab')$_2$ using the semi-rigid bifunctional chelating agent 4-isothiocyanato-cyclohexyl EDTA (4-ICE) and others (17). Using the preorganised ligand approach, the biodistribution in normal and tumor mice of the ^{47}Sc labeled preparations was comparable or better than that of the corresponding ^{111}In labeled antibodies (23). Antibodies prepared using 4-ICE have shown higher tumor uptake with a three to four-fold reduction in the retention of ^{111}In in the liver compared to DTPA-immunoconjugates in mice (24), and similar results were obtained with scandium-47 (23).

Copper labeled DTPA-immunoconjugates are not stable in serum. Even though the serum stability of Cu labeled 4-ICE-immunoconjugates is substantially higher they are still unstable in-vivo and produce high non-specific retention of copper-67. Stable Cu labeled immunoconjugates result only by using derivatives of the macrocyclic polyaminocarboxylates p-aminobenzyl-TETA (25) and DOTA or derivatised cyclic polyamines (cyclams) (26). Preliminary studies in patients with pharmacological doses of ^{67}Cu labeled Lym-1 MAb prepared using parabromo-acetamidobenzyl-TETA have given promising results (15). Little work has been done on ^{153}Sm as an antibody label, however. In one study in mice, ^{153}Sm labeled K-1-21 murine IgG (labeled using DTPA-DA) gave a slightly lower tumor uptake with higher bone and liver uptake compared to ^{131}I or ^{111}In labeled K-1-21 (27). The use of bifunctional chelator 4-ICE did not improve the ^{153}Sm labeled 17-1A biodistribution compared to ^{153}Sm labeled DTPA-17-1A (28). This may be due to the fact that since Sm is a lanthanide with f valence electrons having no specific coordination geometry, it does not need a preorganised chelation cavity. A higher number of coordination sites on the ligand is more important for samarium. The macrocyclic polyaminocarboxylate DOTA (eight coordination sites) produced much better results with samarium-153 (28).

The experience with the above mentioned radiometals has been valuable in terms of understanding the chelation chemistry for attachment to immunoconjugates, and will serve to improve our current methodology to produce stable radioimmunoconjugates with these and other promising radiometals listed in Tables 2 and 3.

Treatment of Metastatic Bone Pain

A number of radiopharmaceuticals appear to offer advantages over narcotic or other conventional treatments for bone pain from osseous metastases in cancer patients (29). This concept is not new, and ^{32}P has been investigated for over three decades for this purpose (30). However, the recent FDA approval of ^{89}Sr chloride (Metastron) has opened up a new era for the development of unsealed sources for bone pain palliation therapy. Introduction of ^{89}Sr has catalysed the development of newer competitive agents that may offer improvements in efficacy or reduced myelosuppression. The radionuclides under investigation include β-emitters ^{186}Re (31) and ^{153}Sm (32), and the conversion-electron emitter tin-117m (33,34). Physical and nuclear properties of the various radionuclides for bone pain palliation therapy are summarised in Table 4.

The primary concern from the therapeutic use of this class of bone-seeking radiopharmaceuticals is the absorbed dose to the red marrow. The energy of the beta particles seems to be an important factor because the dose to the marrow depends on the range of penetration of the particles into the marrow from the deposited radioactivity on to the bone surfaces. In this respect, ^{117m}Sn may offer a distinct advantage because of the discrete limited range (0.2-0.3 mm) of its conversion electrons in tissue (33-35). It remains to be seen which one of these agents eventually will become the agent of choice.

Table 4. Physical Characteristics of Radionuclides for Bone Pain Palliation Therapy

Radionuclide	Maximum Eβ (MeV)	Weighted Average Eβ (MeV)	Average Range (mm)	Half-Life (days)	Gamma Photons (MeV (%)
Strontium-89	1.46	0.583	2.4	50.5	None
Rhenium-186	1.08	0.329	1.05	3.71	0.137 (9.2)
Samarium-153	0.81	0.225	0.55	1.93	0.103 (28)
Tin-117m	0.127[a]	-	0.21[b]	13.6	0.159 (86)
	0.152[a]	-	0.29[b]		

a Monoenergetic conversion electron

b Discrete travel of emitted conversion electron (not an average)

Radionuclides that appear promising for this application (Table 4) are all reactor-produced and there does not seem to be a supply/demand problem for most cases. Tin-117m could be considered an exception since a high-flux reactor is required for producing it in sufficient quantities and there are only a few reactors world-wide with such a capability. However, future production in sufficient quantities now appears feasible (36).

Radiation Synovectomy

Radiation synovectomy is an attractive alternative to chemical or surgical synovectomy for the treatment of inflammatory synovial disease, including rheumatoid arthritis. The procedure entails a single injection of a beta-emitting radiopharmaceutical directly into the synovium to control and ablate inflammation. The injected agents, typically colloids or larger aggregates, are assumed to be rapidly phagocytosed by synoviocytes and then distributed within the synovium, primarily at the surface. Most commonly used agents have comprised radiocolloids or macroaggregates employing high-energy beta emitters, ^{90}Y, ^{198}Au, ^{165}Dy, and ^{186}Re (37). While these agents have shown good treatment efficacy, they are not widely used especially in the United States. All display some degree of leakage of the radionuclide from the joints leading to an increased radiation dose to normal organs. The size of these radiolabelled particles cannot be adequately controlled during formation, and it is assumed that small (<10 μm) particles leak from the synovium over time. However, a new type of particle, made from hydroxyapatite (HA), a natural constituent of bone, has become commercially available in various controlled sizes ranging from 1 - 80 μm. Research interest has thus focused recently on incorporating HA particles into new agents for radiation synovectomy. Initial studies in rabbits with antigen-induced arthritis (AIA) using ^{153}Sm labeled HA, showed minimal leakage of activity (0.09% over four days) from the treated joint compared to leakage rates obtained with other radiocolloid agents (5-45%); results with ^{186}Re-HA, however, showed slightly higher leakage (3.05% over four days) (38).

The presumed heterogeneous distribution of radionuclide within the synovium has limited existing agents to only those labeled with high energy beta emitters. It is presumed that the longer range of these particles is necessary to treat medium to large sized joints. However, low-energy beta emitters may be equally or more effective in reducing inflammation for small to medium joints since a much larger radiation dose could be delivered to the synovium without excessive irradiation of surrounding tissue. This could be analogous to the effectiveness of the short range conversion electrons from ^{117m}Sn for bone pain palliation, compared to the high-energy beta emitter ^{89}Sr (35). The only clinical example to date for treating synovial inflammation using a low-energy beta emitter is the use of ^{169}Er (β^{-}avg. 111 keV) colloids to treat inflammation in the small finger joints (37) Based on various considerations, appropriate sized particles labeled with ^{47}Sc, ^{117m}Sn, ^{153}Sm, and ^{169}Er would seem to be the agents of choice for radiation synovectomy.

Radionuclide Production

A detailed description of production methods, in particular those that can be implemented on an economic scale, is not within the purview of this article. However, it is considered important to provide a summary of the current status in this area including problems and concerns related to isotope availability. Radionuclides are primarily produced using a nuclear reactor or a charged-particle accelerator (mainly cyclotrons), and their properties depend upon a number of factors that include targetry, irradiation conditions and processing chemistry (5,6,39). The production and supply of many routine imaging and some therapeutic radionuclides that have a commercial market have continued at a satisfactory level (5,39).

In terms of the radionuclides listed in Table 2 that are particularly attractive for targeting nuclear antigens (13), only ^{123}I, ^{125}I, ^{67}Ga and ^{201}Tl are available commercially. Although the production methodology for others has been worked out to some extent, they are not readily available in sufficient quantities on a regular basis. A notable exception is ^{117m}Sn which has been discussed above for bone pain palliation therapy in cancer patients. The current specific activity (~8 mCi/mg), however, that is adequate for this application is not high enough for radiobioconjugate development. Its use as a target for nuclear antigens will have to await the development of methods that could provide a no-carrier-added product (40). Additional radionuclides in Table 2 that have been investigated to some extent include ^{124}I (41), ^{211}At (42), and bismuth-212 (43). Their properties are suitable for targeting nuclear antigens using MAb systems or other vehicles that are shown to be internalised into the tumor cells. However, the production, the availability, and the conjugation chemistry of these radionuclides remain to be developed further.

REACTOR PRODUCTION

Table 5 lists some therapeutic radionuclides that can be produced in a nuclear reactor in quantities sufficient for widespread clinical use (4,6). It is noteworthy that many of the β^- or β^{-}/γ emitters discussed in this article are best produced using neutron bombardment reactions.

In reactor production, there are three types of reactions that are employed: (i) neutron capture, (n,γ); (ii) neutron capture followed by decay; and (iii) fission. The n,γ reaction using thermal neutrons is the most widely employed technique. The reasons are that elemental targets can be used and the yields are generally high. However, separation from the bulk of the stable element is not possible and thus the specific activities can be low unless the cross sections are very high. No-carrier added radionuclides are not producible using the n,γ reaction. The other reactions allow improvement in specific activity, and can often be used (n,$\gamma \rightarrow \beta^-$ decay, n, f, etc.) under certain situations such as when an intermediate nuclide decays to the product of interest. In general, high chemical purity reagents and enriched stable element targets have to be employed in reactor production of radionuclides.

Table 5. Reactor Production of Therapeutic Radionuclides

Radionuclide	Nuclear Reaction
Scandium-47	$^{47}Ti(n,p)$
Yttrium-90	$U\ (n,f)\ ^{90}Sr \rightarrow \beta$
Rhodium-105	$^{nat}Ru\ (n,\gamma)\ ^{105}Ru \rightarrow \beta$
Palladium-109	$^{108}Pd\ (n,\gamma)$
Silver-111	$^{110}Pd\ (n,\gamma)\ ^{111}Pd \rightarrow \beta$
Tin-117m	$^{117}Sn\ (n,n',\gamma)\ ^{117m}Sn$
Iodine-131	$^{235}U\ (n,f)$
Praseodymium-142	$^{141}Pr\ (n,\gamma)$
Promethium-149	$^{148}Nd\ (n,\gamma)\ ^{149}Nd \rightarrow \beta$
Samarium-153	$^{152}Sm\ (n,\gamma)$
Gadolinium-159	$^{158}Gd\ (n,\gamma)$
Holmium-166	$^{165}Ho\ (n,\gamma)$
Lutetium-177	$^{176}Lu\ (n,\gamma)$
Rhenium-186	$^{185}Re\ (n,\gamma)$
Rhenium-188	$^{186}W\ (n,\gamma)\ ^{187}W\ (n,\gamma)\ ^{188}W \rightarrow \beta$
Iridium-194	$^{193}Ir\ (n,\gamma)$
Gold-199	$^{198}Pt\ (n,\gamma)\ ^{199}Pt \rightarrow \beta$
	$^{197}Au\ (n,\gamma)\ ^{198}Au\ (n,\gamma)$

Table 6. Accelerator Production of Therapeutic Radionuclides

Radionuclide	Nuclear Reaction
Scandium-47	$^{48}Ti\ (p,2p)$
Copper-67	$^{68}Zn\ (p,2p)$
Bromine-77	$^{79}Br\ (p,3n)\ ^{77}Kr\ \beta^{+} \rightarrow$
Arsenic-77	$^{80}Se\ (p,\alpha)$
Tin-117m	$^{121}Sb\ (p,2p,3n)$
Platinum-193m	192Os (a3n)

ACCELERATOR PRODUCTION

The cyclotron is the most widely used accelerator for producing radionuclides. A wide variety of cyclotrons now exist ranging from "baby" cyclotrons of energies as low as 3 MeV to very large isochronous synchrotrons with energies in excess of 500 MeV. The variety of accelerated particles (p,d,^{3}He,α) and the energy range available make cyclotrons very flexible for radionuclide production. Commercial cyclotrons commonly have a range of 5-30 MeV particles and many are used exclusively for isotope production. Some of the more interesting radionuclides are listed in Table 6.

Certain radionuclides that can be produced only using high-energy linear accelerators (e.g., spallation reactions) or whose production is more cost effective when made this way are either scarce or not available (5). One of the main reasons for this is that high-energy machines are very expensive to build and operate and isotope production is usually in conflict with their primary mission which is physics research (44). Consequently, isotope production in these machines has been undertaken only as an intermittent and parasitic activity. This situation has created considerable concern within the radioisotope research community that includes nuclear medicine as well as basic physical and life science investigators (44,45). This is especially in view of the fact that a number of high-energy produced radionuclides are emerging as being potentially useful and in some cases unique for applications (mostly imaging, some therapeutic) in nuclear medicine. With the recent rapid growth in biotechnological and immunological approaches to treatment of cancer, bone pain, and other diseases, there is an urgent need at least in the U.S. for a continuous and reliable availability of certain high-energy produced radionuclides (5).

At the present time, there are about six high-energy accelerators world-wide that engage in isotope production for distribution. These are located in the U.S. (BLIP and LAMPF), Canada (TRIUMF), Switzerland (PSI), South Africa (NAC), and Russia (45). A few others also have the capability for isotope production but are utilised rarely or very little for this purpose. It must be emphasised that the cost of production is a critical factor and unless there is a commercial market, high-energy produced radionuclides are not produced in any consistent fashion.

GENERATOR SYSTEMS

A number of relatively short-lived therapeutic radionuclides, especially β^- emitters, can be obtained through generator systems. These are listed in Table 7.

The ^{90}Sr/^{90}Y generator system has been utilised for quite some time; it has a number of practical advantages. The chemistry of yttrium, as mentioned earlier, is also favourable for labelling MAbs and other bioactive molecules. A number of therapeutic protocols have employed ^{90}Y with significant success (46). Another generator system, ^{188}W/^{188}Re (18), has also been developed and investigated for antibody labelling and other applications. The results are still preliminary but quite promising. Large-scale production of ^{188}W can be accomplished in a high-flux reactor. The generator system for the alpha emitter ^{212}Bi has been available on an experimental basis only (43). The use of this isotope because of the 1 h half-life is possible only in special situations. The $^{115}Cd/^{115m}In$ generator system should be useful for applications where a short range (it emits a 300 keV conversion electron with ~1 mm range) and a short half-life are advantageous.

Table 7. Generator Systems for Therapeutic Radionuclides

Daughter				Parent	
Radionuclide	$T_{1/2}$	β^-max, MeV	(γ, keV (%)	Radionuclide	$T_{1/2}$
Copper-66	5.1 min	2.63	1039 (9)	Nickel-66	2.3 d
Zinc-69	55 min	0.90	—	Zinc-69m	0.6 d
Yttrium-90	64 h	2.27	—	Strontium-90	28.6 yr
Silver-112	3.2 h	3.94	617 (41)	Palladium-112	0.9 d
Indium-115m	4.5 h	0.83 (5%) 0.30 (49%)[a]	335 (50)	Cadmium-115	2.2 d
Cesium-128	3.6 min	2.89 (β^+)	441 (27) 511 (110)[b]	Barium-128	2.4 d
Iodine-132	2.3 h	2.12	773 (89)	Tellurium-132	3.2 d
Rhenium-188	17 h	2.1	155 (15)	Tungsten-188	69.4 d
Bismuth-212[c]	60 min	—	727 (11)	Radium-224/ Lead-212	3.7d

[a]Conversion electron
[b]γ from β^+ emission
[c]Alpha emitter, also has some β^- emission

The remaining generator systems listed in Table 7 primarily produce daughter radionuclides with short $t_{1/2}$ and high β^- energies. There is an inverse relationship between $t_{1/2}$ and β^- decay energy and therefore, there are only a few radionuclides that have both a several-day $t_{1/2}$ and a high β^- energy. To circumvent this problem one could use the approach of labelling with an intermediate $t_{1/2}$ radionuclide that decays in-vivo to a much shorter $t_{1/2}$ daughter with high β- emission. Since the daughter will be in equilibrium with the parent, it will exert an in-situ cytotoxic effect over a prolonged period, essentially as an "in-vivo generator" (47). However, a number of critical questions will have to be answered before his approach can be applied successfully for radiotherapy (e.g., the fate of the daughter nucleus following the uptake of the parent by the tumor - will it translocate to other tissues before decay? etc.). A theoretical test of the feasibility of this approach has been attempted with encouraging results (48).

Conclusion

There are a number of potential candidate radionuclides for tumor therapy and for other therapeutic applications. This article has attempted to provide a brief discussion of the criteria for selecting radionuclides for specific applications. The choice of the radionuclide best suited for a particular application depends upon a number of factors that include: (1) Half-life; (2) Type of emission (α, β, γ, Auger or conversion electrons); (3) Specific activity; (4) Chemistry; (5) Route of administration; (6) Internal dosimetry; (7) Radiation safety and environmental concerns; (8) Vehicle used as the carrier; (9) In-vivo biopharmacokinetics of the labeled carrier and the free radionuclide; and (10) Cost of production and availability.

The various important therapeutic applications, where radionuclide therapy may have an important role to play in, and the radionuclides that are considered best suited for the application, are summarised in Table 8. It should be noted that this listing is not meant to be exhaustive, and additional radionuclides can be added based on present and future work as well as various other considerations. At times, the cost and availability, especially if the radionuclide is "new" and/or difficult to produce, become issues of paramount importance.

In summary, there are a number of therapeutic radionuclides that are presently under investigation, and some of these may eventually turn out to be ideal or best-suited for specific applications. Although issues relating to cost and availability of many of these are yet to be addressed to everybody's satisfaction, there does not seem to be a dearth of new therapeutic radionuclides. As new needs and applications develop, appropriate radionuclides will follow. The substantial progress of investigations in certain areas, for example, tumor radioimmunotherapy and bone pain palliation, offer renewed hope and promise for the widespread use of internally administered radionuclides for various novel and effective therapeutic approaches.

Table 8. Choice of Radionuclides for Principal Therapeutic Applications

Application	Route of Administration	Best-suited Radionuclide(s)[a]
I. Tumor Therapy		
(i) Solid Tumours a. Large lesions	i.v.	Sc-47, Y-90, I-131, Re-188
	intra-tumoral	Sc-47, Sm-153, Re-188
b. Micrometastases	i.v.	Sc-47, Sn-117m, Sm-153, Auger emitters
(i) Leukemias, lymphomas	i.v.	Sc-47, Cu-67, Sn-117m, I-131
II. Palliation		
(i) Soft tissue	i.v.	Y-90, I-131, Ho-166, Re-188
(ii) Bone pain	i.v.	Sr-89, Sn-117m, Sm-153, Re-186
III. Non-Oncology and Other		
(i) Synovectomy	Regional	Sc-47, Sn-117m, Sm-153, Er-169
(ii) Marrow ablation	i.v.	Sn-117m, Ho-166
(iii) Microspheres	i.v. or regional	Y-90, lanthanides
(iv) Receptor-positive, nuclear antigens	i.v.	Auger, conversion electron, and short-range β^- emitters

[a]Based, partially, on a Therapy Isotope Workshop sponsored by Nordion International, Inc., at the 43rd Annual Meeting of the Society of Nuclear Medicine, Minneapolis, MN, June 11, 1995. The order of listing of isotopes here is based on atomic mass and not necessarily their degree of effectiveness for a particular application.

Acknowledgements

This work was supported by the United States Department of Energy, Office of Health and Environmental Research, under Contract No. DE-AC02-76CH00016. The author is thankful to Ms. Susan Cataldo for excellent secretarial assistance during the preparation of this article.

References

1. Srivastava SC (ed): Radiolabeled Monoclonal Antibodies for Imaging and Therapy, New York, Plenum Press, 1988, 876 pp
2. Britton KE, Mather SJ, Granowska M: Radiolabelled monoclonal antibodies in oncology III. Radioimmunotherapy. Nucl Med Commun 12:333-347, 1991
3. Larson SM, Digvi CR, Scott A, et al: Current status of radioimmunotherapy. Nucl Med Biol 21:785-792, 1994
4. Mausner LF, Srivastava SC: Selection of radionuclides for radioimmunotherapy. Med Phys 20:503-509, 1993
5. Srivastava SC, Mausner LF: Production and supply of radioradionuclides with high-energy particle accelerators: Current status and future directions: in: Proc 21st Japan Conf Radiat and Radionuclides, Feb. 2-4, 1994, Japan Atomic Industrial Forum, B-550, pp 1-11
6. Volkert WA, Goeckler WF, Ehrhardt GJ, et al: Therapeutic radionuclides: production and decay property considerations. J Nucl Med 32:174-185, 1991
7. O'Donoghue JA, Bardies M, Wheldon TE: Relationships between tumor size and curability for uniformly targeted therapy with beta emitting radionuclides. J Nucl Med 36:1902-1909, 1995
8. Adelstein SJ, Kassis AI: Radiobiologic implications of the microscopic distribution of energy from radionuclides. Nucl Med Biol 14:165-169, 1987
9. Jungerman JA, Yu Kin-Hung P, Zanelli CI: Radiation absorbed dose estimates at the cellular level for some electron emitting radionuclides for radioimmunotherapy. Int J Appl Radiat Isot 35:883-888, 1984
10. Humm JL: Dosimetric aspects of radiolabeled antibodies for tumor therapy. J Nucl Med 27:1490-1497, 1986
11. Wessels BW, Rogus RD: Radionuclide selection and model absorbed dose calculations for radiolabeled tumor-associated antibodies. Med Phys 11:638-645, 1984
12. Griffith MH, Yorke ED, Wessels BW, et al: Direct dose confirmation of quantitative autoradiography with micro-TLD measurements for radioimmunotherapy. J Nucl Med 10:1795-1809, 1988
13. Srivastava SC: Criteria for the selection of radionuclides for targeting nuclear antigens for cancer radioimmunotherapy. Cancer Biother Radiopharm 11: 43-50, 1996
14. Srivastava SC, Mease RC: Progress in research on ligands, nuclides, and techniques for labeling monoclonal antibodies. Nucl Med Biol 18:589-603, 1991
15. DeNardo GL, DeNardo SJ, Meares CF, et al: Pilot therapy of lymphoma with fractionated Cu-67-BAT Lym-1. J Nucl Med 34:93P, 1993
16. DasGupta AK, Mausner LF, Srivastava SC: A new separation procedure for Cu from proton irradiated Zn. Int J Appl Radiat Isot 42:371-376, 1991
17. Mausner LF, Kolsky KL, Mease RC, et al: Production and evaluation of Sc-47 for radioimmunotherapy. J Labelled Compds Radiopharm 32:388-390, 1993
18. Ehrhardt G, Ketring AR, Turpin TA, et al: An improved tungsten-188/rhenium-188 generator for radiotherapeutic applications. J Nucl Med 28:656, 1987
19. Carasquillo JA, Kramer B, Fleisher T, et al: In-111 versus Y-90 T101 biodistribution in patients with hematopoietic malignancies. J Nucl Med 32:970, 1991 (abstr)
20. Breitz H, Ratliff B, Schroff R, et al: Phase I studies of 186-Re whole MoAb and $F(ab')_2$ fragment for radioimmunotherapy in solid tumors. J Nucl Med 31:724-725, 1990
21. Roselli M, Schlom J, Gansow OA, et al: Comparative biodistribution of yttrium- and indium-labeled monoclonal antibody B72.3 in athymic mice bearing human colon carcinoma xenografts. J Nucl Med 30:672-689, 1989
22. Adams GP, DeNardo SJ, Deshpande SV, et al: Dual isotope pharmacokinetics of an anti-lymphoma antibody (LYM-1) with a new bifunctional chelating agent. J Nucl Med 31:823, 1990
23. Mausner LF, Joshi V, Kolsky KL, et al: Evaluation of chelating agents for radioimmunotherapy with scandium-47. J Nucl Med 36:104P, 1995 (abstr)
24. Srivastava SC, Mease RC, Meinken GE, et al: Reduction in non-specific uptake of indium-111 from using semi-rigid cyclohexyl EDTA immunoconjugates. J Labelled Compds Radiopharm 35:303, 1994

25. Moi MK, Meares CF, McCall MJ, et al: Copper chelates as probes of biological systems: Stable copper complexes with a macrocyclic bifunctional chelating agent. Anal Biochem 148:249, 1985
26. Macke H, Ruser G, Koch P, et al: New bifunctional chelators for antibody labeling with metallic radionuclides. J Labelled Compds Radiopharm 30:318, 1991
27. Boniface GR, Izard ME, Walken KZ, et al: Labeling of monoclonal antibodies with samarium-153 for combined radioimmunoscintigraphy and radioimmunotherapy. J Nucl Med 30:683-691, 1989
28. Srivastava SC, Mausner LF, Mease RC, et al: Development and evaluation of 67-Cu and 153-Sm labeled conjugates for tumor radioimmunotherapy. Int J Radiopharmcognosy, 33:92-101, 1995
29. McEwan AJB: Radiopharmaceuticals for palliative treatment of painful bone metastases. New Perspectives in Cancer Diagnosis and Management. 2:24, 1994
30. Silberstein EB, Elgazzar AH, Kapilivsky A: Phosphorus-32 radiopharmaceuticals for the treatment of painful osseous metastases. Semin Nucl Med 22:17-27, 1992
31. Maxon HR, Schroder LE, Hertzberg VS, et al: Rhenium-186(Sn)HEDP for treatment of painful osseous metastases: results of a double-blind crossover comparison with placebo. J Nucl Med 32:1877-1881, 1991
32. Goeckler WF, Edwards B, Volkert WA, et al: Skeletal localization of samarium-153 chelates: potential therapeutic bone agents. J Nucl Med 28:495-504, 1987
33. Srivastava SC, Meinken GE, Richards P, et al: The development and in-vivo behavior of tin containing radiopharmaceuticals. I: Chemistry, preparation, and biodistribution in small animals. Int J Nucl Med Biol 12:167, 1985
34. Atkins HL, Mausner LF, Srivastava SC, et al: Human biodistribution of Sn-117m(4+)DTPA: A new agent for palliative therapy of painful osseous metastases. Radiology 186:279-283, 1993
35. Atkins HL, Mausner LF, Srivastava SC, et al: Tin-117m(4+)-DTPA for palliation of bone from osseous metastases: A pilot study. J Nucl Med 36:725-729, 1995
36. J. Lister-James, Diatide, Inc., personal communication, 1996.
37. Deutsch E, Bordack JW, Deutsch KF. Radiation syovectomy revisited. Eur J Nucl Med 20:1113, 1993, and references therein
38. Chinol M, Vallabhajousula S, Goldsmith SJ, Klein MJ, Deutsch KF, Chinen LK, Brodack JW, Deutsch EA, Watson BA, Tofe AJ. Chemistry and biological behavior of samarium-153 and rhenium-186-labeled hydroxyapatite particles: Potential radiopharmaceutical for radiation synovectomy. J Nucl Med 34:1536, 1993
39. Lamb JF, Kramer HH: Commercial production of radionuclides for nuclear medicine, in Rayudu GVS (ed): Radiotracers for Medical Applications Volume I. Boca Raton, FL, CRC, 1983
40. Mausner LF, Mirzadeh S, Maher R, et al: Production of high specific activity 117m-Sn with the Szilard-Chalmers process. J Labelled Compds Radiopharm 16:177-178, 1989
41. Larson SM, Pentlow KS, Volkow ND, et al: PET scanning of I-124-3F9 as an approach to tumor dosimetry during treatment planning for radioimmunotherapy in a child with neuroblastoma. J Nucl Med 33:2020-2023, 1992
42. Zalutsky MR, Garg PK, Friedman HS: Labeling monoclonal antibodies and $F(ab')_2$ with the "-particle-emitting nuclide astatine-211: preservation of immunoreactivity and in-vivo localizing capacity. Proc Natl Acad Sci USA 86:7149-7153, 1989
43. Atcher RN, Friedman AM, Hines JJ: An improved generator for the production of 212-Pb and 212-Bi from 224-Ra. Int J Appl Radiat Isot 39:283-286, 1988
44. Radionuclides for Medicine and the Life Sciences, Adelstein SJ, Manning FJ (ed): Washington, DC, National Academy Press, 1995, pp 1-132
45. Srivastava SC: Is there life after technetium: (What is the potential for developing new broad-based nuclides)?. Semin Nucl Med, 1996 (in press)
46. Hnatowitch DJ, Chinol M, Siebecker DA, et al: Patient biodistribution of intraperitoneally administered yttrium-90 labeled antibody. J Nucl Med 29:1428-1435, 1988
47. Mausner LF, Straub RF, and Srivastava SC: Production and use of prospective radionuclides for radioimmunotherapy. In: Radiolabeled Monoclonal Antibodies for Imaging and Therapy, Srivastava SC, Editor, Plenum, New York, 1988, pp. 149-163
48. Mausner LF, Straub RG, Srivastava SC: The in-vivo generator for radioimmunotherapy. J Labelled Compds Radiopharm 16:498-500, 1989

RADIOPHARMACEUTICALS FOR IMAGING HYPOXIA

Colin M Archer, Barbara Edwards and Nigel A Powell

Introduction

The purpose of this article is to briefly review recent research on radiolabelled agents designed for the purpose of imaging tissue hypoxia in vivo. The text of this article will present a broad brush summary of the subject matter with more detailed information contained in the literature sources referenced. Another review of this subject area has recently been published elsewhere and may offer the reader the chance to gain additional insights into work performed in this area of research [1].

Hypoxia: What is it?

One requirement of all mammalian cells is an adequate supply of oxygen. However in diseases which involve a reduction in the supply of oxygen to a tissue or to cells in a region of the body, the metabolic demands of the affected cells can exceed the amount of energy supplied by the lower oxygen concentrations present. When the supply of oxygen to a cell is exceeded by the metabolic requirements of the cell, that cell is hypoxic. In animals and man the degree of oxygenation of the cells in the body is determined by a combination of the energy required by the cells in order to carry out their normal functions and the amount of oxygen diffusing into the cells from the vasculature. Typically, then, cells in vivo become hypoxic when the supply of blood to the cells becomes reduced.

The normal concentration of oxygen ($pO2$) in the human body varies greatly from tissue to tissue. For instance, typical median $pO2$ values for the kidneys are 70-80 mm Hg [2,3]. In contrast, the normal median partial oxygen pressure in the liver and the brain is approximately 20 mm Hg. Despite the regional variations in $pO2$ levels, tissues or cells where the $pO2$ is below ~5 mm Hg would generally be described as being hypoxic.

Most cells can survive even prolonged periods of hypoxia. However, if the supply of oxygen is reduced sufficiently, the cells will die. The purpose of any radioimaging

S. J. Mather (ed.), Current Directions in Radiopharmaceutical Research and Development, 81–88.

agent for the detection of hypoxia is to identify regions of living tissue which is severely underperfused.

During periods of hypoxia, cells experience a great number of changes. Oxidative phosphorylation decreases while glycolysis increases to help meet the energetic requirements of the cell [4,5]. As a consequence of the increased importance of glycolysis, intracellular concentrations of ATP and hydrogen ions decrease during hypoxia. Intracellular concentrations of ADP and lactate increase during hypoxia. In addition, calcium homeostasis is impaired which leads to an increase in the cytosolic concentration of calcium ions with a concomitant reduction in the amount of calcium in the mitochondria. The operation of the sodium-potassium ATPase system is also effected with consequent potassium loss and sodium loading [6-8].

In hypoxic cells the concentrations of certain proteins can also increase. Intracellular concentrations of oxygen-regulated proteins, glucose-regulated proteins and heat shock proteins have all been shown to increase during hypoxia. In addition, the concentrations of some less abundant proteins can increase during hypoxia. For example, the vascular regulatory proteins erythropoietin and vascular endothelial growth factor (VEGF), the cell cycle regulated protein p53 and, in tumour cells, the metastasis promoting protein cathepsin L are all present in larger concentrations in hypoxic cells than in normally oxygenated cells[9]. The expression of these various proteins during hypoxia can be interpreted as being part of an overall cellular response to a stress condition. This response is intended to increase the cells' chances for survival.

Clinically, hypoxia is encountered in a number of disease states. In fact, the concept of tissue hypoxia originally arises from studies on the radiotherapeutic treatment of tumours and the apparent radioresistance of hypoxic tumours[10]. There are an increasing number of published studies which demonstrate that a significant fraction of certain types of tumours have median pO2's of less than 2.5 mm Hg [3,11-14]. For example, approximately 80% of head and neck squamous cell carcinoma have significant hypoxic fractions while the figure for carcinoma of the uterine cervix is about 50%. The identification of hypoxic tumours in vivo would greatly improve the staging and treatment of these difficult to treat tumours.

Restrictions of the cardiac vasculature can lead to either transient or prolonged hypoxia. In cardiology one important issue is the identification of poorly perfused but viable tissue. A radiodiagnostic agent localising in hypoxic tissues would therefore allow clinicians to differentiate such tissue from necrosed regions effected by, for instance, a severe myocardial stenosis. The diagnosis of tissue at risk of infarction which would benefit from medical intervention to restore blood flow to the poorly perfused tissue is a key target for an in vivo radiodiagnostic hypoxia agent .

Hypoxia Agents

For a number of decades now many researchers have sought to use the increased reductive environment present in hypoxic tumour cells to localise compounds in such tumours which would either increase the efficacy of radiotherapy of such cells or which would deliver cytotoxins specifically designed to kill hypoxic tumour cells to the tumour [15]. An important class of compounds studied as radiosensitisers are substituted 2-nitroimidazoles. 2-Nitroimidazoles have been shown to be susceptible to reductive trapping in cells with low pO2's. These compounds can be reduced in vivo by a number of cytosolic and mitochondrial enzymes under hypoxic conditions initially to form a one-electron reduction product, the nitro radical anion. In the presence of oxygen this radical anion is reoxidised to the original nitroimidazole and no trapping occurs. In hypoxic cells reoxidation does not occur and the nitro radical anion can be further reduced to a number of other products (Figure 1). Intracellular trapping of nitroimidazoles has been hypothesised to result from either the formation of hydrophilic reduction products which cannot diffuse out of the cell, or from the binding of reactive reduction products to either cytosolic macromolecules or to the DNA in the cell's nucleus. This work has been extensively reviewed elsewhere [16-22].

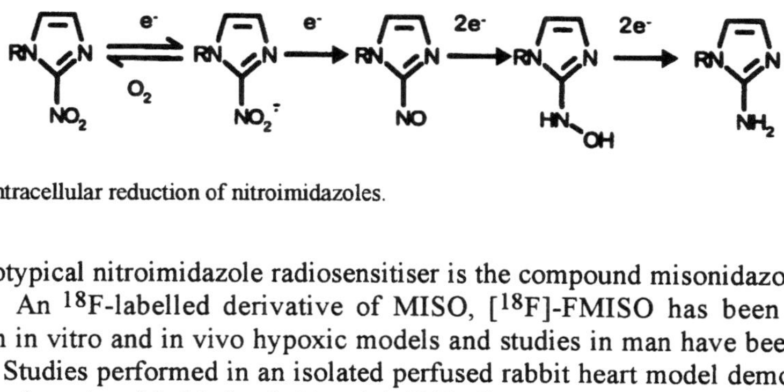

Figure 1. Intracellular reduction of nitroimidazoles.

The prototypical nitroimidazole radiosensitiser is the compound misonidazole (MISO) [23, 24]. An ^{18}F-labelled derivative of MISO, [^{18}F]-FMISO has been prepared, studied in in vitro and in vivo hypoxic models and studies in man have been reported [25-30]. Studies performed in an isolated perfused rabbit heart model demonstrated a hypoxic:oxic ratio of 2.6:1 (peak % ratio) [28]. The compound has shown uptake in hypoxic tumours in man with encouraging results [29, 30]. However, the availability of the compound, as with most positron emitting agents, is likely to remain limited to a few specialist centres.

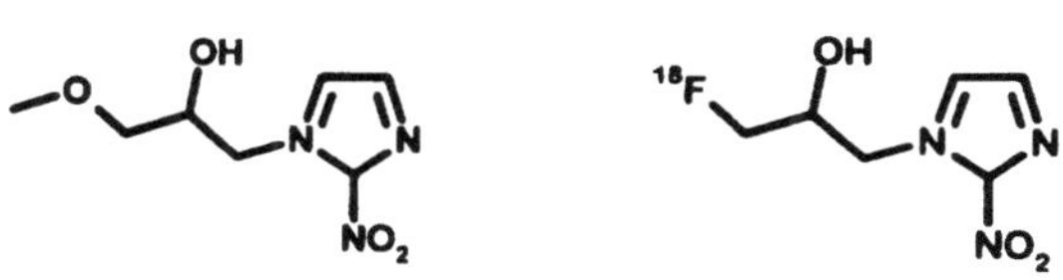

MISO **[^{18}F]-FMISO**

A group of researchers at the University of Alberta and the Cross Cancer Institute have prepared a number of iodine-labelled agents which contain 2-nitroimidazole moieties connected to an radioiodinated sugar group[31-35]. Typically this group have used ^{125}I-labelled compounds for their in vitro work and ^{123}I-labelled material for imaging studies. All of the compounds studied have exhibited oxygen dependent cell uptake in EMT-6 cells and all exhibit some amount of de-iodination in vivo. The lead compound of this series of agents is the iodoarabinoside compound, IAZA. [^{123}I]-IAZA has been administered to a number of patients and a variety of types of tumours have been imaged successfully by the Alberta groups. The drawbacks associated with this approach to hypoxia imaging are the fact that, as is the case for [^{18}F]-FMISO, because of the chemistry involved in the preparation and the radionuclide used, [^{123}I]-IAZA is not likely to be available outside of a limited number of research centres.

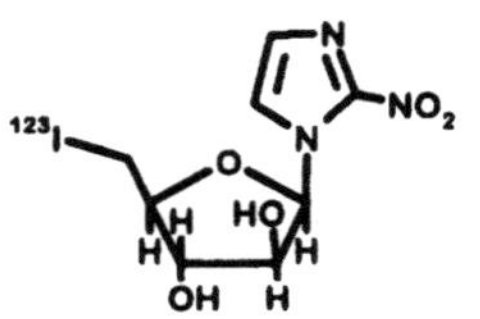

^{123}I-IAZA

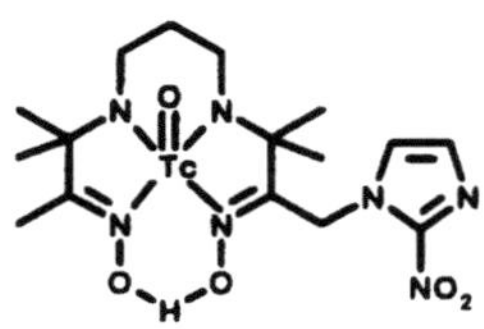

BMS181,321

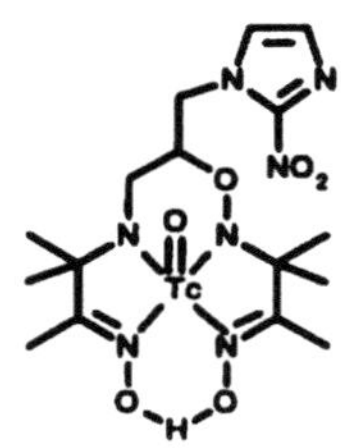

BMS194,796

For most clinical settings, the ideal radionuclide for diagnostic imaging is technetium-99m (^{99m}Tc). It is therefore not surprising, given the relative merits of the nitroimidazole-functionalised ^{18}F and ^{123}I agents discussed above, that researchers have adapted the general approach to the preparation of ^{99m}Tc-labelled hypoxia imaging agents. The research group lead by Linder, Nunn and Rumsey have now described several different ^{99m}Tc-complexes with ligands containing 2-nitroimidazole substituents[36-44]. Their first compounds encouragingly exhibited oxygen specific uptake and retention in vitro and this lead to the identification of the ^{99m}Tc-complex, BMS181,321 as a potential agent for use in vivo[36-38]. However, because BMS181,321 is very lipophilic, its behaviour in vivo is characterised by poor clearance from background tissues, especially from the liver[43,44]. However, BMS181,321 could potentially find use imaging hypoxia in the brain. The same group have recently reported the development of a less lipophilic compound, BMS194,796, which has improved liver clearance relative to BMS181,321[45].

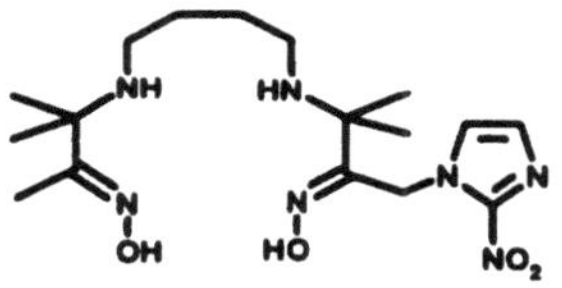

HL91M

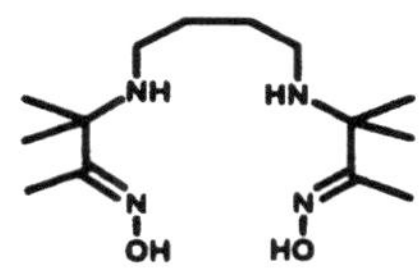

HL91

Our research group has also been involved in the development of new ^{99m}Tc-complexes for hypoxia imaging [46-48]. During an initial programme of work, a useful lead compound, 99mTc-HL91M, was identified on the basis of model studies in isolated perfused rat hearts [46]. However, negative control experiments were performed using the ^{99m}Tc-complex of the same ligand without the nitroimidazole group (^{99m}Tc-HL91) and this complex proved to exhibit more selective retention in hypoxic tissues than ^{99m}Tc-HL91M [46]. Studies also demonstrated that the retention of ^{99m}Tc-HL91 in cell cultures is oxygen dependent and that this complex can be reduced enzymatically by xanthine oxidase. While this complex does not contain a 2-nitroimidazole moiety, studies to date support the hypothesis that the ^{99m}Tc-complex is itself a bioreducible group. Further studies are underway to elucidate the structure and reactivity of this intriguing molecule as well as its potential use as an in vivo radiodiagnostic for imaging hypoxia.

While the biological activity of ^{99m}Tc-HL91 was unexpected and warrants further study, there is literature evidence that there are transition metal-ligand complexes which undergo bioreduction in hypoxic cellular environments. Of particular interest are the copper(II) dithiosemicarbazone complexes shown below which have been reported by Fujibayashi, et al [49,50]. The ^{62}Cu-complexes reported were chosen as markers of hypoxia on the basis that the Cu(II/I) redox couple for these complexes is biologically accessible and, in fact, is very similar to those observed for 2-nitroimidazoles. Like BMS181,321, these copper complexes could find use as brain imaging agents.

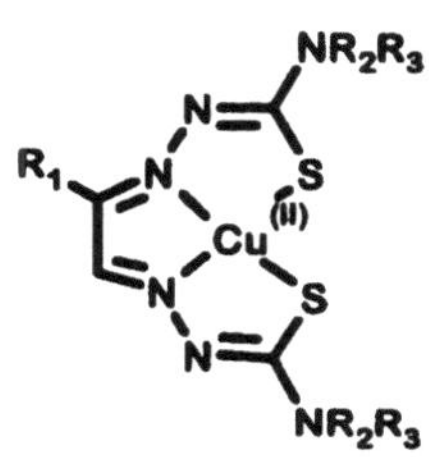

R_1, R_2, R_3 = H, Me

Conclusion

To date only [^{18}F]-FMISO and [^{123}I]-IAZA are in routine clinical use in a few localities. Unfortunately, their use is unlikely to become more widespread because of the specialist expertise required to prepare them. The progress thus far towards useful ^{99m}Tc-based agents is encouraging. However, these new agents will need to be proven in a clinical setting before they can be taken up more widely. As yet, there have been no reports of studies in man with either BMS 181,321 or BMS 194,796. Preliminary human studies have been performed using ^{99m}Tc-HL91 and the results of these will be published elsewhere.

References

1. Nunn A, Linder K, Strauss HW. Nitroimidazoles and imaging hypoxia. Eur J Nucl Med 1995;22:265-280.
2. Ehlry, AM, editor. Determination of tissue oxygen pressure in patients. Oxford: Pergamon Press, 1983.
3. Vaupel P, Kallinowski F, Okunieff P. Blood flow, oxygen consumption and tissue oxygenation of human tumors. In: J Piiper et al., editors. Oxygen transport to tissue XII. New York: Plenum Press, 1990: 895-905.
4. Jones DF, Aw TY, Shan X, Tribble DL. Characteristics of hypoxic cells that enhance their susceptibility to chemical injury. In: Adams GE, Breccia A, Fielden EM, Wardman P, editors. Selective activation of drugs by redox processes. New York: Plenum Press,1990: 1-9.
5. Connett RJ, Honig CR, Gayeski TEJ, Brooks GA. Defining hypoxia: a systems view of VO2, glycolysis, energetics, and intracellular PO2. J Appl Physiol 1990; 68: 833-842.
6. Weiss JN, Shieh RC. Potassium loss during myocardial ischaemia and hypoxia: does lactate efflux play a role? Cardiovascular Res 1994; 28: 1125-32.
7. Wilde AAM, Aksnes G. Myocardial potassium loss and cell depolarisation in ischaemia and hypoxia. Cardiovascular Res 1995; 29: 1-15.
8. Zhang XQ, Pang L, Eyzaguirre C. Effects of hypoxia on the intracellular K+ of clustered and isolated glomus cells of mice and rats. Brain Res 1995; 676: 413-420.
9. Brown JM, Giaccia AJ. Tumour hypoxia: the picture has changed in the 1990's. Int J Radiat Biol 1994; 65: 95-102.
10. Denekamp J, Rojas A. Multifactorial approaches to overcoming clinical radioresistance. In: Kogelnik HD, editor. Progress in radio-oncology V. Bologna: Monduzzi Editore, 1995: 9-19.
11. Vaupel P, Schlenger C, Knoop C, Höckel M. Oxygenation of human tumors: evaluation of tissue oxygen distribution in breast cancers by computerized O2 tension measurements. Cancer Res 1991; 51:3316-3322.
12. Höckel M, Schlenger C, Knoop C, Vaupel P. Oxygenation of carcinomas of the uterine cervix: evaluation by computerized O2 tension measurements. Cancer Res 1991; 51:6098-6102.
13. Nordsmark, M, Bentzen SM, Overgaard J. Measurement of human tumour oxygenation status by a polarographic needle electrode: an analysis of inter- and intratumour heterogeneity. Acta Oncol. 1994; 33: 383-389.
14. Gatenby RA, Kessler HB, Rosenblum JS, et al. Oxygen distribution in squamous cell carcinoma metastases and its relationship to outcome of radiation therapy. Int J Radiat Oncol Biol Phys 1988; 14: 831-838.
15. Brown JM, Siim BG. Hypoxia-specific cytotoxins in cancer therapy. Semin Radiat Oncol 1995; 6: 22-36.
16. Edwards DI. Nitroimidazole drugs - action and resistance mechanisms. I. Mechanisms of action. J Antimicrob Chemother 1993; 31: 9-20.
17. Kedderis GL, Miwa GT. The metabolic activation of nitroheterocyclic therapeutic agents. Drug Metab Rev 1988; 19: 33-62.

18. Woodrooffe AJM, Bayliss MK, Park GR. The effects of hypoxia on drug-metabolising enzymes. Drug Metab Rev 1995; 27: 471-495.
19. Whitmore GF, Varghese AJ. The biological properties of reduced nitroheterocyclics and possible underlying biochemical mechanisms. Biochem Pharmacol 1986; 35: 97-103.
20. Biaglow JE, Varnes ME, Roizen-Towle L, et al. Biochemistry of reduction of nitroheterocycles. Biochem Pharmacol 1986; 35: 77-90.
21. Breccia A, Cavalleri B, Adams GE, editors. Nitroimidazoles: chemistry, pharmacology and clinical application. New York: Plenum Press, 1982.
22. Kirkpatrick DL. Bioreductive antineoplastic agents. Drugs of Today 1990; 26: 91-108.
23. Olive PL, Durand RE. Misonidazole binding in SCCVII tumors in relation to the tumor blood supply. Int J Radiat Oncol Biol Phys 1989; 16: 755-761.
24. Overgaard J, Sand Hansen H, Andersen AP, et al. Misonidazole combined with split-course radiotherapy in the treatment of invasive carcinoma of larynx and pharynx: report from the DAHANCA 2 study. Int J Radiat Oncol Biol Phys 1989; 16: 1065-1068.
25. Martin GV, Caldwell JH, Rasey JS, Grunbaum Z, Cerqueira M, Krohn, KA. Enhanced binding of the hypoxic cell marker [3H]fluoromisonidazole in ischemic myocardium. J Nucl Med 1989; 30: 194-201.
26. Martin, GV, Caldwell JH, Graham, MM et al. Noninvasive detection of hypoxic myocardium using fluorine-18-fluoromisonidazole and positron emission tomography. J Nucl Med 1992; 33: 2202-2208.
27. Caldwell JH, Revenaugh JI, Martin GV, Johnson PM, Rasey JS, Krohn KA. Comparison of fluorine-18-fluorodeoxyglucose and tritiated fluoromisonidazole uptake during low-flow ischemia. J Nucl Med 1995; 36: 1633-1638.
28. Shelton ME, Dence CS, Hwang DR, Welch MJ, Bergmann SR. Myocardial kinetics of Fluorine-18 misonidazole: a marker of hypoxic myocardium. J Nucl Med 1989; 30: 351-358.
29. Koh WJ, Bergman KS, Rasey JS, et al. Evaluation of oxygenation status during fractionated radiotherapy in human non small cell lung cancers using [F-18] fluoromisonidazole positron emission tomography. Int J Radiat Oncol Biol Phys 1995; 33: 391-398.
30. Koh WJ, Rasey JS, Evans ML, et al. Imaging of hypoxia in human tumors with [F-18] fluoromisonidazole. Int J Radiat Oncol Biol Phys 1991, 22: 199-212.
31. Jette DC, Wiebe LI, Flanagan RJ, Lee J, Chapman, JD. Iodoazomycin riboside (1-(5'-iodo-5'-deoxyribofuranosyl)-2-nitroimidazole), a hypoxic cell marker. Radiat Res 1986; 105: 169-179.
32. Mannan RH, Mercer JR, Wiebe LI, Somayaji VV, Chapman JD. Radioiodinated 1-(2-fluoro-4-iodo-2,4-dideoxy-(-l-xylopyranosyl)-2-nitroimidazole: a novel probe for the noninvasive assessment of tumor hypoxia. Radiat Res 1992; 132: 368-374.
33. Mannan RH, Somayaji VV, Lee J, Mercer JR, Chapman JD, Wiebe LI. Radioiodinated 1-(5-iodo-5-deoxy-(-d-arabinofuranosyl)-2-nitroimidazole (iodoazomycin arabinoside: IAZA): a novel marker of tissue hypoxia. J Nucl Med 1991; 32: 1764-1770.
34. Parliament MB, Chapman JD, Urtasun RC, et al. Non-invasive assesment of human tumour hypoxia with 123I-iodoazomycin arabinoside: preliminary report of a clinical study. Br J Cancer 1992; 65: 90-95.
35. Groshar D, McEwan AJB, Parliament MB, et al. Imaging tumor hypoxia and tumor perfusion. J Nucl Med 1993; 34: 885-888.
36. Linder KE, Chan YW, Cyr JE, Nowotnik DP, Eckelman WC, Nunn AD. Synthesis, characterization, and in vitro evaluation of nitroimidazole-BATO complexes: new technetium compounds designed for imaging hypoxic tissue. Bioconjug Chem 1993; 4: 326-333.
37. Rumsey WL, Patel B, Linder KE. Effect of graded hypoxia on retention of technetium-99m-nitroheterocycle in perfused rat heart. J Nucl Med 1995; 36: 632-636.
38. Ng CK, Sinusas AJ, Zaret BL, Soufer R. Kinetic analysis of technetium-99m-labeled nitroimidazole (BMS-181321) as a tracer of myocardial hypoxia. Circulation 1995; 92: 1261-1268.
39. Stone CK, Mulnix T, Nickles RJ, et al. Myocardial kinetics of a putative hypoxic tissue marker 99mTc-labeled nitroimidazole (BMS-181321), after regional ischemia and reperfusion. Circulation 1995; 92: 1246-1253.
40. Rumsey WL, Cyr JE, Raju N, Narra RK. A novel [99m]technetium-labeled nitroheterocycle capable of identification of hypoxia in heart. Biochem Biophys Res Comm 1993; 193: 1239-1246.

41. Rumsey WL, Kuczynski B, Patel B. Detecting hypoxia in heart using phosphorescence quenching and 99m-technetium-nitroimidazoles. In: Hogan MC, et al, editors. Oxygen transport to tissue XVI. New York: Plenum Press, 1994: 99-104.
42. Rumsey WL, Patel B, Kuczynski B, et al. Potential of nitroimidazoles as markers of hypoxia in heart. In: Vaupel P, et al, editors. Oxygen transport to tissue XV. New York: Plenum, 1994: 263-269.
43. Shi CQX, Sinusas AJ, Dione DP, et al. Technetium-99m-nitroimidazole (BMS181321): a positive imaging agent for detecting myocardial ischemia. J Nucl Med 1995; 36: 1078-1086.
44. Rumsey WL, Kuczynski B, Patel B, et al. SPECT imaging of ischemic myocardium using a technetium-99m-nitroimidazole ligand. J Nucl Med 1995; 36: 1445-1450.
45. Wedeking P, Yost F, Wen M, et al. Comparison of the biologic activity of the isomers of the Tc-99m-nitroimidazole complex BMS-194796. J Nucl Med 1995; 36: 17P.
46. Archer CM, Edwards B, Kelly JD, King AC, Burke JF, Riley, ALM. Technetium labelled agents for imaging tissue hypoxia in vivo. In: Nicolini M, Bandoli G, Mazzi U, editors. Technetium and rhenium in chemistry and nuclear medicine 4. Padova: SG Editoriali, 1995: 535-539.
47. Johnson III G, Nguyen KN, Edwards B, Archer CM, Okada RD. HL91-technetium-99m: effects of flow and hypoxia on the myocardial kinetics of a new hypoxia avid imaging agent. Circulation 1995; 92 (Supplement 1): 3801.
48. Johnson III G, Nguyen KN, Edwards B, Archer CM, Okada RD. HL91-technetium-99m: uptake and retention of a new hypoxia avid imaging agent can differentiate ischemic viable from ischemic nonviable myocardium. Circulation 1995; 92 (Supplement 1): 3791.
49. Fujibayashi Y, Taniuchi H, Tajima N, Yonekura Y, Konishi J, Yokoyama A. New non nitroimidazole hypoxia imaging agents, Cu-62-dithiosemicarbazone complexes with low redox potential. J Nucl Med 1995; 36: 49P.
50. Fujibayashi Y, Wada K, Taniuchi H, Yonekura Y, Konishi J, Yokoyama A. Mitochondria-selective reduction of 62Cu-pyruvaldehyde bis(N4-methylthio-semicarbazone) (62Cu-PTSM) in the murine brain; a novel radiopharmaceutical for brain positron emission tomography (PET) imaging. Biol Pharm Bull 1993; 16: 146-149.

This chapter is reproduced with kind permission of Amersham International plc.

GENETIC ENGINEERING OF MONOCLONAL ANTIBODIES

Lorna M.D. Stewart

Introduction

Antibody based medicines present themselves, in principle, as ideal drugs, and can be considered as molecules with two functional parts. One will allow the molecule to target and will confer exquisite specificity while the other links directly into the host defence and repair systems. The former activity is the one which is exploited when antibodies are used to target radiopharmaceuticals.

Developments in antibody engineering over the past two decades have allowed us to manipulate the system in such a way that we can attempt to increase the affinity and to try to reduce the inherent immunogenicity of murine monoclonal antibodies. In the field of targeting of solid tumours, the manufacture of smaller antibody based fragments will facilitate increased tumour penetration. In addition to this, the advent of phage display technology allows the selection of new specificities without the use of animal immunisation.

Hybridoma technology

Antibodies are synthesised in the body by B lymphocytes. A normal B lymphocyte is capable of producing a single type of antibody directed against a specific determinant or epitope on an antigen. After immunisation each antigen-activated B lymphocyte forms a clone of cells each producing an identical antibody and this is termed a monoclonal antibody. Since antigens contain multiple epitopes, exposure to an individual antigen stimulates several B lymphocytes each producing different antibodies. This mixture of antibodies which recognise different epitopes on the same antigen are termed polyclonal.

Monoclonal antibodies with a defined specificity are often more useful than the mixture but purification of individual clones of antibodies can be tedious. This situation was made very much easier by Köhler and Milstein in 1975 [1] who developed a system to fuse immune murine spleen cells with a myeloma cell line to

S. J. Mather (ed.), Current Directions in Radiopharmaceutical Research and Development, 89–98.

produce an immortal hybridoma which will manufacture unlimited quantities of a specific monoclonal antibody which can be purified from the supernatant of growing cells (See figure 1).

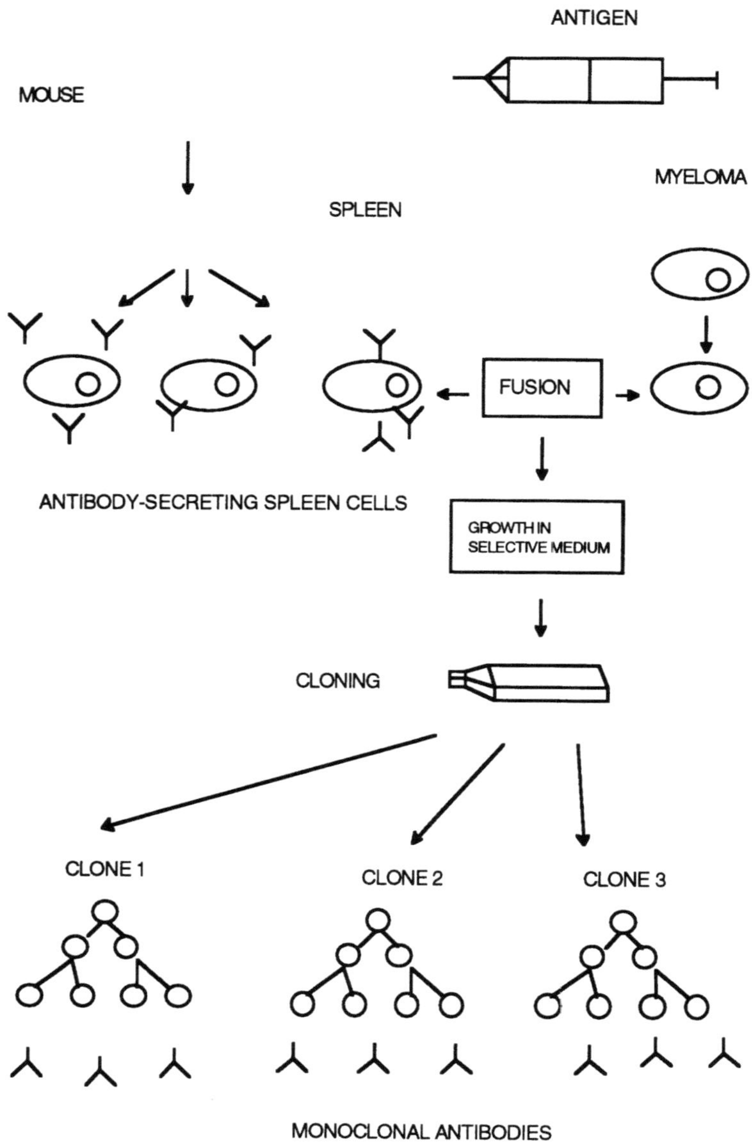

Figure 1 Schematic representation of the fusion process used to develop monoclonal antibodies.

Such monoclonal antibodies are used extensively for immunoassays; immunohistopathology; flow cytology; marrow purging; imaging of infarcts, clots and tumours; in addition to the prevention of allograft rejection; immunotherapy of autoimmune and graft versus host disease. They can be used alone as passive therapy or immunogens or can be used to carry toxic agents such as drugs, toxins or isotopes. However, since these antibodies are murine (mouse) in origin, multiple doses of these antibodies may elicit human anti murine antibody (HAMA) responses by the host [2].

Antibody structure and diversity

A typical antibody molecule of the IgG isotype is composed of two heavy chains and two light chains which come together or form a bivalent structure (see figure 2). The chains are composed of a variable number of domains each containing 110-120 amino acid residues. Each light chain has two domains and each heavy chain has 3 or 4 domains depending on isotype (i.e. IgG, IgM etc.). The heavy and light chains are linked by strong non-covalent forces and by inter-chain disulphide bonds. Similar forces hold the heavy chains together.

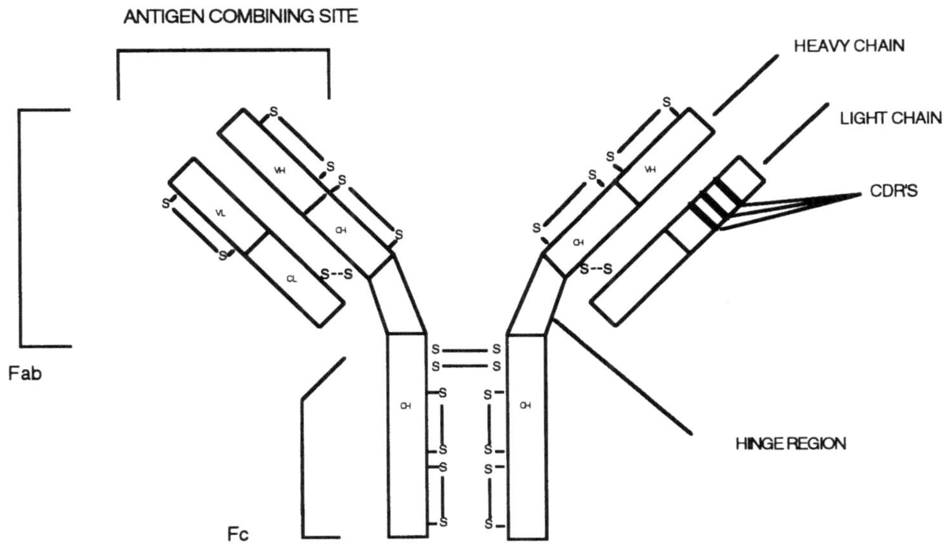

Figure 2. Schematic representation of an IgG molecule

Variability and the antigen binding region reside in the amino terminal domain of both the heavy(V_H) and the light(V_L) chains. The antigen binding site is composed of amino acids from each chain. The variable domains are composed of three hyper-variable regions called complimentarity determining regions (CDR's) which are held in the correct position relative to each other by framework regions which have a more conserved sequence. The remainder of the antibody is composed of domains which we term the constant region (C_H and C_L) since these are identical in antibodies of varying specificity but similar isotype. The ability to recognise a huge variety of epitopes is determined totally by the sequence of amino acids in the V domains and the origin of this diversification stems from the organisation of the genes coding for the amino acids of the antibody chains.

The raw genetic information is carried in the DNA of each cell and this is transcribed into RNA to form a primary transcript which is edited and processed into messenger RNA (mRNA) which codes for the final amino acids of the protein. The huge variety of sequences found within the V domains can be accounted for by two mechanisms. If we consider the light chain, firstly, a number of variable regions and a number of joining regions exist which join together with an individual constant region. The choice of V and J regions used allows for a large number of possible light chain combinations to exist A similar situation occurs with the heavy chain. The heavy chain V region is composed of 3 parts or exons called V, D and J regions. The combination of sequeces from hundreds of possible V regions, at least 20 D regions and 4 J regions combined with inaccuracy of the joining mechanism creates diversity. It has been estimated that random association of units would produce 10^{11} different antibodies. The second method used to create diversity lies in the fact that the variable regions undergo extensive somatic mutation. It has been estimated that recombination and mutation results in the ability to manufacture 10^{30} antibodies with differing specificity.

Rescuing antibody sequence from a hybridoma

Manipulations of the antibody amino acid sequence are carried out at the DNA level. Therefore when a hybridoma expresses an antibody of interest, the DNA sequence must be rescued from these cells. As mentioned above, rearrangement and editing of the DNA occurs prior to the final sequence encoded in the mRNA which will code for the desired antibody, therefore it is the mRNA sequence which is required. The mRNA may be identified by a string of 50-250 adenylate residues located at the end of the sequence, called the poly-A tail. Around 10^6 cells producing the antibody are harvested and lysed. Oligo(dT) cellulose which is complementary to the poly(A) tail is used to pull out the message from the cells. The mRNA is then used as a template to make DNA using an enzyme called reverse transcriptase. This enzyme can generate a cDNA strand based on the mRNA sequence, primed from a synthetic oligonucleotide. This oligonucleotide primer may consist of a string of thymine residues which will hybridise to the poly(A) tail or, if known, it could be an internal sequence. At this stage only small amounts of cDNA exist which can then be amplified using the Polymerase Chain Reaction (PCR).

PCR is used to amplify DNA using two oligonucleotide primers which flank a DNA segment of interest. Excess primers are added which hybridise to opposite ends of a double stranded target sequence and DNA synthesis occurs across the region between the primers. This synthesis takes place in the presence of TAQ polymerase, dNTP's and an appropriate buffer system. The reaction is heated to 94°C to denature the double stranded DNA into single stranded DNA and the temperature is lowered to around 50°C to allow the primers to hybridise to their complementary sequences. The temperature is then raised to 72°C where the polymerase extends the primers. This process doubles the amount of target sequence present and repeated cycles of these temperature changes amplifies the DNA in an exponential manner.

The oligonucleotide primers can incorporate restriction endonuclease sites which will allow the cloning and sequencing of the amplified region. This technique may also be used to create desired mutations in the sequence by incorporation of the mutant sequence within the oligonucleotide primer. The design of primers specific to the end of the variable regions of the heavy and light chains allow amplification of these specific sequences [3,4].

Amplification of these regions from the hybridoma, allows us to clone and obtain the nucleotide sequence of the antibody genes. Knowledge of the sequence of the variable regions of the heavy and light chains allows comparison against known antibody sequences in Kabat's data base [5] and then CDR and framework regions can be assigned. This service is now available on the World Wide Web (http://immuno.bme.nwu.edu/).

Expression

After amplification, sequencing and manipulation, the antibody sequence is usually placed into some sort of plasmid based system which will facilitate protein expression. A variety of cell types are used for protein expression and each has advantages and disadvantages.

The most basic expression systems are bacterial systems. These allow the production of large amounts of protein but post-translational modification of the protein is minimal and very different to that observed in higher organisms. Consequently, this system has been widely used for the expression of single-chain antibody fragments where no constant regions are present and no glycosylation is needed.

The expression systems of choice are those based on higher organisms where the processing of the proteins is identical or very similar to that observed in man. The most frequently used cells are CHO (Chinese hamster ovary) or COS (derived from African green monkey kidney cells).

Alteration of immunogenicity

Most monoclonals are murine in origin and as such will elicit a HAMA response when introduced into humans. This results in the formation of complexes involving the administered antibody, resulting in a reduction of active antibody in the circulation coupled with the possibility of adverse allergic reactions by the patient during this and subsequent administrations. This may not be a problem if only one dose is to be given, e.g. when the antibody is used in imaging, but when multiple doses are to be administered then a reduction in the immunogenicity is desired.

In order to reduce the immunogenicity, murine sequences are replaced with those from a human antibody. The simplest way to do this is to replace the murine constant regions with human constant regions to produce a chimaeric antibody [6]. It is generally believed that the constant regions are the most immunogenic and this basic procedure reduces the immunogenicity without interfering with the ability of the antibody to recognise and bind to its epitope. This procedure is taken a stage further when all murine sequences not directly involved in binding are replaced with human sequences. In this case both the constant regions and the framework regions are replaced [7]. This process is more complicated than the formation of chimaeric antibodies. The murine sequence is compared to all existing human antibody sequences in order to search for antibodies with a high degree of homology in the framework regions (generally 70% homology is required). The sequences are then modelled by computer to identify any residues in the murine sequence outside the CDR's which are involved in maintaining the conformation of the antigen binding site, and these residues are retained in the new sequence. The antibody expressed using this new sequence is termed a humanised antibody and in theory should not be immunogenic to humans, however it should be noted that the CDR's and the junction of murine CDR's to human framework regions creates new sequences which in themselves may be immunogenic.

Veneering of the antibody surface is a third option. This recognises the fact that the framework regions may be important in the presentation of the antigen combining site and that it is beneficial to retain interior and inter-domain contacts. Since antigenicity is dependent on the nature of the surface of the antibody, replacement of only those amino-acids found on the outer surface of the antibody with those normally found in human antibodies should decrease the probability of an immune response directed against the surface [8]. In one case, only 13 amino acids were altered to obtain this 'human' surface [9].

Production of smaller fragments

Smaller fragments based on the antibody structure may result in more effective penetration of tissue boundaries and allow faster blood clearance. Smaller fragments may be produced by digestion of the antibody with enzymes such as papain and pepsin. These digestion's produce monovalent Fab and bivalent F(ab')$_2$ respectively. However, these fragments can also be made by genetic manipulation of the DNA sequences whereby only the domains required are made by the chosen expression system. Genetic manipulation is the usual method employed to make even smaller fragments (fig 3).

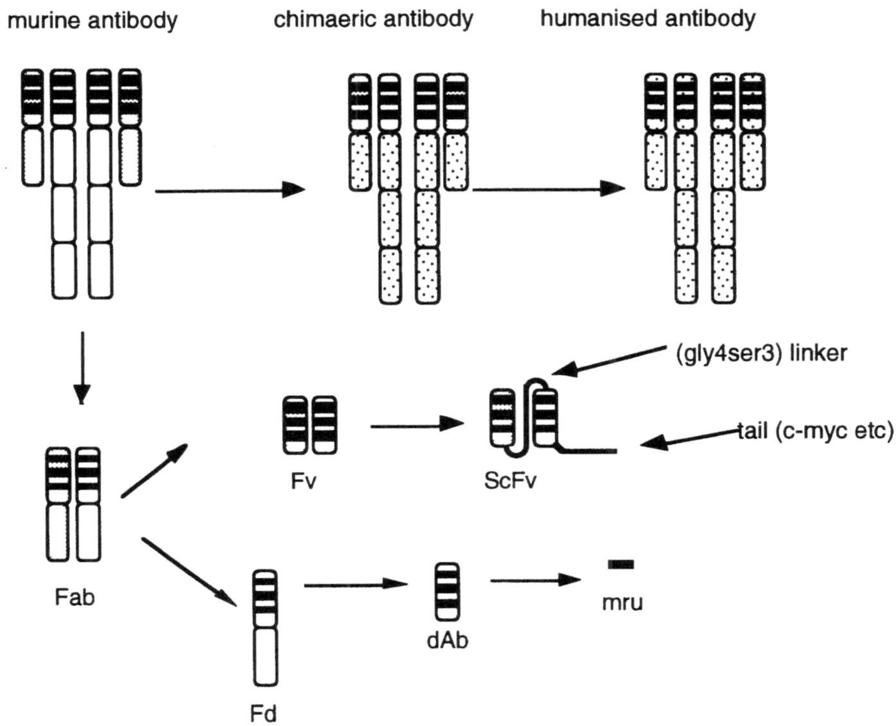

Figure 3. Engineered antibodies and smaller antibody based fragments. Each rectangle represents a domain and the shading indicates, grey - murine light chain; white - murine heavy chain; black - murine CDR's; speckled - human regions; solid black lines - ScFv linker and additional terminal sequences. The lower part of the diagram shows the fragments (see text for descriptions).

The monovalent Fv consists of the variable domains of both the heavy and the light chain. The genetic elements coding for these domains can be placed separately into plasmids which will allow the expression of the proteins in a bacterial system. However the product (Fv) is not stable and may not fold properly. The problems were partially solved by the manufacture of single chain antibodies (ScAb's or ScFv's) [10]. In ScFv's the heavy and light chains are genetically linked by an artificial neutral linker and are expressed as one transcriptional unit which will associate and stabilise the contact between heavy and light chains. The linker is generally a (Gly4Ser)$_3$ sequence which is 15 amino acids long. This flexible peptide linker is designed to span the

3.5nm gap between the carboxyl terminus of the first chain and the amino terminus of the second chain [11]. The order of the chains may be V_L-V_H or V_H-V_L. The linker facilitates the pairing of the two chains and minimises aggregation problems encountered when the chains are expressed individually. An array of additional sequences may be added to the carboxyl terminus of this construct to aid in labelling, detection and purification of the construct. These include additional cysteine residues for site specific functionalisation with thiol reactive agents, enzyme or toxin/protoxin sequences to be used directly or as part of an ADEPT system [12], immunogenic sequences such as c-myc which enable production of the fragment to be followed (these sequences can be removed later) and polyhistidine tags which will allow purification on a metal affinity column.

Other fragments which can be produced are the Fd and dAb, where the variable domain and the first constant domain of the heavy chain or only the heavy V domain are expressed. The success of this strategy is dependent on the antibody used. The diversity encountered in the antibody chains is far greater for the heavy chain than the light. In consequence some interactions with epitopes are primarily made through the heavy chain residues. Production of this fragment may be problematic due to the hydrophobicity of the face which usually interacts with the light chain.

Even smaller fragments, called minimal recognition units (mru) can be made. These comprise of one of the CDR sequences and can be classed almost as binding peptides.

The most useful of all these fragments has tended to be the single chain antibody, and this is the unit most commonly used in the phage display technology which allows the selection of antibodies with increased affinities and new specificities.

Surface Display Systems

Filamentous phage may be used to display small peptides on their surface by the insertion of synthetic DNA encoding the peptide into the genome of the phage. The protein can either be expressed fused to the major coat protein, pVIII, or to the minor coat protein, pIII, depending on where the sequence was inserted. Genes coding for single-chain antibody fragments have been cloned into the amino terminus of pIII and the ScFv is expressed as a fusion protein at the tip of the phage which has been secreted into the medium (Fig 4.). The expression of antibody fragments on the surface of bacteriophage allows the screening and analysis of a large number of colonies for antigen binding activity [13 ,14].

This technology utilises the biology of M13 bacteriophage which infect the bacterium Escherichia coli in a non-lytic manner which means that infected cells do not lyse but secrete phage particles into the growth medium. The phage particle attaches to the f-pilus of the host cell via the protein coded for by gene III on the phage surface. On entry into the host cell, the phage coat protein is removed and the single stranded phage DNA is converted into double stranded DNA which can be replicated and eventually packaged into new phage particles. In phage display technology, the gene coding for the joined heavy and light chains is linked to the gene III and is expressed as a fused protein displayed at the tip of the phage which is secreted into the medium (fig.4).

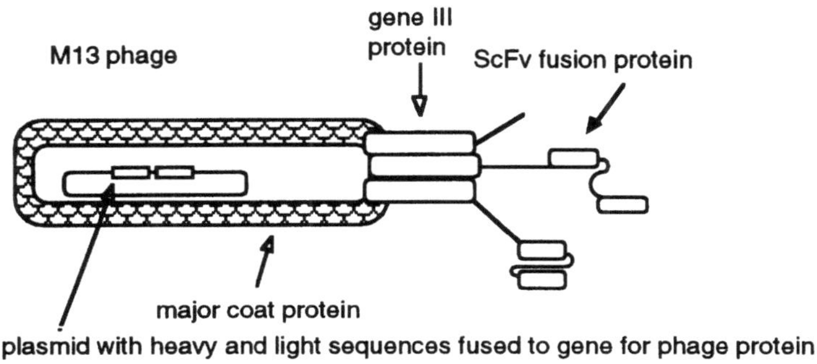

Figure 4. Diagram of M13 phage used to display antibody fragments fused to the phage gene III protein.

The ScFv bound to the surface of the phage can then be captured by its ability to bind its specific antigen bound to a plate. The whole phage/ScFv can then be detected on the plate by an enzyme labelled antibody directed against the major coat protein of M13.

The source of the genes used to construct the ScFv can determine the use of the system. Use of this technology in conjunction with PCR to rescue the sequences of the heavy and light chain may be used as a rapid method to isolate and confirm an antibody sequence from a known source such as a hybridoma. In order to bypass the production of hybridomas, the source of template for retrieval of antibody sequences may be a hyper-immunised mouse spleen followed by selection against the desired antigen. More recently it has been shown that a library of sequences derived from mRNA obtained from peripheral blood lymphocytes from non-immunised human donors could be used to isolate human antibodies specific for target antigens. The antibodies derived in this manner tend to have lower affinity than natural human antibodies, or murine counterparts derived by the traditional methods. An attempt to rectify this can be made by allowing the antibodies to go through a process of affinity maturation and antigen directed selection to enrich for higher affinity variants [15] Oligonucleotide directed mutagenesis of the CDR regions of selected antibodies can lead to the production of higher affinity antibodies. Chain-Shuffling may also be used in an attempt to increase the affinity of the antibody [16]. Here, the original light or heavy chain is retained and new partner chains from another source are combined and assessed for any improvement in binding.

Conclusion

Continual emergence of new techniques in the field of molecular biology associated with the extraction and manipulation of sequences coding for whole or partial antibody genes ensures that many new exciting developments will occur over the next few years. The possibility of obtaining human antibodies from non-immunised donors and increasing the affinity to selected antigens already exists. In addition to this, the increasing role of the biomolecular modeller to analyse interactions and suggest modifications to antibody/antigen associations will allow us to fine-tune these interactions and even to design small binding peptides.

References

1. Kohler G, Milstein C. Continuos cultures of fused cells secreting antibodies of predetermined specificity. Nature 1975;250:52-53
2. Khazaeli MB, Conry RM, LoBuglio AF. Human immune response to monoclonal antibodies. J.Immunother. 1994;15:42-52
3. Larrick JW, Danielsson L, Brenner CA, Abrahamsonn M, Fry K, Borrebaek CAK. Rapid cloning of rearranged immunoglobulin genes from human hybridoma cells using mixed primers and polymerase chain reaction. Biochem.Biophys.Res.Commun. 1989;160:1250-1256
4. Orlandi R, Güssow DH, Jones PT, Winter G. Cloning immunoglobulin variable domains for expression by the polymerase chain reaction. Proc.Natl.Acad.Sci.USA. 1989;86:3833-3837
5. Kabat EA, Wu TT, Reid Miller M Perry HM, Gottesman KS. Sequences of proteins of immunological interest 1991 (DHHS, Washington DC) 5th edition.
6. Morrison SL, Johnson MJ, Herzberg CA, et al. Chimaeric human antibody molecules: Mouse antigen binding domains with human constant domains. Proc. Natl.Acad.Sci.USA 1984;81: 6851-6855
7. Reichmann L, Clark M, Waldermann H, Winter G. Reshaping human antibodies for therapy. Nature 1988;332:327
8. Padlan EA. A possible procedure for reducing the immunogenicity of antibody variable domains while preserving their ligand binding properties. Mol. Immunol. 1991;28:489-498
9. Roguska MA, Pedersen JT, Keddy CA et al. Humanization of murine monoclonal antibodies through variable domain resurfacing. Proc.Acad.Sci.USA. 1994;91:969-973
10. Bird RE, Hardman KD, Jacobson JW, Johnson S. et al. Single-chain antigen-binding proteins.Science.1988;242:423-426
11. Huston JS, McCarthy J, Tai M-S,et al. Medical applications of single chain antibodies. Intern.Rev.Immunol. 1993;10:195-217
12. Bagshawe KD. Antibody directed enzyme prodrug therapy (ADEPT). In: J.D.Fortner and J.E.Rhoads,editors. Accomplishments in Cancer Research. London: Chapman and Hall Medical, 1991:154-170
13. McCafferty J, Griffith AD, Winter G, Chiswell DJ. Phage antibodies: filamentous phage display of antibody variable domains. Nature. 1991;348:552-554
14. Hoogenboom HR, Griffith AD, Johnson KS, Chiswell DJ, Hudson P, Winter G. Multisubunit proteins on the surface of 'filamentous phage: methodologies for displaying antibody (Fab) heavy and light chains. Nuc.Acid.Res. 1991;19:4133-4137
15. Hawkins RE, Russel SJ, Winter G. Selection of phage antibodies by binding affinity, mimicking affinity maturation. J,Mol.Biol. 1992;226:889-896
16. Jespers LS, Roberts A, Mahler SM, Winter G, Hoogenboom HR. Guiding the selection of human antibodies from phage display repertoired to a single epitope of an antigen. Bio/technology. 1994; 12:899-903

THE DEVELOPMENT OF RADIOPHARMACEUTICALS FOR IMAGING CNS RECEPTORS

Hank F. Kung

Introduction

Receptors are special protein molecules that recognize or selectively bind to drugs, hormones or neurotransmitters (see figure 1). There are various types of receptors, including hormone, peptide, biogenic amine and ion channel. Ligands are chemical molecules that fit the receptor binding sites. The extent of ligand-receptor interaction is usually expressed in terms of binding affinity; it represents the binding constant at equilibrium (K_d, dissociation constant; or K_i, inhibition constant). When a ligand is bound to a receptor (R) located in the cell membrane, the ligand-receptor complex triggers responses of secondary messengers (i.e., induce protein kinase activity). There is a large number of CNS receptors responsible for different types of neuronal function.

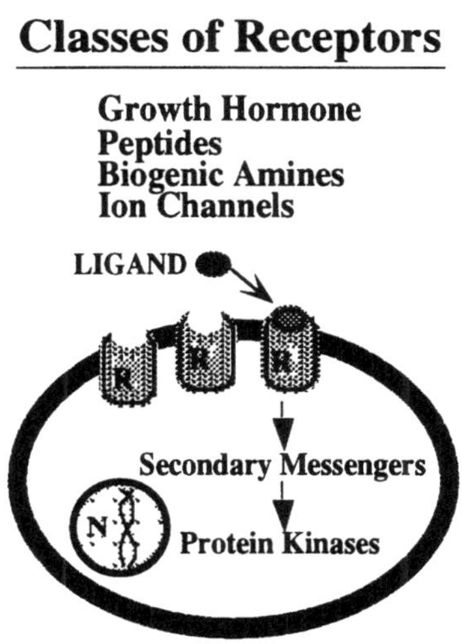

Figure 1. Classes of receptors in the cell membrane.

S. J. Mather (ed.), Current Directions in Radiopharmaceutical Research and Development, 99–113.

It would be nearly impossible to cover all of the radiopharmaceuticals available for CNS receptor imaging in one chapter. Instead, this chapter will use the dopaminergic neurotransmitter as a model system to describe the design and development of new radiopharmaceuticals for CNS receptor imaging.

The CNS dopaminergic system in the mammalian brain has been the subject of extensive study in the past three decades. Not only is this system necessary for normal brain function, it is also the apparent action site for various neuroleptic drugs for treatment of schizophrenia and other mental disorders. There is a wealth of pharmacological information on postsynaptic dopamine (DA) receptors [1,2]. The neurotransmitter, dopamine, is synthesized *in situ* by converting tyrosine to 3,4-dihydroxyphenylalanine (DOPA; catalyzed by tyrosine hydroxylase, TH), after which aromatic amino acid decarboxylase (AADC) catalyzes the conversion of DOPA to dopamine. There are several potential secondary messenger linkers, the most prominent of which is the formation of cyclic adenosinemonophosphate (cAMP), triggered by the activation of adenylyl cyclase. Responding to an initial neuronal signal (electrical pulse), the neurotransmitter is released into the synaptic cleft, where it binds to the postsynaptic receptors. As a conservation measure, the free dopamine in the synaptic cleft is taken up by the reuptake transporters on the presynaptic neuronal sites and is repackaged inside the presynaptic vesicles before being released again. The dopamine can also be metabolized by degradation enzymes such as catecholamine methyl transferase (COMT) and monoamine oxidases (MAOs), through which the concentration of free dopamine is carefully controlled. The concentration of the neurotransmitter is directly proportional to the firing rate of the neuron.

In recent years, the application of molecular biology techniques to express receptors in cloned cells has dramatically expanded the understanding and complexity of CNS molecular pharmacology. Cloning of postsynaptic dopamine receptors has yielded at least five different dopamine receptor subtypes, D1, D2, D3, D4 and D5 [3,4]. a diversity far beyond the traditional classification of two subtypes, D1 and D2. The majority of the CNS neurotransmitter receptor systems, with the exception of ion channels, belong to the G-protein-coupled super-receptor family. The receptors present themselves in the G-protein-coupled state or G-protein-uncoupled state [5]. It is generally believed that the agonists bind to G-protein-coupled receptors and elicit secondary messengers. Recent reports on the G-protein-coupling at normal and disease states of various CNS receptors clearly suggest that G-protein-coupling may be involved in regulating receptor affinity states as well as determining the apparent receptor density. In a neurotransmitter network such as the dopaminergic system (illustrated in Fig. 2), an agonist (i.e., dopamine and other structurally related chemicals) can bind to postsynaptic receptors and induce secondary messenger(s). This is sometimes called a "non-covalent catalyst," in contrast to enzyme-catalyzed reactions, which involve covalent bond formations. Antagonists differ from agonists in that they can inhibit the binding of agonists by binding to the receptors themselves without inducing a secondary messenger response.

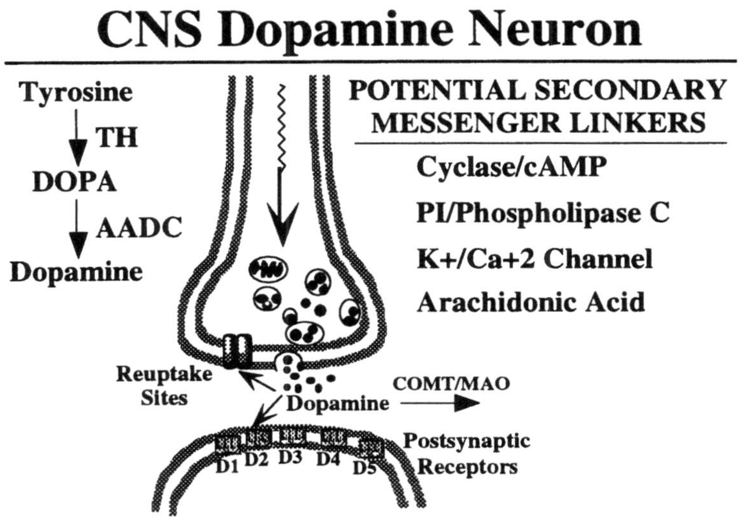

Figure 2. A schematic drawing of the CNS dopamine neuron.

Progress on evaluating receptor function in the CNS using *in vivo* imaging has demonstrated that this is a promising field of research that may contribute to improved diagnosis and patient management [6,7]. Normally, C-11 ($T_{1/2}$ = 20 min, b^+) and F-18 ($T_{1/2}$ = 120 min, b^+) labeled agents are used for PET imaging, while I-123 ($T_{1/2}$ = 13 h, 159 KeV) labeled agents are used for SPECT imaging. These agents are designed to study the localization of CNS receptors and to reflect their quantitative density *in vivo*. The procedures extend beyond what is currently being performed routinely in nuclear medicine clinics using Tc-99m HMPAO (Ceretech®)[8] and ECD (Neurolite®) [9] to measure regional brain perfusion. *In vivo* PET and SPECT radiotracer imaging techniques provide powerful tools for evaluating CNS receptor function in normal or disease states. Normally, the overriding factors in selecting ligands for the pharmacological evaluation of CNS receptor or binding sites are selectivity, affinity and specific activity. However, when choosing appropriate PET and SPECT ligands, several additional factors, such as radiochemistry (preparation time for short-lived labeled agents), suitable modeling for tracer uptake kinetics and retention, and metabolism, must also be considered.

Since C-11, F-18 and I-123 labeled CNS receptor imaging agents are based on cyclotron produced isotopes, which are expensive, a similar Tc-99m labeled agent (Tc-99m costs approximately US $1/mCi) would be highly desirable for routine clinical study. Even though I-123 labeled agents are available for a limited amount of CNS receptor imaging in conjunction with SPECT, Tc-99m labeled agents would broaden the prospect of the receptor imaging because they are more suitable for routine clinical use. Nearly every hospital nuclear medicine service is equipped with some type of SPECT camera optimized for detecting Tc-99m. Although it is a formidable challenge to incorporate a Tc complex moiety into a small receptor ligand and at the same time maintain the binding affinity of the original ligand, the potential benefits for a large number of patients in need of nuclear medicine diagnostic procedures are enormous. Recent advances in technetium chemistry have provided a basic foundation for building molecules with appropriate binding properties (see discussion below) [10,11].

Basic properties for cns receptor radiopharmaceuticals

In addition to the challenges of meeting particular properties required for radiopharmaceuticals, such as the ability to be labeled with a suitable isotope with an appropriate gamma emission and physical half-life, the basic requirements for CNS receptor imaging agents are:

i) stable *in vitro* and *in vivo*
ii) neutral and lipophilic
iii) able to pass through the intact blood-brain barrier by simple diffusion
iv) display selective and specific receptor binding
v) exhibit regional cerebral distribution *in vivo* reflecting receptor density and feasible for kinetic modeling
vi) suitable for routine clinical use

Dopamine d2 receptor ligands

The most extensively studied PET ligands for dopamine D2 receptors are [^{11}C]raclopride and N-methylspiperone (NMSP). PET imaging of dopamine D2 receptors using [^{11}C]raclopride has been investigated in humans [12-14]. The binding constants (K_d = 7.1 nM, B_{max} = 15 pmol/ml) were measured in living human brain using an equilibrium model and Scatchard plots. The dopamine D2 receptor density values were comparable to those determined earlier with N-methylspiperone (K_d = 0.097 nM, B_{max} = 16.6 pmol/g) [15]. However, different receptor concentrations were reported based on quantitative *in vivo* imaging studies of schizophrenic patients with [^{11}C]N-methylspiperone [15] and [^{11}C]raclopride [16] [^{11}C]N-methylspiperone showed a higher dopamine D2 concentration, and raclopride displayed no change in dopamine D2 receptor density. The discrepancy may be a result of variations in the differential effects of endogenous dopamine concentration between raclopride and NMSP [17,18]. In addition, differences due to methodology and/or patient population have been suggested [19] When the same patients were studied with either raclopride or NMSP, the D2 receptor density appeared to be the same [15,16].

The most widely used SPECT imaging agent for dopamine D2 receptors is (S)-2-hydroxy-3-iodo-6-methoxy-N-[(1-ethyl-2-pyrrolidinyl)methyl]benzamide (IBZM).

This agent was initially reported in 1988 [20] The radioiodination was achieved by an oxidative iodination reaction using peracetic acid as the optimal oxidant. Binding studies using rat striatal membrane preparations showed that it bound to dopamine D2 receptors with high affinity (K_d = 0.4 nM). Initial *in vivo* imaging study suggested that it concentrated in the basal ganglia area of human brain, where dopamine D2 receptors are concentrated [21] It is important to note that after subtypes of the D2-like family (D2, D3 and D4) were cloned [1]. IBZM showed high affinity to D2 and D3 receptors (K_d = 0.26 and 0.29 nM, respectively). However, the affinity to dopamine D4 receptors is relatively low (K_i > 200 nM).

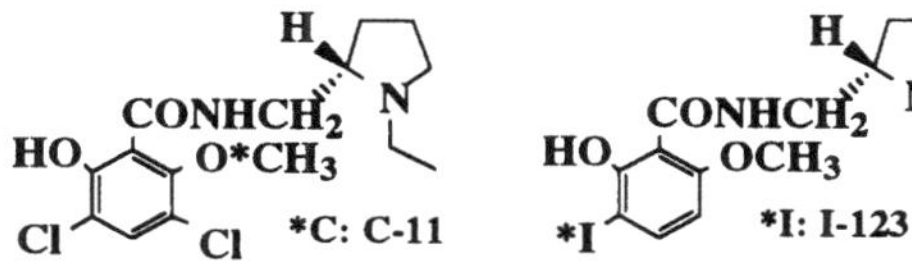

Raclopride **IBZM**

Figure 3. Chemical structures of raclopride and IBZM, the most commonly used dopamine D2 receptor imaging agents for PET and SPECT, respectively.

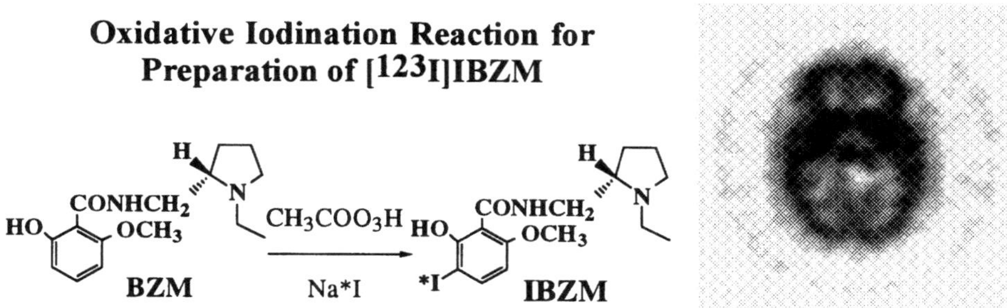

Figure 4. The oxidative iodination reaction used for the preparation of [^{123}I]IBZM is described. A transaxial SPECT image of dopamine D2 receptors in a normal subject after an iv injection of 5 mCi of [^{123}I]IBZM (30-80 min). High accumulation of IBZM was observed in the basal ganglia, where dopamine D2 receptors are concentrated. It is important to keep in mind that the distribution reflects binding to both D2 and D3 receptors.

IBZM has been used widely in Europe since 1990 because it is commercially available (Cygne bv, Belgium). Using this agent, it is possible to facilitate the diagnosis of movement disorders such as Parkinson's, Huntington's, and Wilson's diseases [22-29]. The IBZM/SPECT studies in the literature use the ratios of basal ganglia/cerebellum or basal ganglia/frontal cortex as indicators for dopamine D2 receptor binding. The values range from 1.2 to 2.0, depending on the type of camera used and the method of data calculation. Introduction of kinetic modeling, either with a three-compartment model, graphic analysis method or slow infusion method to achieve a steady state, will improve the quantification of D2 receptors [25,28]

Imaging agents for dopamine reuptake sites

Cocaine is an alkaloid that has been used as a local anesthetic and abused as a CNS stimulant [30,31]. One of its major mechanisms of action in the CNS is the blocking of dopamine reuptake sites, which are responsible for reinforcing action. PET imaging using [^{11}C]-N-methyl labeled cocaine indicated that, after an IV injection, the uptake and retention of cocaine in the brain coincided with the subjective euphoric effects [32]. The regional brain distribution of cocaine is largely concentrated in the basal ganglia, where the dopamine neurons are located. [^{11}C]-N-methyl labeled cocaine is a very useful PET ligand for studying the pharmacology and drug effects of cocaine itself; however, additional modifications on the cocaine molecule have led to very interesting derivatives that display much higher binding affinity and selectivity to dopamine reuptake sites. These derivatives may be more suitable than GBR12,935 [33] in developing PET and SPECT ligands for imaging dopamine reuptake sites (dopamine transporters). The dopamine reuptake site ligands are useful in evaluating changes in dopamine reuptake sites *in vivo* and *in vitro*, especially for patients with Parkinson's disease (PD), which is characterized by a selective loss of dopamine neurons in the basal ganglia and substantia nigra. Recent publications describing the use of [^{11}C]-CFT (WIN35,428) and [^{123}I]-β-CIT suggest a strong correlation between the decrease in localization of dopamine reuptake sites in the anterior putamen area and PD symptoms [34-36]. The results provide an impetus toward the further development of these agents for diagnosing and monitoring the treatment of PD patients. Currently, [^{123}I]-β-CIT is being widely investigated for this purpose. However, one of the drawbacks of [^{123}I]-β-CIT is the time required (>18 h) for reaching optimal uptake ratio in the target area, the basal ganglia (BG), vs. the nontarget area, the frontal cortex (CTX). Because of the need for agents with faster equilibrium times, new ligands such as IPT [37-40] and CIT-FP [41] both of which reach equilibrium in less than one hour, will play an important future role as the agents of choice.

Table 1. Binding affinity (IC_{50}, nM) of cocaine and various tropane derivatives for dopamine (DA) reuptake sites.

Compounds	X	DA[a]
WIN35,428 (CFT)	F	15.7
β-CIT (RTI-55)	I	1.26
FP-CIT		1.20
Cocaine		102
IPT		0.25[b]

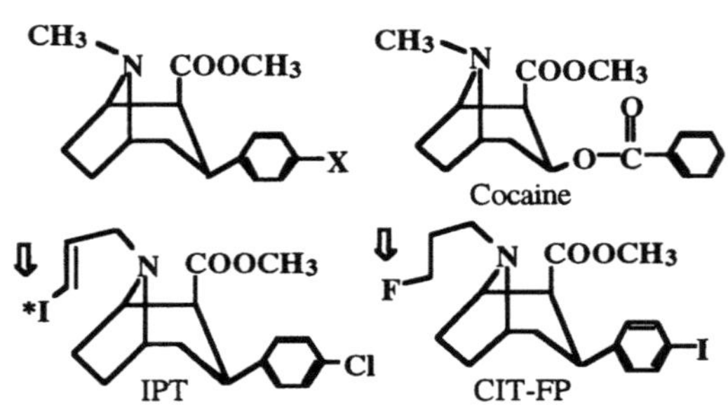

a. [^{3}H]WIN35,428 (CFT)
b. K_d

To improve the kinetics of the dopamine transporter ligand for SPECT imaging, a new iodinated cocaine derivative, N-(3'-iodopropen-2'-yl)-2b-carbomethoxy-3b-(4-chlorophenyl) tropane (IPT), was evaluated [37-40] It is useful as a probe for *in vitro* and *in vivo* labeling of dopamine (DA) and serotonin (5-HT) reuptake sites in rat brain. Saturation binding analysis of [^{125}I]IPT in rat striatal homogenates, in two different buffer solutions, Tris-HCl and phosphate, demonstrated one-site binding with affinities (K_d) of 0.25 ± 0.02 and 0.16 ± 0.02 nM and densities (B_{max}) of 939 ± 161 and 1982 ± 137 fmol/mg protein, respectively. Both *ex vivo* and *in vitro* autoradiographic studies revealed high densities of [^{125}I]IPT binding sites in caudate nucleus, putamen, olfactory tubercle and nucleus accumbens, areas known to be rich in dopaminergic innervation. Moderate accumulation of activity was also observed in the substantia nigra. Furthermore, systemic administration of IPT to rats increased the locomotor activity, a behavioral effect consistent with the *in vitro* and *in vivo* characteristics of compounds acting at dopaminergic sites. These results demonstrate that [^{125}I]IPT is a useful ligand for *in vitro* labeling of dopamine reuptake sites and is selective for labeling dopamine reuptake sites. The initial Phase I evaluation in normal volunteers done in our laboratory clearly indicated that [^{123}I]IPT shows maximum uptake (3.6% injected dose in brain at 40 min) and a BG/CTX ratio of 26 at 2 h after an IV injection [39] (See figure 5). In addition, the agent displayed a marked decrease in uptake in PD patients [42].

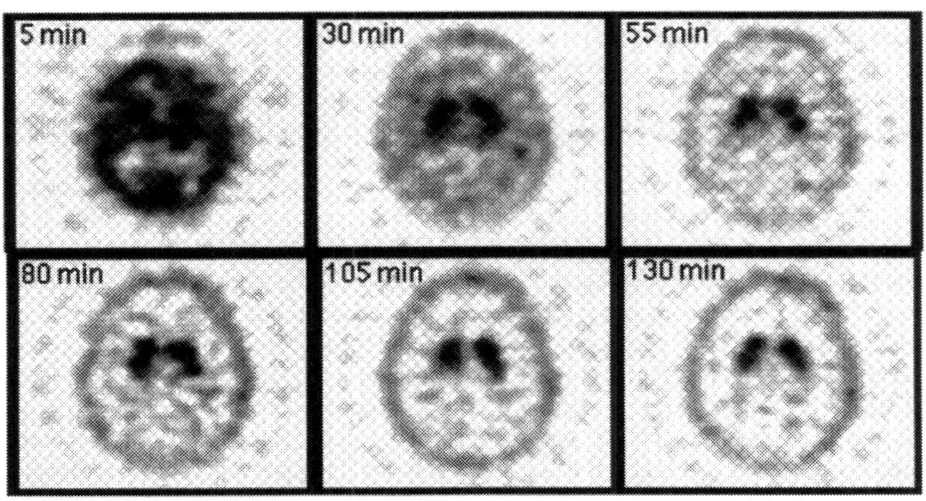

Figure 5. An [^{123}I]IPT transaxial section of a SPECT image (5 min/frame) of the brain after a bolus injection of 4.74 mCi in a 67 year old male subject. The images show a high density of IPT localization in the basal ganglia area, where dopamine reuptake sites are in high concentration.

Development of technetium-99m labeled dopamine transporter imaging agents

Despite its attractive physical properties, technetium is a difficult metallic element for designing suitable SPECT ligands. Technetium is a transition metal and requires a complexing agent to stabilize it at different valence states [11]. Valence states can vary from plus 7 (as pertechnetate) to zero (0), depending on the reaction conditions and chelating agents used during preparation. After complexation, the molecules invariably become big and bulky, which is the limiting factor in designing a molecule targeted to a specific biological process(es). Additional requirements for Tc-99m labeled complexes as CNS receptor imaging agents are: i) small (mol. weight < 750), with good lipophilicity (partition coefficient ~50 - 1,000); ii) high binding affinity (K_d < 10 nM) and high selectivity; iii) minimum brain uptake in rats should be 0.5% dose/organ at 2 min post IV injection.

It is well established that when Tc-99m pertechnetate (TcO_4^-) is reduced in the presence of a reducing agent, such as stannous chloride, and a "soft" chelating ligand, such as N_2S_2 and NS_3, a $[Tc^VO]^{+3}N_2S_2$ or $[Tc^VO]^{+3}NS_3$ center core is formed. Several recent reports demonstrated that it is possible to incorporate $[Tc^VO]^{+3}N_2S_2$ into potential receptor-selective imaging agents for muscarinic receptors [43], vesamicol sites [44] and steroid hormone receptors [45-50]. Muscarinic receptor ligands with other types of Tc-99m complexes have also been reported [51]. However, these Tc-99m imaging agents have had limited success in *in vivo* studies. Generally, these agents can be classified into two categories: **pendent approach**, in which the Tc-99m complexing moiety hangs from the main body of the molecule responsible for binding to the pocket of the receptor-ligand binding site; or **integrated approach**, in which the Tc-99m complex is integrated as part of the receptor specific ligand (Fig. 6).

Initially, our laboratory used the pendent approach to design a series of tropane derivatives in which chelating groups, N_2S_2 and NS_3, were attached peripherally to the portion of the molecule responsible for binding to the receptor site. The rationale for selecting the N_2S_2 and NS_3 ligands as the basic chelating systems for complexing reduced Tc-99m was: i) ligand systems consisting of soft donor atoms, N and S, form highly stable $[Tc^VO]^{+3}$ complexes with pyramidal structures; ii) predictably, two or three protons are removed during the complex formation, countering the +3 charges at the center Tc and creating a complex with an overall net charge of zero; iii) the ionizability of the S-$\underline{H}$ and the amine N-$\underline{H}$ groups determines the final net charge; therefore, they have a strong influence on the ultimate biodistribution of these imaging agents (Fig. 7) [52,53].

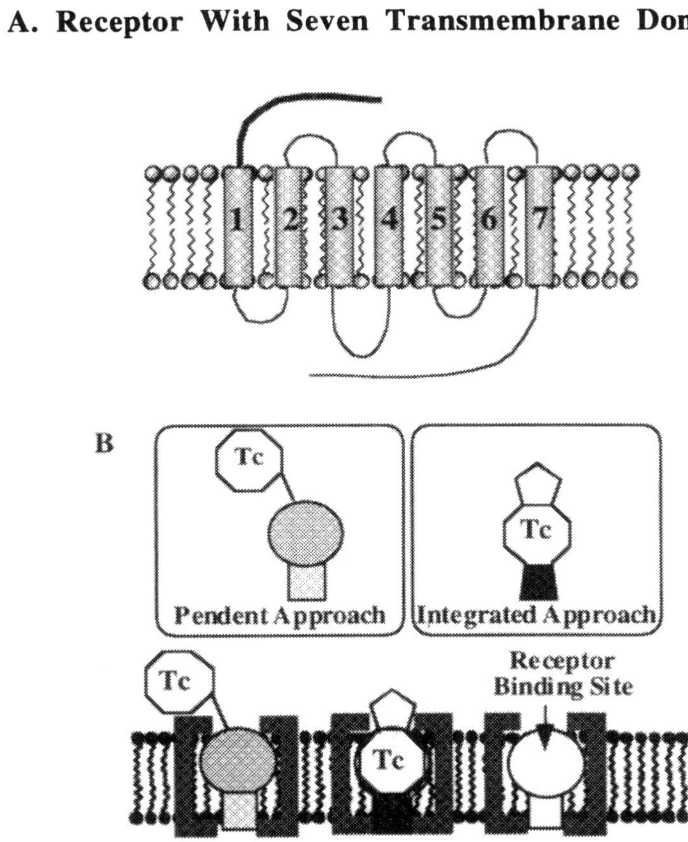

Figure 6. A. A schematic drawing of a receptor with seven transmembrane domains. B. Comparison of different approaches in designing Tc-99m-based receptor ligands. In the pendent approach, the Tc-99m complex moiety is outside the receptor binding region, while the integral approach incorporates the Tc-99m into the ligand that is directly involved in the receptor binding sites.

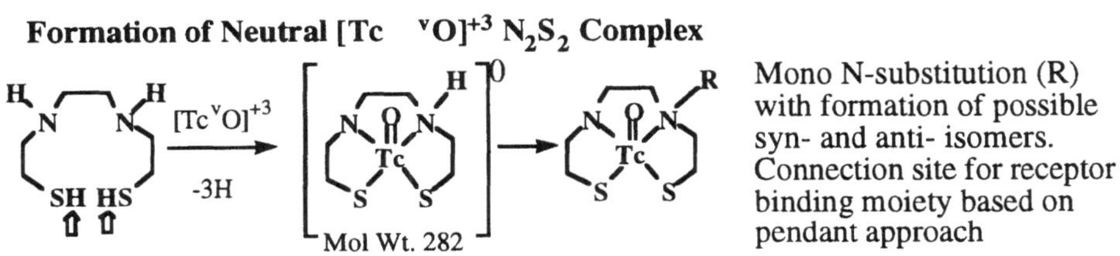

Figure 7 Formation of $[Tc^{V}O]^{+3}$ complexes based on the N_2S_2 (bisaminoethanethiol; BAT) ligands

When a tropane derivative containing a N_2S_2 chelating group to incorporate $[Tc^{V}O]^{+3}N_2S_2$ was labeled with technetium, it was clearly demonstrated by high pressure liquid chromatography that the complexation resulted in the formation of two isomers, most likely the syn and anti isomers. Both isomers showed low brain uptake (0.1% dose/organ in rats at 2 min after injection). However, both isomers displayed selective uptake in the striatal area, suggesting that the localization is consistent with the dopamine transporter distribution [54].

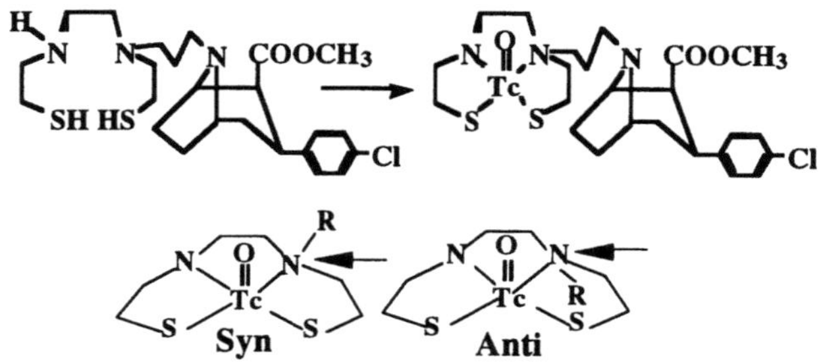

Figure 8. Preparation of a tropane derivative, with a N_2S_2 chelating group to incorporate $[Tc^VO]^{+3}N_2S_2$, as a potential dopamine transporter imaging agent. The N-alkyl substituted $[Tc^VO]^{+3}N_2S_2$ complex may form the syn and anti isomers.

Another approach for designing neutral and lipophilic agents is based on "3+1" NS_3 complexes (See figure 9A). These new NS_3 ligands and their neutral Tc complexes showed high brain uptake and retention in animals [55-57] (See figure 9B). Surprisingly, the hetero-bimolecular complexes of NS_3 as well as heterodimeric, NS plus NS, complexes (as steroid analogs) [45-46] are quite stable *in vivo* and *in vitro*.

A

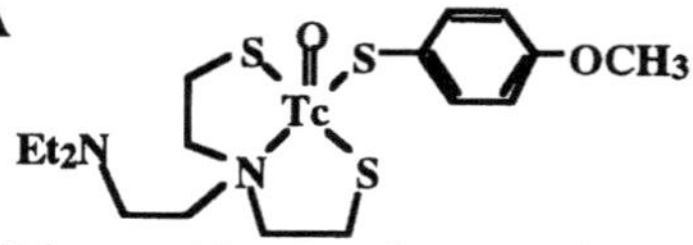

i) hetero-bimolecular complexes by NS_3
ii) neutral, lipophilic and stable complexes
iii) Tc-NS_3 complexes penetrating intact BBB

B

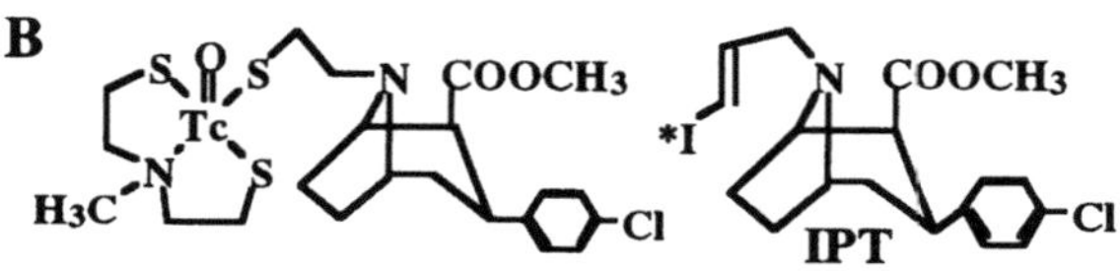

i) minimum molecular weight
ii) neutral, stable and lipophilic
iii) pendent approach

Figure 9. A. Formation of $[Tc^VO]^{+3}$ complexes based on hetero-bimolecular NS_3 ligands [55]. B. Design of dopamine transporter imaging agent based on pendent approach.

Based on the "3+1" approach described above, a Tc-99m labeled cocaine analog potentially useful for *in vivo* imaging of dopamine transporters was demonstrated [58] (Fig. 9B). A novel N-ethanethiol tropane derivative containing a neutral heterodimeric $Tc^{V}O$ aminobisethanethiol and a monothiol complex moiety, [^{99m}Tc]-IPT, was prepared in high purity (Fig. 10A). *In vivo* biodistribution of [^{99m}Tc]-IPT after an IV injection showed specific uptake in the striatum of male Sprague-Dawley rats. X-ray crystallography of a similar rhenium complex, Re-IPT, displayed an expected structure, with a pyramidal Re=O core and a N-methyl group at the anti position to the Re=O functionality (Fig. 10B). *In vitro* binding in rat striatal membrane homogenates, using a comparable compound, [^{125}I]IPT, as the ligand, showed an excellent binding affinity for the Re-IPT complex. The inhibition constant (K_i) of Re-IPT complex was 0.31 ± 0.03 nM (as compared to the parent ligand, [^{125}I]-IPT; K_d = 0.2 nM). This is the first example of a Tc-99m complex that displays selective dopamine transporter binding. Further studies are warranted to fully characterize this series of new Tc-99m complexes that may be very important as a tool for early detection of Parkinson's disease.

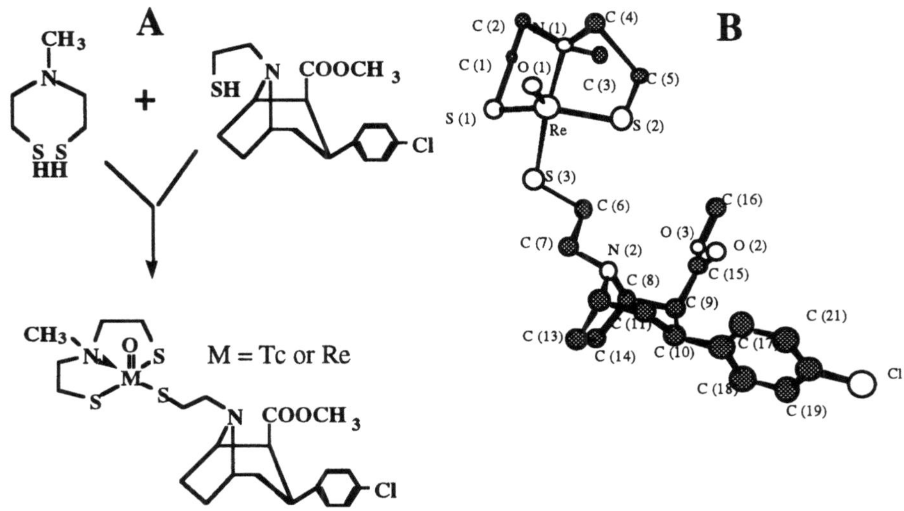

Figure 10. A. Preparation of Tc- or Re-IPT complexes. B. X-ray crystallography structure of Re-IPT complex [modified from ref 58].

Conclusion

A large number of SPECT and PET imaging agents for the evaluation of CNS receptor function in normal or disease states have been reported. Development of the receptor selective imaging agents requires the consideration of various chemical and biological parameters. Factors such as radiochemistry (preparation time for short-lived labeled agents), kinetics of receptor uptake and retention and metabolism must be considered in addition to selectivity, affinity and specific activity. The development of additional Tc-99m labeled agents will broaden the prospect of SPECT CNS receptor imaging, because they are more suitable for routine clinical use than agents labeled with I-123, since most nuclear medicine services in hospitals are equipped with a SPECT camera optimized for detecting Tc-99m. The challenge of incorporating a technetium complex moiety into a small receptor ligand while maintaining the original ligand's binding affinity is formidable, yet justified, because the potential benefits for a large number of patients using nuclear medicine diagnostic procedures are enormous. With advancements in the development of highly selective receptor ligands, noninvasive imaging procedures will achieve wider application both in pharmacological research and diagnosis of CNS disorders.

Acknowledgments

The author would also like to thank Dr. Mei-Ping Kung, Ms. Susan West and Mr. Andrew Beckwith for their assistance in preparing this manuscript. This work is partially supported by grants awarded by the National Institutes of Health (NS-18509, MH-43880 and NS-24538).

References

1. Strange PG. Multiple dopamine receptors: relevance for neurodegenerative disorders [review]. Biochem Soc Trans 22(1):155-159, 1994.
2. Waddington JL, O'Boyle KM. Drugs acting on brain dopamine receptors: a conceptual re-evaluation five years after the first selective D_1 antagonist. Pharmacol Ther 43:1, 1989.
3. Sibley DR, Monsma FJ, Jr., Shen Y. Molecular neurobiology of dopaminergic receptors. Int Rev Neurobiol 35:391-415, 1993.
4. Strange PG. New insights into dopamine receptors in the central nervous system. Neurochem Int 22(3):223-236, 1993.
5. Vanleeuwen DH, Eisenstein J, O'Malley K, Mackenzie RG. Characterization of a chimeric human dopamine D_3/D_2 receptor functionally coupled to adenylyl-cyclase in Chinese hamster ovary cells. Mol Pharmacol 48(2):344-351, 1995.
6. Eckelman WC. The status of radiopharmaceutical research. Nucl Med Biol - Int J Rad Appl Inst Part B 18(7):iii-vi, 1991.
7. Fowler JS, Wolf AP. Recent advances in radiotracers for PET studies of the brain. Ann Rep Med Chem, 1990.
8. Matsuda H, Li YM, Higashi S, Sumiya H, Tsuji S, Kinuya K, Hisada K, Yamashita J. Comparative SPECT study of stroke using Tc-99m ECD, I-123 IMP, and Tc-99m HMPAO. Clin Nucl Med 18(9):754-758, 1993.
9. Léveillé J, Demonceau G, Walovitch RC. Intrasubject comparison between technetium-99m-ECD

and technetium-99m-HMPAO in healthy human subjects. J Nucl Med 33(4):480-484, 1992.
10. Jurisson SS, Berning D, Jia W, Ma D-S. Coordination compounds in nuclear medicine. Chem Rev 93(3):1137-1156, 1993.
11. Steigman J, Eckelman WC. The Chemistry of Technetium in Medicine. Washington, D.C.: National Academy Press, 1992.
12. Farde L. Selective D_1 and D_2 dopamine receptor blockade both induces akathisia in humans--a PET study with [^{11}C]SCH23390 and [^{11}C]raclopride. Psychopharmacology (Berl) 107(1):23-29, 1992.
13. Farde L, Wiesel FA, Stone-Elander S, Halldin C, Nordström AL, Hall H, Sedvall G. D_2 dopamine receptors in neuroleptic-naive schizophrenic patients. A positron emission tomography study with [^{11}C] raclopride. Arch Gen Psychiatry 47(3):213-219, 1990.
14. Volkow ND, Fowler JS, Wang GJ, et al. Reproducibility of repeated measures of carbon-11-raclopride binding in the human brain. J Nucl Med 34:609-613, 1993.
15. Wong DF. PET studies of neuroreceptors in schizophrenia. Commentary on "The current status of PET scanning with respect to schizophrenia." Neuropsychopharmacology 7(1):69-72, 1992.
16. Sedvall G. The current status of PET scanning with respect to schizophrenia. Neuropsychopharmacology 7(1):41-54, 1992.
17. Seeman P, Guan H-C, Niznik HB. Endogenous dopamine lowers the dopamine D_2 receptor density as measured by [^{3}H]raclopride: implications for positron emission tomography of the human brain. Synapse 3(96-97), 1989.
18. Young LT, Wong DF, Goldman S, Minkin E, Chen C, Matsumura K, Scheffel U, Wagner HN, Jr. Effects of endogenous dopamine on kinetics of [^{3}H]N-methylspiperone and [^{3}H]raclopride binding in the rat brain. Synapse 9(3):188-194, 1991.
19. Andreasen NC, Carson R, Diksic M, Evans A, Farde L, Gjedde A, Hakim A, Lal S, Nair N, Sedvall G, Tune L, Wong D. Workshop on schizophrenia, PET, and dopamine D_2 receptors in the human neostriatum. Schizophr Bull 14(3):471-484, 1988.
20. Kung HF, Kasliwal R, Pan S, Kung M-P, Mach RH, Guo Y-Z. Dopamine D_2 receptor imaging radiopharmaceuticals: synthesis, radiolabeling and *in vitro* binding of (R)-(+)- and (S)-(-)-3-iodo-2-hydroxy-6-methoxy-N-[(1-ethyl-2-pyrrolidinyl)-methyl]-benzamide. J Med Chem 31(5):1039-1043, 1988.
21. Kung HF, Alavi A, Chang W, Kung M-P, Keyes JW, Jr., Velchik MG, Billings JJ, Pan S, Noto R, Rausch A, Reilley J. *In vivo* SPECT imaging of CNS D_2 dopamine receptors: initial studies with iodine-123-IBZM in humans. J Nucl Med 31:573-579, 1990a.
22. Brücke T, Wenger S, Asenbaum S, Fertl E, Pfafflmeyer N, Müller C, Podreka I, Angelberger P. Dopamine D_2 receptor imaging and measurement with SPECT. Adv Neurol 60:494-500, 1993.
23. Ichise M, Toyama H, Fonazzari I, Ballinger JR, Kirsch JC. Assessment of subjects with and at risk for developing Huntington's disease by I-123 IBZM and Tc-99m HM-PAO SPECT [abstract]. J Nucl Med 33:970, 1992.
24. Knable MB, Jones DW, Coppola R, Hyde TM, Lee KS, Gorey J, Weinberger DR. Lateralized differences in iodine-123-IBZM uptake in the basal ganglia in asymmetric Parkinson's disease. J Nucl Med 36(7):1216-1225, 1995.
25. Laruelle MA, Abi-Dargham A, van Dyck CH, Rosenblatt W, Zea-Ponce Y, Zoghbi SS, Baldwin RM, Charney DS, Hoffer PB, Kung HF, Innis RB. SPECT imaging of striatal dopamine release after amphetamine challenge. J Nucl Med 36(7):1182-1190, 1995.
26. Schlosser R, Schlegel S. D_2 receptor imaging with [^{123}I]IBZM and single photon emission tomography in psychiatry: a survey of current status. J Neural Transm - Gen Sect 99(1):173-185, 1995.
27. Schwarz J, Tatsch K, Arnold G, Gasser T, Trenkwalder C, Kirsch CM, Oertel WH. [^{123}I]-iodobenzamide-SPECT predicts dopaminergic responsiveness in patients with de novo Parkinsonism. Neurology, 1992.
28. Seibyl J, Woods S, Zoghbi SS, Baldwin RM, Dey HM, Goddard AW, Zea-Ponce Y, Zubal G, Germine M, Smith EO, Heninger GR, Charney DS, Kung HF, Alavi A, Hoffer PB, Innis RB. Dynamic SPECT imaging of dopamine D_2 receptors in human subjects with iodine-123-IBZM. J Nucl Med 33:1964-1971, 1992.

29. Tatsch K, Schwartz J, Oertel WH, Kirsh CM. Dopamine D_2 receptor imaging with [^{123}I]IBZM SPECT to differentiate idiopathic from other Parkinson syndromes [abstract]. J Nucl Med 33:917-918, 1992.
30. Carroll FI, Lewin AH, Boja JW, Kuhar MJ. Cocaine receptor: biochemical characterization and structure-activity relationships of cocaine analogues at the dopamine transporter. J Med Chem 35(6):969-981, 1992.
31. Carroll FI, Mascarella SW, Kuzemko MA, Gao Y, Abraham P, Lewin AH, Boja JW, Kuhar MJ. Synthesis, ligand binding, and QSAR (CoMFA and classical) study of 3b-(3'-substituted phenyl)-, 3b-(4'-substituted phenyl)-, and 3b-(3',4'-disubstituted phenyl)tropane-2b-carboxylic acid methyl esters. J Med Chem 37:2865-2873, 1994.
32. Fowler JS, Volkow ND, Wolf AP, Dewey SL, Schlyer DJ, Macgregor RR, Hitzemann R, Logan J, Bendriem B, Gatley SJ. Mapping cocaine binding sites in human and baboon brain *in vivo*. Synapse 4(4):371-377, 1989.
33. Fowler JS, Volkow ND, MacGregor RR, Logan J, Dewey SL, Gatley SJ, Wolf AP. Comparative PET studies of the kinetics and distribution of cocaine and cocaethylene in baboon brain. Synapse 12(3):220-227, 1992.
34. Frost JJ, Rosier AJ, Reich SG, Smith JS, Ehlers MD, Snyder SH, Ravert HT, Dannals RF. Positron emission tomographic imaging of the dopamine transporter with [^{11}C]-WIN 35,428 reveals marked declines in mild Parkinson's disease. Ann Neurol 34(3):423-431, 1993.
35. Innis RB. Single photon emission tomography imaging of dopamine terminal innervation: a potential clinical tool in Parkinson's disease [editorial; review]. Eur J Nucl Med 21(1):1-5, 1994.
36. Wong DF, Yung B, Dannals RF, Shaya EK, Ravert HT, Chen CA, Chan B, Folio T, Scheffel U, Ricaurte GA, et al. *In vivo* imaging of baboon and human dopamine transporters by positron emission tomography using [^{11}C]WIN35,428. Synapse 15:130-142, 1993.
37. Goodman MM, Kung M-P, Kabalka GW, Kung HF, Switzer R. Synthesis and characterization of radioiodinated N-(3-iodopropen-1-yl)-2b-carbomethoxy-3b-(4-chlorophenyl)tropanes: potential dopamine reuptake site imaging agents. J Med Chem 37:1535-1542, 1994.
38. Kung M-P, Essman WD, Frederick D, Meegalla SK, Goodman MM, Mu M, Lucki I, Kung HF. IPT: a novel iodinated ligand for the CNS dopamine transporter. Synapse 20(4):316-324, 1995.
39. Mozley PD, Stubbs JB, Kim H-J, McElgin WT, Kung M-P, Meegalla SK, Kung HF. Dosimetry of an iodine-123-labeled tropane to image dopamine transporters. J Nucl Med 37(1):151-159, 1996.
40. Malison RT, Vessotskie JM, Kung M-P, McElgin WT, Romaniello G, Kim H-J, Goodman MM, Kung HF. Striatal dopamine transporter imaging in non-human primates with iodine-123-IPT SPECT. J Nucl Med 36(12):2290-2297, 1995.
41. Neumeyer JL, Wang S, Gao Y, Milius RA, Kula NS, Campbell A, Baldessarini RJ, Zea-Ponce Y, Baldwin RM, Innis RB. N-w-Fluoroalkyl analogs of (1*R*)-2b-carbomethoxy-3b-(4-iodophenyl)-tropane (b-CIT): radiotracers for positron emission tomography and single photon emission computed tomography imaging of dopamine transporters. J Med Chem 37(11):1558-1561, 1994.
42. Lever SZ, Baidoo KE, Mahmood A, Matsumura K, Scheffel UA, Wagner HN, Jr. Novel technetium ligands with affinity for the muscarinic cholinergic receptor. Nucl Med Biol 21(2):157-164, 1994.
42. Tatsch, K. Unpublished results.
44. Del Rosario RB, Jung Y-W, Baidoo KE, Lever SZ, Wieland DM. Synthesis and *in vivo* evaluation of a [$^{99m/99}$Tc]-DADT-benzovesamicol: a potential marker for cholinergic neurons. Nucl Med Biol 21(2):197-203, 1994.
45. Chi DY, Katzenellenbogen JA. Selective formation of heterodimeric bis-bidentate aminothiol-oxometal complexes of rhenium(V). J Am Chem Soc 115(15):7045-7046, 1993.
46. Chi DY, O'Neil JP, Anderson CJ, Welch MJ, Katzenellenbogen JA. Homodimeric and heterodimeric bis(amino thiol) oxometal complexes with rhenium(V) and technetium(V): control of heterodimeric complex formation and an approach to metal complexes that mimic steroid hormones. J Med Chem 37(7):928-937, 1994.
47. DiZio JP, Anderson CJ, Davison A, Ehrhardt GJ, Carlson KE, Welch MJ, Katzenellenbogen JA. Technetium- and rhenium-labeled progestins: synthesis, receptor binding and *in vivo* distribution of an 11 beta-substituted progestin labeled with technetium-99 and rhenium-186. J Nucl Med 33(4):558-569, 1992.

48. DiZio JP, Fiaschi R, Davison A, Jones AG, Katzenellenbogen JA. Progestin-rhenium complexes: metal-labeled steroids with high receptor binding affinity, potential receptor-directed agents for diagnostic imaging or therapy. Bioconj Chem 2(5):353-366, 1991.
49. O'Neil JP, Carlson KE, Anderson CJ, Welch MJ, Katzenellenbogen JA. Progestin radiopharmaceuticals labeled with technetium and rhenium: synthesis, binding affinity, and *in vivo* distribution of a new progestin N_2S_2-metal conjugate. Bioconj Chem 5(3):182-193, 1994a.
50. O'Neil JP, Wilson SR, Katzenellenbogen JA. Preparation and structural characterization of monoamine-monoamide bis(thiol) oxo complexes of technetium(V) and rhenium(V). Inorg Chem 33(2):319-323, 1994b.
51. Jurisson SS, Pirro J, DiRocco RJ, Rosenspire KC, Jagoda E, Nanjappan P, Eckelman WC, Nowotnik DP, Nunn AD. Boronic acid adducts of technetium dioxime (BATO) complexes derived from quinuclidine benzilate (QNB) boronic acid stereoisomers: syntheses and studies of their binding to the muscarinic acetylcholine receptor. Nucl Med Biol 22(3):269-281, 1995.
52. Kung HF. New technetium 99m-labeled brain perfusion imaging agents. Semin Nucl Med 20(2):150-158, 1990.
53. Kung HF, Liu B-L, Francesconi LC, Ohmomo Y, Billings JJ, Kung M-P. Metal N_2S_2 complexes in radiopharmaceutical development. J Lab Compds Radiopharm 30:29-30, 1990b.
54. Meegalla, SK. Unpublished results.
55. Mastrostamatis SG, Papadopoulos MS, Pirmettis IC, Paschali E, Varvarigou AD, Stassinopoulou CI, Raptopoulou CP, Terzis A, Chiotellis E. Tridentate ligands containing the SNS donor atom set as a novel backbone for the development of technetium brain imaging agents. J Med Chem 37(20):3212-3218, 1994.
56. Spies H, Fietz T, Glaser M, Pietzsch H-J, Johannsen B. The "n+1" concept in the synthesis strategy of novel technetium and rhenium tracers. In Technetium and Rhenium in Chemistry and Nuclear Medicine, Volume 4. Nicolini M, Bandoli G, Mazzi U. Padova, Italy: S. G. Editoriali:243-246, 1995.
57. Spies H, Pietzsch H-J, Hahn FE, Kintzel O, Lügger T. Trigonal-bipyramidal technetium and rhenium complexes with tetradentate NS_3 tripod ligands. Angew Chem Int Ed Engl 33:1354-1356, 1994.
58. Meegalla SK, Plössl K, Kung M-P, Stevenson DA, Liable-Sands LM, Rheingold AL, Kung HF. The first example of a Tc-99m complex as a dopamine transporter imaging agent. J Am Chem Soc 117(44):11037-11038, 1995.

IMAGING THE FUNCTIONS OF THE CELL NUCLEUS

Leonard I. Wiebe

Introduction

The identification of exploitable molecular targets for nuclear medicine has evolved steadily over the past four decades. This chapter presents an overview of some of the molecular targets that have been, and could be, utilized for diagnostic imaging of the cell nucleus functions. This will include radiopharmaceuticals that directly and indirectly provide information about intracellular DNA-related processes, as well as about DNA and chromosomes. To develop this theme, the nature of the membrane barriers lying between an intravenously-injected radiopharmaceutical and the nucleus will be reviewed, and an overview of nucleic acid metabolism will be presented. A full discussion of the metabolic and physiological traps for these radiopharmaceuticals, although essential to the design of nucleus-directed probes, lies beyond the scope of this paper. Approaches to imaging nucleus-associated molecular targets in the extracellular, cytoplasmic and nucleoplasmic compartments will be reviewed and the chapter will close with a description of cell nucleus imaging applications in gene therapy.

Many of the early clinical nuclear medicine imaging radiopharmaceuticals provided anatomical images based on physiological function. Some utilized blood capillary diameter (e.g. micro- and macro-aggregates) for regional uptake, whereas others responded to physiological functions such as renal clearance (e.g. iodo-aromatic acids and hydrophilic 99mTc-chelates) and hepatic clearance (e.g. higher molecular weight iodo-organics and lipophilic 99mTc-chelates). Although of lesser interest to the nuclear medicine community, there was also substantial scientific interest, beginning in the late 1950's, in nucleoside antimetabolites that were directed towards DNA synthesis. An example is the use of IUDR to delineate tissues that had high mitotic indices [1]. The science of nuclear imaging made steady progress in the 1960's, but the 1970's were the golden age of radiopharmaceutical development. Metabolic reactions, molecular transporters, enzymes and receptors became targets for new radiopharmaceuticals. Advances in other imaging modalities such as x-ray CT, magnetic resonance imaging (MRI) and ultrasound have pushed nuclear medicine further into metabolic imaging. Progress in the chemistry and instrumentation of positron emission tomography (PET)

S. J. Mather (ed.), Current Directions in Radiopharmaceutical Research and Development, 115–135.

have made in vivo, in situ mapping of metabolic processes possible. Among the imaging techniques, the sensitivity of both PET and SPECT makes them uniquely suitable for studying molecular targets. These radiopharmaceuticals have changed the nature of diagnostic imaging in nuclear medicine, and given it a future.

Molecular biology and genetic engineering made exponential advances in the 1970's, and the resulting immunological applications took radiopharmaceutical research by storm in the 1980's. Even today, a substantial fraction of publications dealing with experimental and clinical radio-pharmaceutical science addresses radiolabelled monoclonal antibodies and monoclonal antibody fragments. Although there is no verdict on the ultimate success of immunologically-based imaging, the capital and resource investment was not trivial, and in many instances the successes may have been outweighed by the disappointments. None-the-less, immunology research has stimulated strong therapy programs and there continue to be new innovations for the delivery and application of immunologicals, including gene therapy techniques. There is also an evolution towards the development of antibody fragments for diagnosis and therapy. The radiopharmaceutical use of chemotactic peptides follows their chemotherapeutic lead. The subsequent development of small, rigid peptidomimetic structures from structure-function analysis of active peptides will undoubtedly revive small-molecule focus in diagnostic imaging.

At the close of this millennium the buzz-words of therapeutic medicine are certain to be gene therapy. In theory gene therapy represents the first opportunity to eliminate a disease by addressing the root-cause within the host genome or in the genome of the causative agent. The body's metabolic machinery creates a permanent cure in situ. Enzyme deficiencies such as adenosine de-aminase (ADA immune deficiency syndrome), infectious diseases such as HIV and cancer are only examples of a myriad of conditions that may be curable by gene therapy [2]. Although gene structure and function is steadily being unravelled and the genetic basis of many diseases has already been identified, the technology of delivering a therapeutic gene to the site of action is far from perfect. In fact, gene delivery is still in its infancy [3]. Loss of gene expression and loss of the gene itself are additional major barriers to success. Clearly, radiopharmaceutical scientists and nuclear medicine physicians have an opportunity to participate in the development of this important subject.

There are a number of fundamental issues that are inherent in the successful implementation of an intracellularly-targeted pharmaceutical or radiopharmaceutical. In the first instance, the advent of macromolecular (radio)pharmaceuticals has greatly amplified the underlying challenges in drug delivery. When one considers the location of the genetic apparatus deep within the cells of the organism, and the protection nature has afforded these targets, it is understandable that the delivery of any pharmaceutical to the cell nucleus demands careful planning, ingenuity and good fortune.

The fundamental nature of cells

It is generally held that the seventeenth century observations of Robert Hooke underpin the nineteenth century concept of Schleiden and Schwann, that cells are the morphological units of life. Although there are schematic representations of 'typical' cells, there are no single representations that can be applied to all cells. It is nevertheless possible to classify cells on the basis of the presence or absence of a nuclear membrane. Thus, prokaryote cells have no membrane surrounding their DNA, and eukaryote cells have this 'nuclear' membrane; the former are usually unicellular organisms, whereas the eukaryote may be either unicellular or multicellular organisms. For obvious reasons this discussion will focus on the eukaryote, although one should not overlook the importance of prokaryotes and viruses as sources of biomolecules that can be harnessed as targets, substrates and facilitators. Indeed, prokaryotes are the source of some genes currently used in gene therapy.

It is common knowledge that the cell consists of an outer membrane that encapsulates an aqueous environment, the cytoplasm, and that the cytoplasm contains a number of structures. The most common subcellular organelles include the endoplasmic reticulum, the Golgi apparatus, the nucleus, lysosomes, peroxisomes and mitochondria, all held in the appropriate juxtaposition by a cytoskeleton comprised of several classes of fibrous proteins (filaments). The smooth endoplasmic reticulum (SER) manufactures lipids and rough endoplasmic reticulum (RER) includes the ribosomes that translate mRNA into protein. The Golgi apparatus traffics ER products (proteins and nucleic acids) between the ER and other cellular membranes. Lysosomes and peroxisomes contain hydrolytic enzymes and catylase, respectively, the mitochondria are energy generators and the nucleus contains the genetic code for the cell.

CELLULAR MEMBRANES: BASIC STRUCTURE AND FUNCTION

Eukaryote cells have a large number of subcellular features that are defined by, or that consist of, membranes. It is less well known, and indeed frequently ignored, that the external membrane, called the cell or plasma membrane, together with the intracellular membranes, may constitute up to 60% of the total mass of the cell. These membranes are amphoteric, with hydrophobic cores and hydrophilic surfaces; they serve not only to encapsulate an aqueous environment, but to perform a number of specific functions that are important to the homeostasis of the cell and the organism. Membranes stand in the way of any effort to influence or measure cell function, if that measurement necessitates the insertion of indigenous and/or exogenous substances. Molecular probes that are to be delivered into subcellular organelles will obviously encounter additional membrane barriers. Clearly the importance of these membrane barriers cannot be overstated in terms of their impact on the delivery of any intracellular molecular probes, and especially for probes directed towards the nucleoplasm. An understanding of the challenges and opportunities likely to be encountered is critical to the design and delivery of the (radio)pharmaceutical.

Cell membranes are frequently thought of only as simple lipophilic barriers that can be crossed by diffusion. A simplistic view of the membrane as a symmetrically arranged lipid bilayer of phospholipids may lead to critical underestimation of the challenges that exist. The membranes are anything but simple; for example, within its phospholipid bilayer the plasma membrane contains small molecules such as cholesterol, and proteins with multiple trans-membrane domains. In other words, although a barrier to simple diffusion, the membrane may also facilitate (frequently energy-dependent) passage of specific permeants and it may serve as a lipophilic reservoir for some compounds. Such a membrane-depot effect has been postulated for the azomycin nucleoside hypoxia tracers (e.g. the IAZA family). These relatively lipophilic nucleosides show good correlation for radiosensitizer potency and cytotoxicity if one compensates for differences in lipophilicity (partition coefficient) and membrane mass [4]. This observation is consistent with a membrane depot concept and with model partition studies using liposomes.

Membranes consist mainly of phospholipids, glycolipids and sterols. Phospholipids, which have lipophilic tails and negatively-charged phosphate heads are the most predominant (25-35% by weight). Choline phosphate glycerol esters are examples of this class of membrane constituent. Other major components include glycolipids (up to 3%), which have oligosaccharide heads on a fatty chain such as sphingosine, and sterols (up to 10%), which are exemplified by cholesterol. Interestingly, the standard approach to determine the lipophilicity of small-molecule drugs is based on water (buffer):octanol (vegetable oil) partition coefficients, but it has been shown that for at least some drugs, better activity correlation's can be obtained if liposomes comprised of a complex of phospholipids and cholesterol are used in place of the simple biphasic partition systems [5]. The heterogeneity of membranes is also seen when one considers the differences between the internal (cytoplasmic) and external faces. Lipids on the cytoplasmic face are more charged and have lower phase transition temperatures (greater degree of unsaturation). Glycolipids are found only on the external face of the plasma membrane.

Typical plasma membranes usually contain approximately equal amounts of protein and lipid, whereas internal membranes have up to 75% by weight protein. These proteins are predominantly trans-membrane structures, with hydrophilic (protruding) and hydrophobic (imbedded) domains. They may be fixed or internalized, and they can have a broad range of function that include signal transduction and transport. Again proteins are not symmetrically distributed to the two faces of the membrane. The faces will feature different protruding sequences for transmembrane proteins, and also completely different surface-associated proteins.

Membrane budding to form vesicles is an important mechanism for moving proteins and other macromolecules across membranes. Budding may be endocytotic and serve to move substances into the cytoplasmic space, or exocytotic for externalization of cell products. The transport process involves a sequence of budding, migration of the vesicle and finally fusion of the vesicle with another membrane.

Two subcellular structures have special membranes and interestingly, both structures contain nucleic acids. The cell nucleus and the mitochondria are formed by an envelope that is comprised of a double lipid-bilayer membrane, one inner membrane and one outer membrane, each with two faces. These membranes are rich in trans-membrane proteins, many of which function as transporters. These proteins have asymmetric distribution, reaching from the cytosol to the intermembrane space or from the intramembrane space to the lumen of the envelope, but not directly from the cytoplasm to the nucleoplasm. The chemical contents of the cytoplasm, the intermembrane space and the lumen of the envelope are held distinct from each other through selective transport of proteins and other substances.

During cell division, internal membranes are broken down into vesicles, thereby halting all cell processes not directly involved in division and ensuring equal delivery of all cell components to both daughters. The nuclear envelope is also dismantled, but mitochondria are passed on to the progeny by virtue of their distribution in the cytoplasm. The establishment of structural elements (e.g. microtubules and fibres) precedes sorting of chromosomes and brings cell division to its conclusion. Reassembly of internal membranes and the nuclear envelope mark completion of the cell cycle.

MITOCHONDRIA

The evolutionary origin of the mitochondrion has attracted much interest because of the structure of its nucleic acids and its metabolism. Endosymbiosis involving insertion of a primitive bacterium into a eukaryotic cell has been postulated as a likely explanation, but regardless of its origin, the mitochondrion does contain genetic code. Mitochondrial code displays systematic changes from the universal code and although relatively small (~16.5kb), it encodes about half of its proteins. The importance of mitochondrial nucleic acid metabolism to drug design cannot be overemphasized. A recent clinical trial of an antiviral 2'-fluoro-arabino pyrimidine nucleoside, for example, resulted in a number of unpredictable deaths that have been attributed to its unanticipated insertion into hepatic mitochondrial DNA and causing intractable lactic acidosis [6]. This effect was not observed in other species.

The outer membrane of the mitochondrial envelope defines the perimeter of the organelle. The highly convoluted inner membrane forms the cristae, creating an intermembrane space and the lumen (matrix space). The matrix contains an enzyme-rich, gel-like medium. The overall process of ATP synthesis occurs in the matrix and the membrane-bound enzymes in the cristae.

THE NUCLEUS

The nuclear envelope differs from the mitochondrial envelope in that the inner and outer nuclear membranes are essentially concentric and held in juxtaposition by adhesion points. The outer membrane is continuous with the endoplasmic reticulum and the intermembrane space is continuous with the lumen of the endoplasmic reticulum. A major function of the nuclear membrane is to segregate DNA-regulatory proteins from DNA when the cell is not in the process of dividing.

The nuclear intermembrane space is called the perinuclear space and the lumen is called the nucleoplasmic space. The nuclear membranes are perforated by numerous nuclear pores, formed by protein complexes (~90Å; ~10^8 daltons), that transport proteins into the nucleus. Most cells also contain a nucleolus, which packages RNA and ribosomal proteins into immature ribosomes for export to the cytoplasm.

Nuclear targets for imaging in clinical nuclear medicine

STRUCTURAL ELEMENTS

Although structural elements in themselves are not thought of as targets for imaging, their assembly and disassembly are realistic targets. Tubulin is a structural protein that forms microtubules. These fibres form the centrosome-oriented cytoplasmic scaffold for cellular organelles when the cell is in the G1 (premitotic) phase of the cell cycle. During division, microtubules are involved in functions such as formation of the mitotic spindle. The constant rebuilding (often called dynamic instability) of microtubules has made them the site of action for traditional drugs such as colchicine and the modern cancer chemotherapeutic agent taxol [7]. The enzymes involved in hydrolysis (e.g. converting 'plus end' GTP to GDP) and polymerization of GTP-tubulin subunits are potential targets for imaging-based investigations. Other fibrous proteins could equally-well be of interest, as in the case of actin filaments which are involved in muscle contraction and which form the contractile ring that separates the daughter cells at the completion of division.

DNA BINDING

There are several families of anticancer drugs that bind with DNA to induce their effect. A number of acridines, ellipticines and ethidium bromide, among others, are known for their ability to bind tightly but reversibly to the double helix of DNA. The binding process involves charge transfer between nucleic acid bases and the aromatic portions of the reagent, H-bonding and electrostatic effects in a process known as intercalation. Although a number of manifestations arise from the intercalation of these agents, one of the effects is to interfere with the function of topoisomerases, enzymes that alter the topological state of circular DNA (Type-1 topoisomerases relax supercoiled DNA; Type-2 topoisomerases, also known as gyrases, induce DNA supercoiling).

RECEPTOR PROTEINS

There are four main categories of protein receptor in the cell. Transmembrane signal transduction proteins are represented by receptors for polypeptide growth factors (e.g. epidermal-GF; platelet-derived-GF; transforming-GFα) that upon stimulation of the extracellular segments, activate their cytoplasmic segments to initiate a specific function (e.g. substrate protein phosphorylation). Transmembrane protein receptors may also stimulate the release of second messengers such as cAMP. A second receptor class is exemplified by the acetylcholine receptor that regulates ion channels. These receptor types are unlikely targets for imaging radio-pharmaceuticals directed towards nuclear processes.

The steroid receptor proteins are frequently-targeted protein receptors. They are cytosolic receptors that, once occupied, are transported into the nucleus, where they bind to response elements and eventually induce or supress transcription of their associated genes. Thus, radiopharmaceuticals that bind to these receptors with high specificity and high affinity represent an important approach to imaging the cell nucleus. Steroid receptor based imaging has been actively pursued by Katzenellenbogen [8] and others, and is discussed in detail elswhere in this book by Mike Welch.

Nucleoside transporters in the plasma membrane represent a special case where the transporter may not be directly linked to nuclear biochemistry, but the metabolic interactions of the transported nucleosides may be manifest in the nucleus, the mitochondria and the cytoplasm. Non-physiological nucleosides can, of course, also bind competitively or irreversibly with the transporter to induce transport inhibition, thereby skewing nucleic acid-related metabolism. Clearly, a radiolabelled transport inhibitor would not provide direct information about nuclear processes. Radionucleosides that are not transporter-dependent permeants could not be effective diagnostics unless other mechanisms of permeation were available (e.g. diffusion for non-polar molecules). The nucleoside transporter field has broadened substantially in the last decade. A brief summary of salient issues is presented in the following paragraphs, but a full discussion lies beyond the scope of this treatise. Interested readers are referred to a recent review by Cass [9].

NUCLEOSIDE TRANSPORTERS

The most intensively studied plasma membrane nucleoside transporter was first characterized in the early 1970's. It is an equilibrative transporter that lies on the extracellular face of the plasma membrane, and is prominent in red cells. This transporter operates in association with a superficial, exposed nucleoside binding site. There are, however, more transporters; at present, a total of seven nucleoside transport systems are known. Specific roles have not been ascribed to these transporters and their inter-relationship is also not known. A physiological interpretation of the effect or importance of any single transport process is therefore complex at best, but the importance of transport is undisputed, since cells utilize and secrete nucleosides as part of their normal function.

The nucleoside transporter proteins isolated to date show substantial heterogeneity in structure and mechanism of action. Some are concentrative (energy-dependent; require Na+ gradient), some are equilibrative (Na+ independent) and others have permeant specificity that may include nucleotides. The physiological distribution of these sub-types is not uniform. The equilibrative systems have virtually ubiquitous distribution among cells, but the concentrative systems are found only in certain specialized cell types, while both classes appear to be present in cancer cells. Classification of these systems is still undergoing revision and expansion. At the present time, there are unanswered questions about transporter structure and function. The degree of interspecies protein homology for a given transporter type is unknown and structural differences between inhibitor-sensitive and inhibitor-independent transporters of a given functional type has not been determined [e.g. differences between the equilibrative nitrobenzylmercaptopurine riboside (NBMPR)-sensitive and the equilibrative NBMPR-insensitive transport systems. The structure of NBMPR is shown in Figure 1. The relationships among nucleoside transporters and other transporter systems (e.g. the relationship of the equilibrative NBMPR-sensitive transporter to the facilitative glucose transporter) are also not clear.

The transport of nucleosides into the nucleus and the mitochondrion from the cytoplasm is of particular interest. Although nucleosides obviously enter both of these organelles, direct evidence for the existence of a specialized transport mechanism has not been reported. There is some indirect evidence that the Golgi apparatus is involved and that there are nucleoside transport proteins in the external membrane of the mitochondrial envelope. Passage of nucleosides into the lumen of the nucleus may be as simple as passage through the nuclear pores, or as complex as the multifaceted process of plasma membrane permeation.

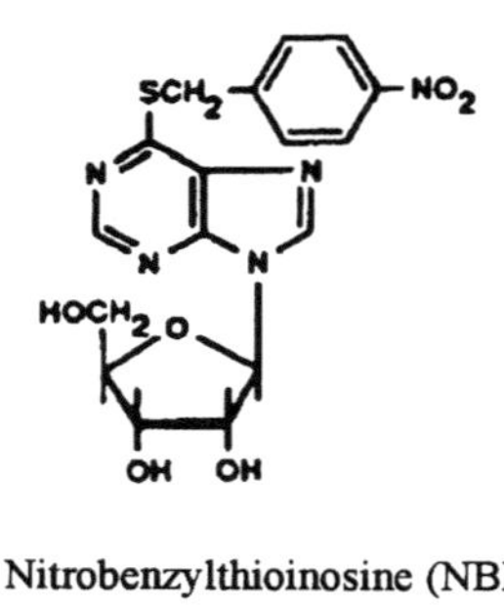

Figure 1. Nitrobenzylthioinosine (NBMPR).

The interactions of representative compounds from several classes of antiviral and antitumor radiolabelled nucleosides with the NBMPR-sensitive equilibrative transport system in fresh murine erythrocytes have been reported[10]. 3D-QSAR studies of the protein binding site have also been reported [11]. The in vivo use of NBMPR to block the equilibrative nucleoside transport of therapeutic nucleosides did not favourably modulate their biodistribution in a murine tumor model, perhaps due in part to the severe hypotensive effects of the transport inhibitor [12,13]. A radiolabelled NBMPR analogue has been reported [14].

NUCLEIC ACID PRECURSORS, INTERMEDIATES AND METABOLIC ENZYMES

The anabolic and catabolic metabolism of nucleic acids presents innumerable targets for nucleus imaging radiopharmaceuticals. The de novo synthesis and salvage pathways for the nucleobases, and the interconversion pathways for deoxyriboside and riboside nucleosides and nucleotides, are replete with enzymes that can be targeted by labelled nucleosides and nucleotides, as either substrates or inhibitors [15]. Interpretation of the action and localization of both indogenous and exogenous nucleosides within this milieu is further complicated by allosteric inhibition, pool effects and cell cycle phenomena. As a result, enzyme targets must be selected with care, and evaluation of activity must include identification of highly specific interactions with the intended target and with other specific but not-targeted enzymes. Chemical structures of major nucleoside constituent molecules are depicted in Figure 2.

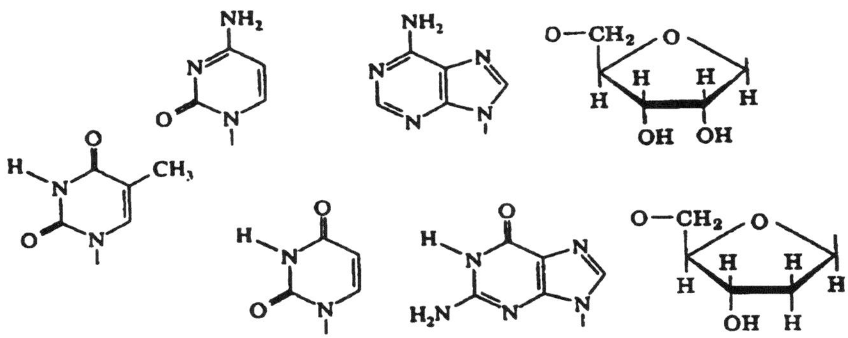

Figure 2. Nucleobase and sugar building blocks of nucleic acids; fron left to right, thymine, cytosine, uracil, adenine, guanine, ribose, and deoxyribose.

In most cases, nucleobases, nucleosides and even monophosphate and diphosphate nucleotides are precursors for the active form, the nucleotide triphosphates. In anabolic metabolism, for example, 5-fluorouracil is a substrate for uracil and/or thymidine phosphorylase followed by the respective kinase, or a pyrimidine phosphoribosyl transferase to be converted to its ribo- or 2'-deoxynucleotide monophosphate, respectively. As the deoxyuridine monophosphate it can function as a strong-binding inhibitor of thymidylate synthase [16]. The ribonucleotide or deoxyribonucleotide can be a substrate, undergoing elaboration by uridylate or thymidylate kinase to the respective triphosphate nucleotide before the appropriate polymerase can insert it as a point mutation into RNA [17] or DNA [18], respectively. Both processes are believed responsible for its antitumor activity. Other nucleosides such as radiolabelled thymidine and iodo(deoxy)uridine are substrates for the respective ribo- or deoxyribo-nucleoside kinases and polymerases, leading to their incorporation into the nucleic acids.

Nucleobases and Nucleosides as Nucleus-imaging Probes

Although nucleosides and nucleobases could be thought of as useful for assessing cellular transport function, most literature studies are aimed at their participation, either as substrates or inhibitors of enzymes in the nucleic acid pathways, including insertion into a nucleic acid. These processes, for both DNA and RNA, are nuclear processes. Their uptake has most often been interpreted, rather simplistically, in terms of nucleic acid turnover and cell cycling (mitotic rate). As a result, the major objective for using these agents is as diagnostic radio-pharmaceuticals for cancer imaging.

There is a large body of literature dealing with the development of nucleobase and nucleoside radiopharmaceuticals. The work began in the early 1950's with the synthesis of 5-halogeno-2'-deoxyuridines that were bioisosteric with thymidine and therefore seen as agents that would have both therapeutic and diagnostic impact on DNA synthesis [1]. The 5-iodo- and 5-bromo- analogues (IUDR and BUDR, respectively) are still in use. In fact, IUDR is currently experiencing its third rediscovery in nuclear medicine, with numerous papers addressing radiolabelling methodology [19,20] and biological evaluation of the radioiodonucleosides [21-23]. Similar histories accompany 5-fluorouracil [24,25] and its nucleosides [26,27], and ^{11}C-thymidine [28](Figure 3).

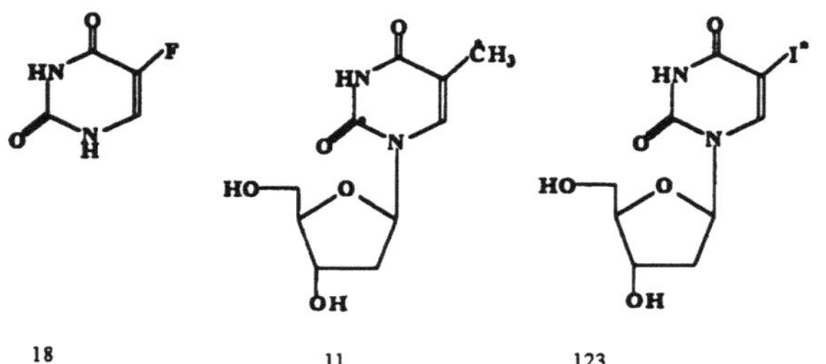

^{18}5- FU 2- or CH_3[^{11}C] thymidine 5-[^{123}I] iodo deoxyuridine

Figure 3. 'Classical' nucleoside radiopharmaceuticals.

There are several difficult problems associated with the use of nucleosides that reflect cell turnover to study pathologies such as cancer. The first is that there are several organ systems that normally have very high mitotic indices, some far outstripping the growth rate of all but the most aggressive tumors. Hematopoietic regeneration and replacement of intestinal epithelial cells, for example, occurs with doubling times measured in days, compared to doubling times of weeks or months for solid tumors. As a result, there may be substantial radiation doses to, and strong image signals from, non-target tissues, rendering interpretation difficult if not impossible. The second problem lies in nature's tight control over nucleoside metabolism. These controls are not limited to 'pool' effects and feed-back inhibition. The aggressive catabolism by indigenous enzymes can severely compromise data quality and interpretation. Phosphorolytic cleavage of the glycosidic bond, followed by ring degradation provides a complex picture from the point of view of basic pharmacokinetics as well as from the perspective of their selective redistribution and reutilization.

Imaging with Nucleotide Polymers (Oligonucleotides)

Recombinant techniques have opened the door to developing specific DNA or RNA fragments that will react with RNA or DNA to form a complex. These fragments, called oligonucleotides, bind specifically with regions of a complimentary nucleic acid strand, thereby inhibiting expression of that nucleic acid code. For example, a DNA-derived oligonucleotide will be selected for its specific binding (duplex formation) to messenger RNA that codes for a specific target protein. In this case, the binding will be in the cytoplasm; it is extranuclear and does not reflect nuclear processes directly. If the oligonucleotide is derived from RNA it will form a DNA triplex (by binding in the major groove), and will therefore reflect nuclear function. Applications of this technology to nuclear medicine imaging have been reviewed by Dewanjee [29,30] and are the subject of a chapter by Don Hnatowich, elsewhere in this volume.

Aptamers represent a special class of oligonucleotides that bind to specific proteins rather than to their complimentary RNA or DNA sequences. They are synthesized using combinatorial chemistry, with selection of active species through competitive binding to the target protein. These unique compounds were introduced by Spiegelman in the early 1970's [31] Radiolabelled aptamers for diagnostic imaging were recently introduced by Dougan [32]. Although these probes could theoretically be either deoxyribo- (DNA) or ribo- (RNA) aptamers targeting proteins in the nucleus, in the cytoplasm or extracellularly, the serum is considered to be the only realistic compartment where they will function. The DNA aptamers are more stable in vivo than the RNA aptamers. In this seminal work Dougan targeted thrombin; it is in the appropriate compartment and it is of considerable interest for both diagnosis and therapy. The thrombin binding aptamer is a 15-mer DNA oligonucleotide. Reports of approaches to radiolabelling, and preliminary data with labelled aptamer, are anticipated [33].

Both antisense oligonucleotides and aptamers present special challenges for use in clinical therapy and diagnosis. In the first instance, and perhaps critically important, there is the question of stability. When injected intravenously, these probes immediately face very rapid degradation by circulating nucleases. In imaging applications, this instability and the difficulties with membrane permeation create a serious challenge to delivering sufficient radioactivity into cells to generate an imaging signal. Although the mechanism of the plasma membrane permeation is not known, there is evidence that some uptake does indeed occur. Passage across the nuclear envelope may pose less of a problem, given that the cell routinely moves RNA from the nucleoplasm into the cytoplasm. Molecular design approaches to help overcome some of these difficulties have been proposed [34].

Finally it must be acknowledged that the possibility of incorporating an imaging radiometal such as technetium-99m at a non-critical region of the oligomer without destroying its specificity or avidity is a major advantage of the oligonucleotide approach. This is much less likely to be possible with nucleoside/nucleobase probes, given the tight specifications for interaction with their molecular targets. In terms of clinical use, the small molecules may by limited to positron-emitter or radioiodine labelling; this is not a scientific disadvantage, but it presents serious limitations to widespread clinical use.

Imaging in gene therapy

The transfer of genes to human cells constitutes an unique opportunity for therapy. The process of gene therapy, quite simply, is to transfer a gene and its associated expression factors to a population of somatic cells. In this way the body can produce the molecular components required for alleviation of the condition, thereby eliminating the necessity for exogenous drug therapy. The approach is particularly attractive for congenital disorders and cancer. The insertion of genetic messages into humans in a clinical trial was undertaken for the first time in 1990. Since that time, the Recombinant DNA Advisory Committee of the US FDA has approved more than twenty gene therapy protocols for clinical trials. Today these and other protocols account for almost 200 clinical trials, world-wide. There appear to be no doubts in the minds of leaders in the field that the process needs substantial improvement, that there are risks, that to date there has not been any unequivocal cure and that the technical questions are sure to be resolved. Although current human studies focus on somatic and not germinal cells, the potential for utilization of the techniques for hereditary alterations (perhaps socially unacceptable purposes) will fuel ethics debates for a much longer time.

BASIC CONCEPTS IN GENE THERAPY

An understanding of gene therapy has its beginnings in the vocabulary. The first terms that cause some confusion and that are frequently used interchangeably and technically incorrectly are the words transduction and transfection. Gene transduction refers to the acquisition and transfer of eukaryotic genes by retroviruses, whereas transfection describes the incorporation of the gene into the eukaryote via non-viral vectors. A cloning vector, used to transport the inserted genetic material for production purposes, is usually a plasmid or bacteriophage, and a transfer vector is a material process (usually a virus) that can transfer the therapeutic gene into the host's DNA. The promoter sequence is a section of DNA that can bind to RNA polymerase and initiate gene transcription, while a long-terminal repeat (LTR) is a promoter sequence found at both ends of a gene that regulate its transcription. Reporter genes are genes inserted together with the therapeutic gene to facilitate evaluation of the efficiency of gene transfer and expression. Expression includes both transcription (synthesis of RNA from DNA) and translation (synthesis of protein according to the RNA code). Other terms include ecotropic and amphotropic (vectors), referring to vectors that function either only in a single species (usually rodent) or in many species (man included), respectively.

Gene therapy begins with selection and isolation of the gene(s) to be inserted into the target cell. The gene donor can be a eukaryote, prokaryote or virus. Once isolated, the gene must be delivered to the target cell. This step represents a special case of drug delivery. The naked gene is a DNA strand; it is highly subject to hydrolysis by circulating nucleases, and because it is charged and very hydrophilic, its entry into the cell is impaired by the plasma membrane.

The most popular and effective delivery vectors to date are viruses that have been engineered to render them replication incompetent. Retroviruses are a natural choice because of their natural ability to insert their DNA directly into host cell DNA. They are limited, however, by the DNA load they can carry (6-7 kb), and their ability to transfect only those cells in active cell division. Adenoviruses can carry larger loads (15-25 kb), are not cell cycle selective, and do not actively insert their DNA into nuclear DNA. They are cytoplasmic and generally considered less dangerous with respect to risk of infection through re-establishment of replication competency. Modifications to the adenovirus vectors include not only removal of as much DNA as possible in order to render them replication incompetent, but to alter their tropism and diminish their immunogenecity.

Non-viral vectors have much larger delivery capacities than the viral carriers. They can be administered repeatedly and have the additional advantage of being non-infectious. Their disadvantages include low efficiency of transfection and non-selectivity for targets. The most common non-viral vectors are cationic liposomes, molecular conjugates, DNA vaccines administered in more traditional formulations or via the 'gene gun', and other types of macromolecular/DNA complexes (e.g. using lipids, charged carbohydrates and even inorganic salts).

Gene insertion can be done in vitro or in vivo. In the former approach, target cells are harvested from the patient (e.g. stem cells from cord blood for a blood cell disease, or hepatocytes for a liver disease) and the gene is inserted under laboratory conditions. After a suitable incubation period to allow for replication of these transformed or transfected cells, they are re-injected into the patient at the appropriate tissue site. In in vivo delivery, the target cells undergo gene insertion by strategic (perhaps stereotactic) implantation/injection of the transducing or transfecting vector. The gene-transferring vector could be naked DNA, a plasmid (a small, autonomously replicating DNA molecule found in bacteria), an altered virus or a producer cell.

Approaches in gene therapy have been classified [35] according to the transferred gene's mechanism of action. Currently, protocols fall into one of 5 categories: 1) replacement of deficient or defective genes in hereditary diseases such as ADA deficiency and cystic fibrosis. Enzyme replacement for genetic disease, 2) cytokine production to potentiate the host's immune defence against cancer, 3) the use of drug resistance genes such as the multidrug resistance gene to protect sensitive tissues (e.g. bone marrow) to enable the use of otherwise toxic doses of a drug, 4) the use of drug sensitivity genes such as viral thymidine kinase to induce selective cell sensitivity to a drug (e.g. to ganciclovir) in a cell that would normally be non-responsive to such therapy and 5) treatment of viral diseases that integrate their DNA into host DNA. In this case the host DNA is abnormal and can be treated as a genetic disease. In the case of HIV infection this therapy would be targeted towards T-cells, with several potential sites for action. Of these, model 4), involving the use of sensitivity genes, will be discussed in greater depth in the final section of this chapter.

A detailed description of the techniques, their applications and their limitations must be left to molecular biologists in the field. Interested readers are referred to a number of excellent short literature reviews, overviews and comments [2,3,36-38] or to references for further reading.

A ROLE FOR GENE THERAPY IMAGING

It is clear that gene therapy begins as a nuclear process, although mitochondrial DNA could equally well be a target. It is also certain that despite the current difficulties in its use, gene therapy is unlikely to go away. The question for nuclear physicians and radiopharmaceutical scientists, then, is whether or not they will have a role in gene therapy, and if yes, on what basis and with which objectives.

There are two obvious questions, at least in present day approaches in gene therapy, that are best answered using radiotracer imaging. One question to be answered relates to expression of the transferred gene. If the transferred gene is not being expressed, then there can be no therapeutic benefit. Determination of gene expression in vitro is a relatively easy matter. One can incorporate a second gene (if the therapeutic gene functions by invoking a different response) that encodes an enzyme function that is easily measured (e.g. luminescence-based assay, tracer uptake, colorimetric indicator), or one can measure the products of expression of the therapeutic gene (e.g. cytokine). These techniques are not applicable in vivo except by tissue biopsy or, if the product of expression is externalized and reaches the vascular space, by blood analysis. The short-comings of biopsy includes its invasive nature, the statistically heterogenous nature of the sample obtained and the inaccessibility of some sites.

A second important rational for imaging is the ability to sample all sites, virtually simultaneously. This is particularly important where expression can cause site-specific toxicity. An example would be gene transfer to a solid tumor using a retrovirus vector; because retroviruses can insert their DNA only if the cell is dividing, the gene transfer 'take' will occur only in the tumour cells that are undergoing active cell division. If the vector were to be inadvertently deposited in marrow or the intestinal epithelium (both of which have high mitotic rates), expression in these tissues could be highly undesirable at best, and even lethal, depending on the therapeutic protocol. There is currently no better way to control for unwanted dissemination than by nuclear imaging.

The major role of nuclear imaging is therefore to monitor the gene therapy protocol. In theory it can alert the therapist of impending increases in risk, it can indicate whether or not a therapeutic response should be expected (is there expression?), it may indicate a point at which the therapeutic gene should be switched off and finally, it may indicate the time when no further improvement is to be expected. In other words, gene therapy imaging can be an integral part of a gene therapy protocol.

GENE THERAPY IMAGING RESEARCH

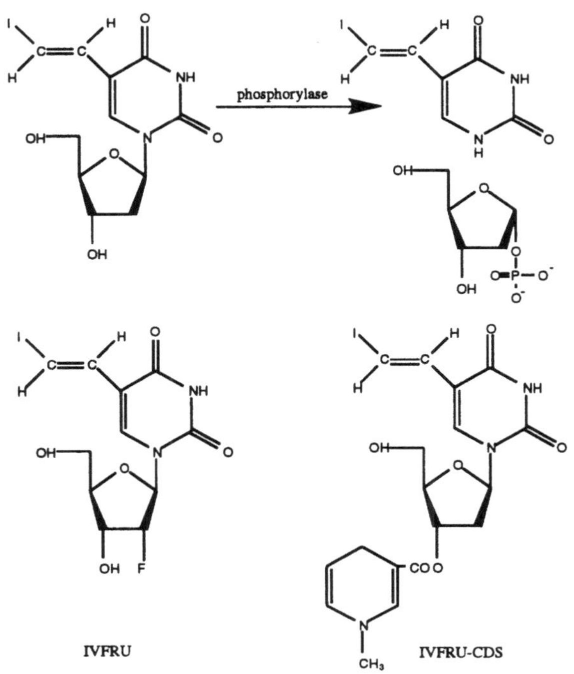

Figure 4. Catabolism of IVDU to its nucleobase and deoxy sugar phosphate (top), (E)-5-(2-Iodovinyl)-1-(2'-deoxy-2'-fluoro)-ribofuranosyl uracil (IVFRU) (bottom left) and its 'chemical delivery system' prodrug (right).

At the present time three gene therapy imaging-oriented projects have been reported. All three projects involve the drug sensitization approach, but have either different gene targets or use different radiopharmaceuticals. The in vitro and in vivo study (including scintigraphic imaging) of the herpes simplex virus type-1 thymidine kinase (HSV-TK+) gene target, using IVFRU (Figure 4) and related nucleosides has been the subject of our research [39-45]. The second approach is also based on the HSV-TK+ target and reports in vitro and in vivo 14C-autoradiography data using FIAC [46]. The third reports in vitro data for cytosine deaminase gene studies using tritiated 5-fluorocytosine [47]. The third approach relates to the exploration of the IVFRU-/-HSV-TK+ research model as described below.

Much of our work has utilized the KBALB-STK cell line kindly made available by Scott Freeman. Development of this HSV-TK+ transduced cell line has been reported [48]. Briefly, wild-type KBALB cells were exposed to Moloney murine leukemia virus producer-cell supernatants containing replication incompetent ecotopic retrovirus. The KBALB-STK cell line was transduced with a vector containing both the HSV-TK+ gene and a neomycin resistance gene, whereas the control cell line (KBALB-LBL) contains only the transferred neomycin-resistance gene [48] (Figure 5).

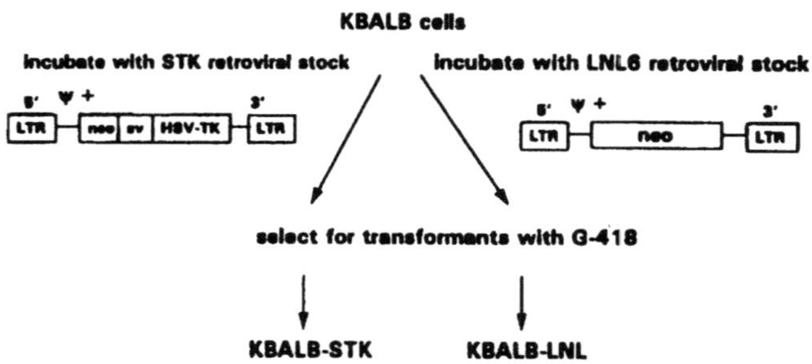

Figure 5. Development of the KBALB-STK and KBALB-LNL sarcoma cell lines. The cell line was developed by Freeman (48). This schematic is presented courtesy of K. Morin.

For our in vitro studies, KBALB-STK cells are grown to confluence, at which time radioiodo-IVFRU (or other labelled nucleosides) is added, The cells are incubated for fixed intervals after which the supernatant is removed and uptake is determined by radiometry. Typical results for test and control cells are shown in Figure 6.

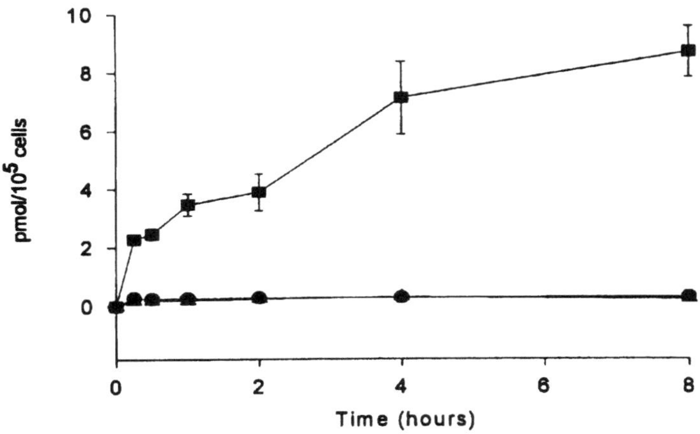

Figure 6. Uptake of radiolabelled IVFRU by KBALB (), KBALB-LNL () and KBALB-STK () cells in vitro.

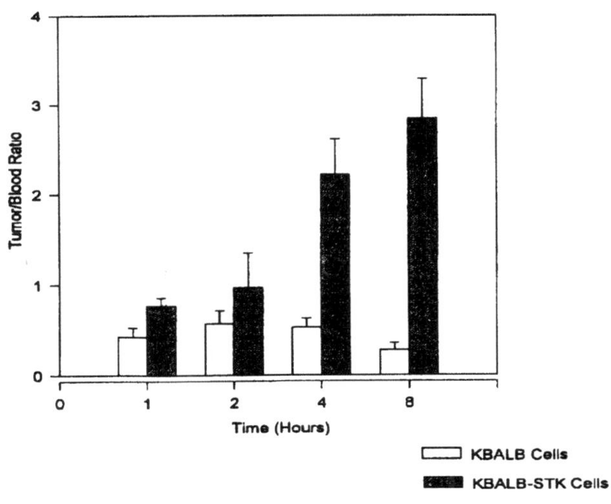

Figure 7. Tumor:blood radioactivity ratios in vivo in mice bearing implanted KBALB or KBALB-STK tumors, after intravenous injection of 131I-IVFRU.

In vivo studies are based on a murine model in which the test or control cell lines are implanted subcutaneously in the flanks of Balb\c mice. Palpable tumors develop rapidly and within about two weeks the tumors weigh about 200 mg, the experimental size used for both quantitative (dissection-based) and imaging biodistribution studies. Typical tumor:blood ratios of radioactivity are presented in Figure 7.

Representative scintigrams are shown in Figure 8. The scintigrams show complete absence of radioactivity in the region occupied by the KBALB-STK tumor following treatment of the host animal with otherwise non-toxic doses of ganciclovir. The HSV-TK+ gene has clearly imparted selective drug sensitivity to ganciclovir, and this sensitivity is reflected by the HSV-TK+-selective radiopharmaceutical (*IVFRU). KBALB-STK tumors treated with ganciclovir in these studies are completely destroyed with no evidence of remission; similarly, there is no uptake once the tumor is dead, even though resorption of the tumor may not be complete for many days after therapy has stopped.

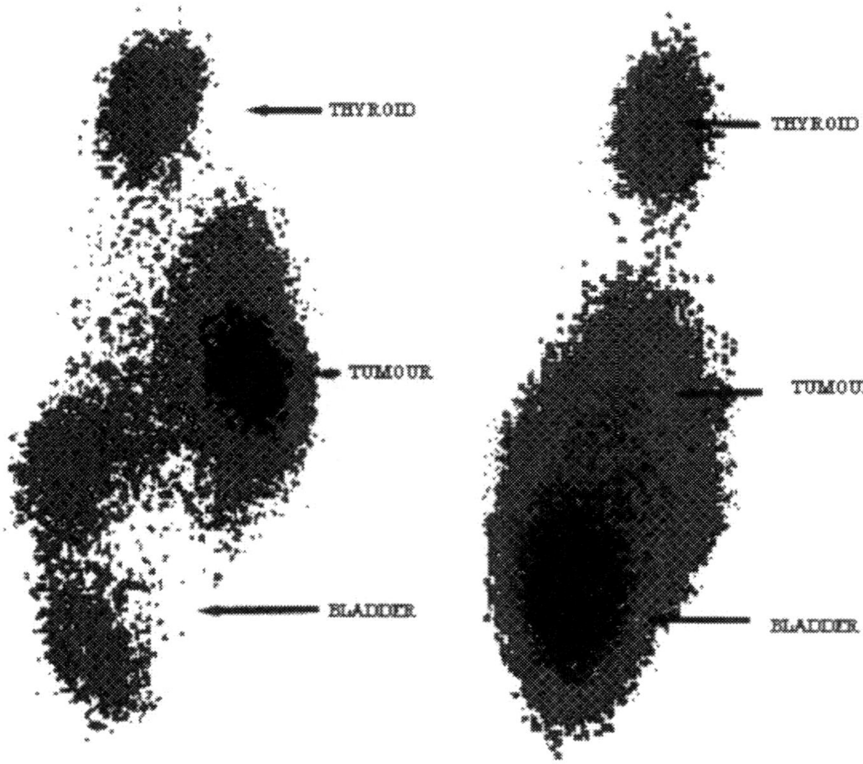

Figure 9. Scintigrams of a Balb\c mouse bearing an implanted KBALB-STK tumor, before (left) and after (right) gancivlovir therapy.

Summary

Approaches to nuclear medicine imaging protocols that will provide information on events occurring in the cell nucleus have been introduced. These approaches have been presented in consideration of the biological barriers present in the cell, with emphasis on the biological membranes separating the nucleoplasm from the extracellular space.

Emphasis has been placed on the applications of gene therapy in the imaging of cell nucleus function. The use of cytoplasmic (antisense probes) and extracellular-oriented (aptamers) oligonucleotide-based imaging agents, has been described and other approaches to visualising nucleus biochemistry have been identified. Steroid receptors (cytoplasmic and nucleoplasmic), cell cytoskeleton and DNA structure have been identified as potential targets that could provide image-based information about the cell nucleus.

The subject material for this topic is huge, evolving rapidly and growing. As a result, the information presented in this chapter, the recommended readings and the cited literature can only whet the appetite of the professionally-interested reader.

Acknowledgements

The information presented here is based on a broad base of support and collaboration. The gene therapy imaging program is the result of an enjoyable and effective collaboration with Professor Edward Knaus and Mr. Kevin Morin. Dr. Scott Freeman contributed cell lines upon which to base our early work, and Drs Jan Balzarini and Erik De Clercq collaborated in critical biochemical studies. Much of this chapter reflects two decades of collaborative research with Prof. Knaus; all members of the 'nucleoside' group, past and present are recognized for their contributions. The financial support of the Medical Research Council of Canada is gratefully acknowledged.

Further reading

Alberts B, Bray D, Lewis J, Raff M, Roberts K, Watson JD. Molecular biology of the cell. New York: Garland Publishing, Inc, 3rd Ed. 1994.

Culver KW. Gene therapy: a handbook for physicians. Mary Ann Liebert, Inc, Publishers 1995

Lewin B. Genes IV. Oxford: Oxford University Press 1990.

Stein WD. Transport and diffusion across cell membranes. Toronto: Academic Press, Inc 1986.

Voet D, Voet JG. Biochemistry, 2nd edition. New York: John Wiley & Sons, Inc 1995.

William DE, editor. Chemistry of antitumor agents. New York: Blackie 1990.

References

1. Prusoff WH. Synthesis and biological activity of iododeoxyuridine, an analogue of thymidine. Biochim Biophys Acta 1959; 32:295-296.
2. Blau HM, Springer ML. Molecular Medicine. Gene therapy - a novel form of drug delivery. The New Engl J Med 1995; 333:1204-1207.
3. Crystal RG. Transfer of genes to humans: early lessons and obstacles to success. Science 1995; 270:404-410.
4. Wiebe LI, Mannan RH, Mercer JR, Haverland GW, Chapman JD. Structure-activity relationships among nitroimidazole nucleosides used as markers of tissue hypoxia. 7th Int Symp Radiopharmacol; 1991 June; Boston.
5. Betageri GV, Rogers JA. The liposome as a distribution model in QSAR studies. Int J Pharmaceut 1988; 46: 95-102.
6. Marshall E. Drug trial death deemed unavoidable. Science 1994; 264:1530.
7. Rowinsky ER, Wright M, Monsarrat B, Lesser, JG. Taxol; Pharmacology, metabolism and clinical implications. Cancer Surveys 1993, 17: 283-304.
8. Dehdashti F, Mortimer JE, Siegel BA, et al. Positron tomographic assessment of estrogen receptors in breast cancer: comparison with FDG-PET and in vitro receptor assays. J Nucl Med 1995; 36:1766-1774.
9. Cass CE. Nucleoside transport. In: Georgopapadakou NH, editor. Drug transport in antimicrobial and anticancer chemotherapy. New York: Marcel Dekker, 1994: 403-451.
10. Xu L, Gati WP, Knaus EE and Wiebe LI. Structure-activity relationships (SAR) in pyrimidine nucleoside transport. In: Maddalena DJ, Snowdon GM Boniface GR, editors. Advances in radiopharmacology. Wollongong: University of Wollongong Printery Services, 1990: 283-298.
11. Vishwanadhan VN, Ghose AK, Weinstein JN. Mapping the binding site of the nucleoside transporter protein: a 3D-QSAR study. Biochim Biophys Acta 1990; 1039:356-366.
12. Wiebe LI, Knaus EE, Gati WP, Iwashina T, McQueen L. Drug-induced perturbations in the in vivo distribution of oncological radiotracers. 1.5-Fluoro-6-3H-2'-deoxyuridine influenced by Nitrobenzylthioinosine-5'-phosphate (NBMPR-P). Int J Nucl Biol Med 1986; 13:257-259.
13. Wiebe LI, Knaus EE. Drug-induced perturbations in the in vivo distribution of oncological radiotracers. 2. 5-[125I]Iodo-2'-deoxyuridine influenced by nitrobenzylthioinosine-5'-phosphate (NBMPR-P). Int J Appl Radiat Isotopes 1990; 41:159-162.
14. Gati WP, Wiebe LI, Knaus EE, Paterson ARP. [125I]Iodohydroxy-nitrobenzylthioinosine: a new high affinity nucleoside transporter probe. Biochem Cell Biol 1987; 65: 467-473.
15. Henderson JF, Paterson ARP. Nucleoside metabolism. New York: Academic Press, Inc 1973.
16. Dananberg PV, Lochshin A. Fluoropyrimidines as tight-binding inhibitors of thymidylate synthetase. Pharmacol Therap 1981; 13:69-90.
17. Kufe D, Major P. 5-Fluorouracil incorporation into human breast carcinoma RNA correlates with cytotoxicity. J Biol Chem 1981; 256: 9802-9805.
18. Major P, Egan E, Herrick D, Kufe DW. 5-Fluorouracil incorporation into DNA of human breast carcinoma cell lines. Cancer Roes 1982; 42: 3005-3009.
19. Silvester DJ, White ND. Preparation of very high specific activity iododeoxyuridine, iodouridine and iodouracil labelled with iodine-125, -131 or -132. Nature 1963; 200:65-66.
20. Keough WG and Hofer KG. An improved method for synthesis and purification of 124I or 131I labelled carrier free 5-iodo-2'-deoxyuridine. J Label Comp Radiopharm 1978; 14:83-90.
21. Hampton EG, Eidinoff ML. Administration of 5-iododeoxyuridine-131I in the mouse and rat. Cancer Res 1961; 21:345-352.
22. Robins AB, Taylor DM. Iodine-123-iododeoxyuridine: a potential Indicator of Tumour response to treatment. Int J Nucl Med Biol 1981; 8: 53-63.
23. Van den Abbeele AD, Tutrone RF, Berman RM et al. Tumor-targetting potential of radioiodinated iododeoxyuridine in bladder cancer. J Nucl Med 1996; 37:315-320.
24. Heidelberger C, Chaudhuri NK, Danenberg P et al. Fluorinated pyrimidines, a new class of tumor inhibitory compounds. Nature 1957; 179:663-666.
25. Fowler JS, Finn RD, Lambrecht RM, Wolf AP. The synthesis of 18F-5-fluorouracil. J Nucl Med 1973; 14: 63-64.

26. Abrams, DN, Knaus EE, Lentle BC, Wiebe LI. Tumor uptake of radiolabelled pyrimidine bases and pyrimidine nucleosides in animal models. II. 6-3H-5-fluoro-2'-deoxyuridine. Int J Nucl Med Biol 1979; 6: 103-107.
27. Dimitrakopoulou A, Strauss LG, Clorius JH et al. Studies with positron emission tomography after systemic administration of fluorine-18-uracil in patients with liver metastases from colorectal carcinoma. J Nucl Med 1993; 34: 1075-1081.
28. Shields AF, Mankoff D, Graham MM et al. Analysis of 2-carbon-11-thymidine blood metabolites in PET imaging. J Nucl Med 1996; 37:290-296.
29. Dewanjee M. Detecting cancer in the body. Chemtech 1994; 24: 21-24.
30. Dewanjee M. Radiolabelled antisense probes: diagnosis and therapy. Diagn Oncol 1993; 3: 189-208.
31. Kramer FR, Mills DR, Cole PE, Nishihara T, Spiegelman S. Evilution in vitro: sequence and phenotype of a mutant RNA resistant to ethidium bromide.. J Mol Biol 1974; 89: 719736.
32. Dougan H, Hobbs JB, Lyster DM, Weitz JI. Radiohalogenated DNA aptamers. J Label Comp Radiopharm. 1995; XXVII: 324-325.
33. Dougan H. personal communication.
34. Cohen JS, editor. Oligonucleotides; antisense inhibitors of gene expression. London: McMillan 1989.
35. Whartenby KA, Marrogi AJ, Freeman SM. Gene therapy. Clinical potential and relationships to drug treatment. Drugs 1995; 50: 951-958.
36. Anderson WF. Gene therapy. Sci Amer 1995; September:124-128.
37. Miller AD. Human gene therapy comes of age. Nature 1992; 357: 455-460.
38. Thayer AM. Large pharmaceutical firms place long-term bets on gene therapy. C & E News 1995; December: 15-20.
39. Wiebe LI. Radiopharmaceuticals-perspectives and future prospects. A state-of-the-art review lecture. 6th World Conf Nucl Med. November 1994; Sydney, Australia.
40. Morin KW, Wiebe LI, Knaus EE, Balzarini J, De Clercq E. Metabolic Imaging of gene therapy. Europ J Nucl Med 1994; 21: 489 (abstr).
41. Morin KW, Wiebe LI, Knaus EE. Transfection imaging. A novel approach to detect gene expression in gene therapy of cancer. Alberta Cancer Board Ann Gen Mtg. November 1994; Calgary, Canada.
42. Wiebe LI, Knaus EE, Morin KW. HSV-Thymidine Kinase: a molecular target for transfection imaging in gene therapy of cancer. Antiviral Res 1995; 26: A307.
43. Wiebe LI. Radiopharmaceuticals to monitor transfection in gene therapy. 6th Eur Symp Radiopharmacy and Radiopharmaceuticals March 1995; Graz, Austria.
44. Balzarini J, Andrei G, Kumar R, Knaus EE, Wiebe LI, De Clercq E. The cytostatic activity of 5-(1-azidovinyl-2'-deoxyuridine (AzVDU) against Herpes simplex virus thymidine kinase gene-transfected FM3A Cells is due to inhibition of thymidylate synthase and enhanced UV light (λ: 254 nm) exposure. FEBS Letters 1995; 373· 41-44.
45. Balzarini J. Morin KW, Knaus EE,. Wiebe LI, De Clercq E. Novel (E)-5-(2-Iodovinyl)-2'-deoxyuridine derivatives as potential cytostatic agents against Herpes simplex virus-thymidine kinase Gene-transfected tumors. Gene Therapy 1995; 2: 317-322.
46. Tjuvajev JG, Stockhammer G, Desai R, et al. Imaging gene expression of transfected genes in vivo. Cancer Res 1995; 55:6126-6132.
47. Haberkorn U, Oberdorfer F, Gerbert J, et al. Monitoring gene therapy with cytosine deaminase: in vitro studies using tritiated 5-fluorocytosine. J Nucl Med 1996; 37: 87-94.
48. Freeman SM. Personal communication. Also see Freeman, SM, Abboud CN, Whartenby KA et al. The by-stander effect: tumor regression when a fraction of the tumor mass is genetically modified. Cancer Res. 1993; 53: 5274-5283, and Moolten, FL Tumor chemosensitivity conferred by inserted herpes thymidine kinase genes: papadigm for a prospective cancer control strategy. Cancer Res. 1986; 46: 5276-5281.

STEROID HORMONE RECEPTORS AS TARGETS FOR DIAGNOSTIC IMAGING

Michael J. Welch, Joanna B. Downer and John A. Katzenellenbogen

Introduction

A century ago the connection between body function and cancer was first reported. In 1896, Beatson released his study of several premenopausal women who had remarkable regression of advanced breast cancers following ovariectomy, and voiced the proposal that there must be some substance in these organs contributing to the growth of the cancers. [1] The search for the factors affecting tumor death and growth had begun. Subsequent scientific advances in the areas of chemical synthesis, biology and physiology, and assay techniques brought substantial progress in the fight to understand and conquer cancer.

During the 1930's a vast amount of knowledge was gained as nonsteroidal estrogens were first prepared. The high biological activity of diethylstilbestrol, a synthetic nonsteroidal estrogen, was first reported in 1938. [2,3] These compounds mimic the behavior of estrogen in the body and were the first steps in directed design of therapeutic agents. The structure of estradiol, a metabolite of naturally occuring estrone, had been elucidated and scientists moved closer to identifying other steroids such as testosterone, progesterone, and glucocorticoids. By far the fastest results were obtained in the study of estrogens and antiestrogens and their receptors. [4]

The advances in synthetic organic chemistry and biochemical methods of protein extraction and purification during the 1940's enabled production of large quantities of both authentic and labeled (^{14}C and ^{3}H) steroids. In turn, these developments led to the ability to study in greater detail the function and effects of steroid hormones and their analogs on receptors and cancer. The year 1959 brought the first physical evidence of a mechanism to concentrate estrogen in a target organ, as tritiated estradiol was selectively taken up and retained by target tissues. [5] In the mid 1960's estrogen receptors were first purified from rat uteri [6,7,8] and some of the physical properties of estrogen receptors were identified. [9]

S. J. Mather (ed.), Current Directions in Radiopharmaceutical Research and Development, 137–156.

Also in the 1960's a potential new therapy for one of the most common cancers was first developed. Tamoxifen, a nonsteroidal antiestrogen shown to be extremely effective in breast cancer therapy, was first synthesized and evaluated in 1966 by Harper and Walpole. [10] In the early 1980's a now famous antiprogestin, RU 486, was first discovered to have high affinity for the progesterone receptor (PgR). [11,12] Since that time, RU 486 has been studied as a once-a-month contraceptive for women [11,13], and has also been used to increase knowledge about the progesterone receptor [12,14].

In the early 1970's a number of reports demonstrated that low levels of estrogen receptors in breast tumors are indicative of a poor response to tamoxifen or other endocrine therapy. [15-19] In addition, studies showed that approximately 60-70% of breast cancer tumors are estrogen receptor positive by analysis of biopsied tissue. [20] Endocrine therapy of breast cancers has been shown to be quite effective in approximately half of estrogen receptor positive patients. The response to endocrine therapy can be more accurately predicted after quantification of both estrogen (ER) and progesterone receptor (PgR) status. ER and PgR rich tumors are the most likely to respond well to endocrine therapy, while ER and PgR receptor poor tumors rarely respond to such therapy. Regardless of response to endocrine therapy, patients with ER and PgR rich tumors have better overall prognoses [21].

Cancers of other systems, such as prostate cancer in males, are not as predictable as breast cancer with respect to receptor content. [22-24] A number of investigators have reported response relative to androgen receptor (AR) content, but in most cases the predictability has not been as good as that seen with ER and PgR in breast cancer. [22-32] Most prostate cancers are in fact AR and PgR positive, but over time the tumors frequently become hormone independent [33] despite initial positive responses to hormonal manipulation. Because of this scenario, imaging of AR in prostate cancer may not only assist treatment selection but may also provide additional means of clarifying the physiology and development of the disease.

Estrogen receptor ligands are useful for imaging prior to hormonal therapy or to monitor effectiveness during therapy since therapeutic agents such as tamoxifen will occupy ER sites resulting in decreased uptake of the radioligand. In order to evaluate tumor response to therapy based on changing tumor size or receptor content, a radiolabeled progestin analog would permit imaging of PgR rich tumors while antiestrogen therapy continues. Thus size of the tumor and number and density of PgR could be compared throughout the course of treatment. Radiolabeled AR ligands would permit similar imaging of cancers that tend to be AR positive, such as prostate cancer. During courses of therapy involving flutamide, a potent antiandrogen, again a progesterone receptor ligand would be preferred for imaging. The endogenous steroids with the highest affinity for their respective ligands are shown in Figure 1.

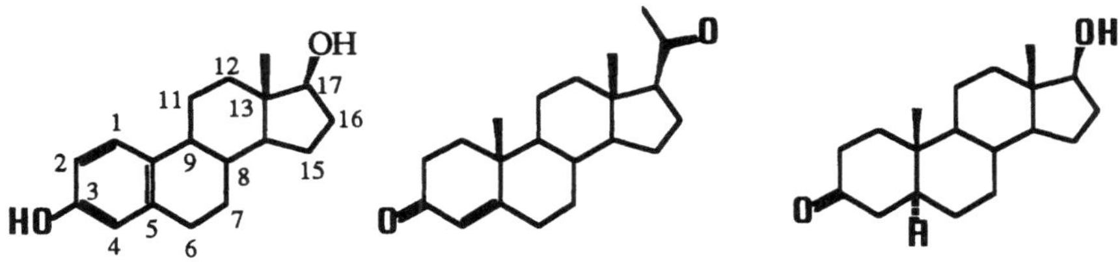

Estradiol-17β Estrogen Receptor | Progesterone Progesterone Receptor | 5α-Dihydrotestosterone Androgen Receptor

Figure 1. Endogenous High Affinity Steroids

The high prevalence of hormone dependent cancers and even higher rate of steroid receptor positive cancers demonstrates that labeled steroid hormones should be remarkably useful for imaging. The fact that it is possible to predict responsiveness to hormonal therapy is a tremendous asset. Quantitation of receptor number and density within a tumor before biopsy can accelerate adminstration of the most beneficial treatment to any given patient. In addition to these benefits, diagnostic imaging using radiolabeled receptor-targeted ligands permits localization of both primary and metastatic tumors and *in vivo* staging of carcinomas. As a result of these advantages, there are a number of ongoing studies to develop and evaluate more effective imaging agents.

Characteristics of Imaging Nuclides

Carbon-11. Even though carbon-11 has a very short half-life (20 minutes), it has been a very useful agent for radiolabeling targets for positron emission tomography (PET). A number of easily made one-carbon starting materials can produce a multitude of labeled products upon reaction with appropriate targets. Strategic placement of the carbon label in the proposed final pharmaceutical can enable rapid synthesis. The short half-life of C-11 does not allow involved chemistry following incorporation of the activity, but development of well designed substrates permits manufacture of complicated molecules with a carbon-11 label. Specific activity and radiochemical purity of carbon-11 compounds depend upon the ^{11}C-synthon produced following the nuclear reaction, but in general are high.

Fluorine-18. Fluorine-18 is a positron emitting isotope used extensively in production of diagnostic imaging agents for use in PET. The half-life of 109.7 minutes makes F-18 convenient not only for chemical manipulations but also allows time for biological distribution of agents while retaining sufficient activity for imaging. Because its atomic size is close to that of hydrogen, fluorine can frequently be substituted for hydrogen in many molecular structures with either no change in activity or in some cases even an increase in the desired biological activity.

Bromine Radioisotopes. Bromine isotopes are frequently used in radiolabeling also. Bromine-75 and bromine-76 are positron emitters while bromine-77 is a gamma emitter and is used in single photon emission computed tomography (SPECT). Bromine-75 has a half-life close to that of F-18 (96.7min vs 109.7min). The half-lives of Br-76 and Br-77 are much longer (16.2hr and 57.0hr) which can complicate patient handling but may be advantageous for therapeutic applications.

Iodine Radioisotopes. Iodine has also been used as a labeling agent for steroid hormones. Many syntheses involve I-125 for use with a gamma counter, but I-123, which is acceptable for SPECT imaging, could be substituted. I-123 has a half-life of 13.2 hours. Due to its very large size, iodine substitution usually has a pronounced effect on the molecule.

Technetium-99m. Despite the advantages of using halogens to radiolabel steroids, interest in using metals has increased over recent years. Halogens can be incorporated with a relatively small overall modification of addition or substitution of a single atom and the strength inherent in a covalent attachment. However, the limited access to PET scanners and cyclotrons, as well as the price and availability difficulties of nuclides of bromine and iodine, has led to the investigation of the use of metal radionuclides as labeling agents for steroid hormones. The ready availability of technetium-99m has made this nuclide particularly attractive. In general, Tc-99m is incorporated onto a biologically active molecule through a chelate. New methods under investigation involve integration of the metal into the steroid ring structure or formation of an organometallic complex.

Estrogens Labeled With Halogens

A large number of compounds based on the structures of both estradiol and hexestrol have been labeled with fluorine-18. A summary of some of the estrogen compounds is shown in Table 1. Several features can be noted from the data presented in this Table. First, the relative binding affinity to the estrogen receptor (RBA), given relative to estradiol as 100, varies by almost 2 orders of magnitude. In addition, the nonspecific binding (measured as the octanol/water partition coefficients relative to estradiol as unity) varies by almost an order of magnitude. In spite of these large differences, the absolute uptake in target tissue in an animal model (expressed as % injected dose/gram in mature rat uterus) varies by only a factor of 3, with the target to blood ratio having slightly greater variation. The compound studied most extensively, 16a-fluoro-estradiol-17b (FES), has a relatively low target uptake (6.6%) with an intermediate uterus to blood ratio of 50. Despite its initial appearance as a mediocre agent in rats, human studies have demonstrated that it is the best of the agents synthesized to date. A possible explanation for this involves binding of the steroid to a plasma protein, sex hormone binding globulin (SHBG), which is found in humans but not in rats. (See later section for discussion.)

Table 1. Selected Fluorine-18 Substituted Estrogens

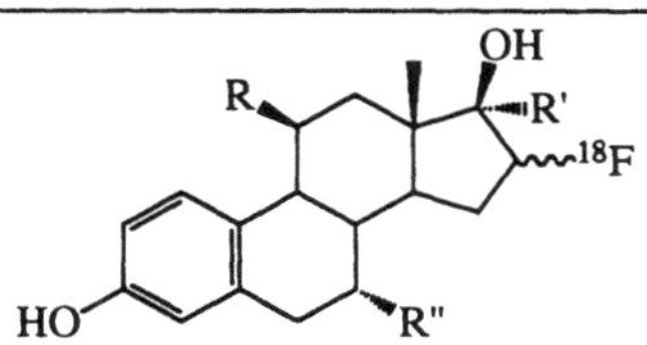

16	11β-R	17α-R'	7α-R''	RBA (ER,25°)	NSB	SHBG[a] binding	%ID/g (Ut,1hr)	Ut/Bl (1hr)
αF	–	–	–	(52)	0.70	9.5	6.6	50
	OMe	–	–	26	0.22	0.502	5.8	49
	Et	–	–	1630	1.62	2.24	12.6	17
	–	C≡CH	–	108	0.82	0.43	11.2	154
	OMe	C≡CH	–	145	0.38	0.098	12.9	145
	Et	C≡CH	–	372	1.54	2.44	9.9	169
	–	–	CH_3	(126)	1.19	0.89	5.7	8.7
	–	C≡CH	CH_3	(146)	0.81	0.168	6.1	101
βF	–	–	–	12	0.63	8.9	5.0	5.6
	OMe	–	–	13	0.39	0.088	6.1	42
	Et	–	–	253	1.60	0.550	5.6	52
	–	C≡CH	–	28	1.04	0.616	7.5	17
	OMe	C≡CH	–	78	0.67	0.035	18.3	75
	Et	C≡CH	–	461	2.43	11.03	8.2	34
	–	–	CH_3	(35)	0.97	0.58	4.4	11
	–	C≡CH	CH_3	(119)	2.26	0.46	3.3	39

[a]Obtained using third trimester pregnancy serum:Data from Reference 34

Table 2. Estrogens Labeled with Bromine and Iodine

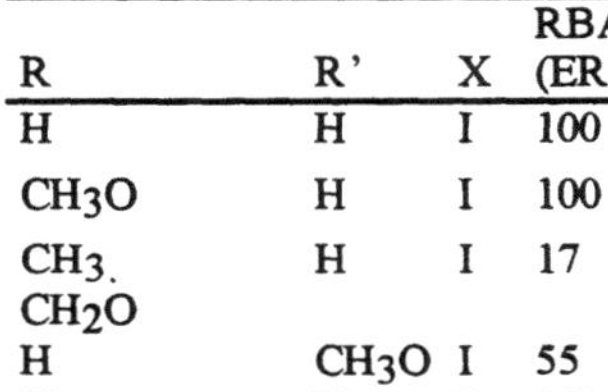

R	R'	X	RBA (ER,0°)	%ID/g (Ut 1hr)	Ut/NT[a]	Ref
H	H	I	100	0.31[b]	9.4[b]	35
CH_3O	H	I	100	40[c]	24[c]	36
CH_3. CH_2O	H	I	17	5.3	13	37
H	CH_3O	I	55	12	10	37
H	H	Br	140	8.4	16	38
CH_3O	H	Br	20	12	26	38

[a]Non-target (NT) for all I labeled estrogens is muscle; for Br labeled compounds NT is the average of lung, muscle, spleen and esophagus.
[b]by sub-cutaneous injection in 200-250 g rats
[c]by intraperitoneal injection

Table 2. Estrogens Labeled with Bromine and Iodine (continued)

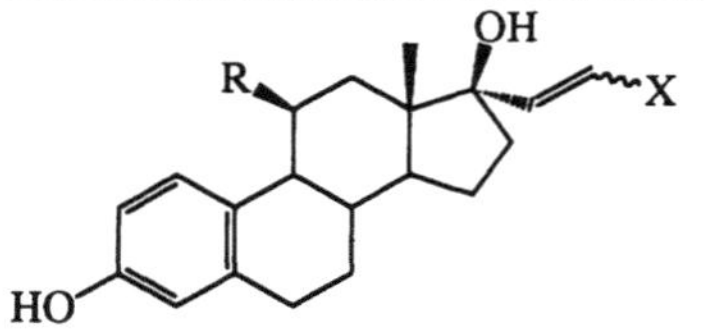

R	X	RBA (ER,0°)	%ID/g (UT,1hr)	Ut/Mus c (1hr)	Ref
H	(Z)I	47	4.0	9.5	39
H	(E)I	33	1.6	3.1	39
		NR	8.0	9.9	40
βCH3O	(E)I	NR	15	13	40
		50-150	8.9	7.9-21	41
αCH3O	(E)I	NR	5	4.9	42
H	(E)Br	NR	6.4-7	11, 35[a]	43
βCH3O	(E)Br	NR	20[a]	40[a]	44

[a]At 2 hr after intraperitoneal injection

In addition to the use of fluorine-18, the use of heavy halogens has also been studied. Many investigators have synthesized steroidal and nonsteroidal estrogens labeled with bromine and iodine radionuclides. A review of these compounds has recently been published. [34] Some of the more promising of these agents are shown in Table 2. The size of the halogen used has a pronounced effect on the binding affinity of the ligands. Comparisons of halogens and their effects on the affinity of estradiol and hexestrol for the ER are compiled in Table 3.

Table 3. Substitutions of Estrogens Which Retain Binding Selectivity Index.

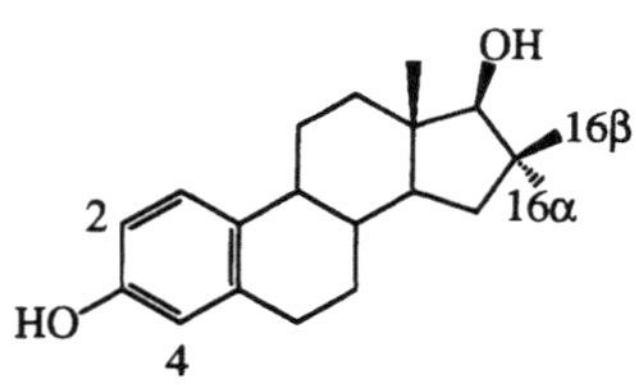

Estradiol (BSI=100):

Location	I	Br	Cl	F
2	<0.03	0.44	–	81
4	<0.03	3.7	–	103
16α	59	91	79	110
16β	–	3.1	–	57

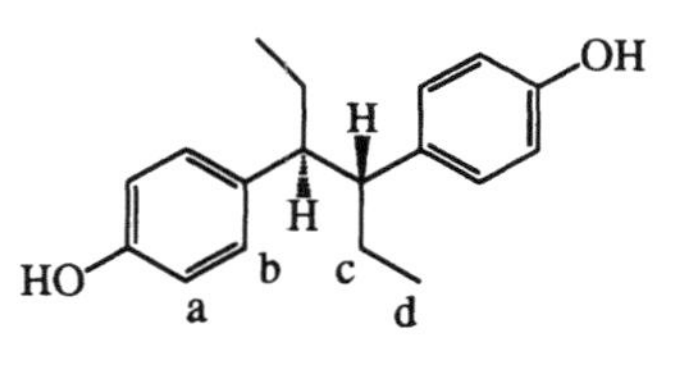

Hexestrol (BSI=104):

Location	I	Br	Cl	F
a	1.4	2.6	–	73
b	3	–	–	55
c	76	110	163	80
d	12	21	–	89

For each compound, the number listed represents the Binding Selectivity Index, or BSI, which is the ratio of relative binding affinity to non-specific binding. [45,46,47]

Labeling of Estrogens With Carbon-11

Carbon-11 labeled estrogens have great potential for use in sequential PET studies. Two estrogens have been labeled with carbon-11 and the tissue uptake described [48,49], however, the biodistribution of these compounds appears to be inferior to that of the halogen nuclides discussed previously. Investigations are continuing.

Progestins Labeled With Radiohalogens

Several progestins have been labeled with fluorine, bromine and iodine. A summary of these compounds is given in Table 4. As can be seen from this table, many of these compounds have very high binding to the progestin receptor. The fluorinated compounds show high target uptake in the uterus of immature rats primed with estradiol and also demonstrate significant selectivity. The compounds labeled using iodine and bromine have not yet been evaluated *in vivo* despite possessing acceptable RBAs.

Table 4. Affinity and Distribution of Progestins Labeled with Radiohalogens

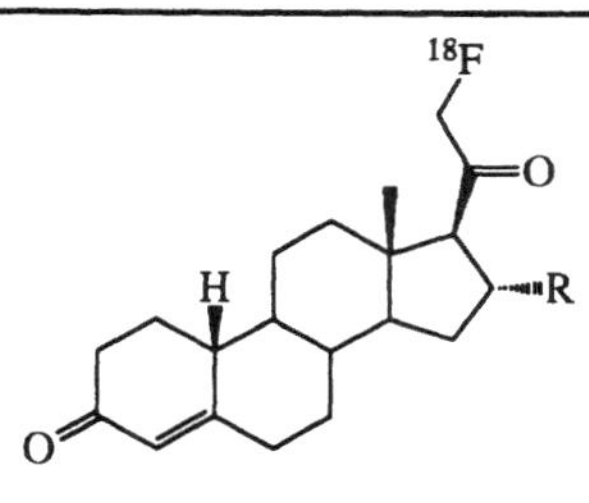

R=	CH_3	CH_2CH_3
RBA (0°)	-	700
%ID/g (Ut,1hr)	1.4	4.6
Ut/musc (1hr)	7	41

References 50, 51

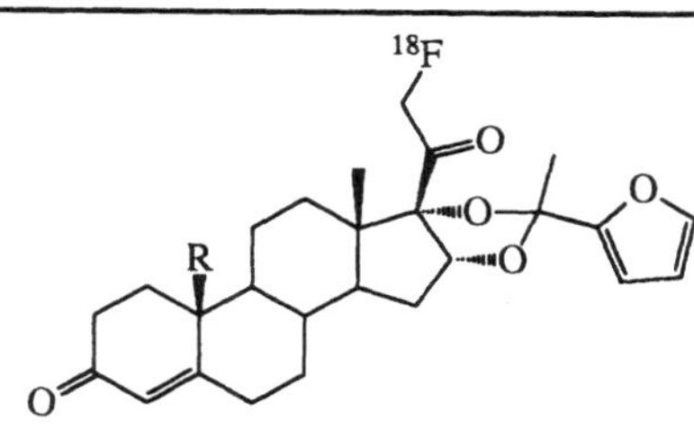

R=	H	CH_3
RBA (0°)	190	173
%ID/g (Ut,1hr)	6.5	6.8
Ut/musc (1hr)	12	12

Reference 53

Table 4. Radiohalogenated Progestins, continued

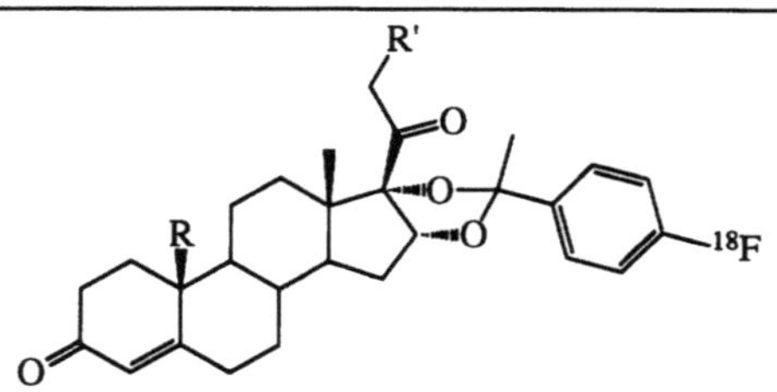

R, R'=	CH_3, H	H, OH
RBA (0°)	53	240
%ID/g (Ut,1hr)	3.1	3.7
Ut/musc (1hr)	3.9	8.2

Reference 52

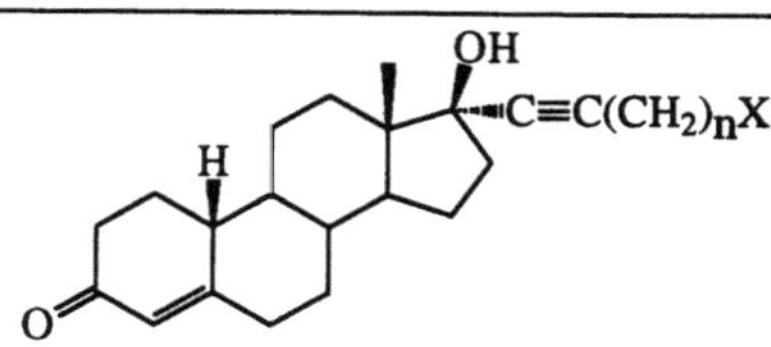

	RBA for X=	
n	Br	I
RBA (0°)	53	240
%ID/g (Ut,1hr)	3.1	3.7
Ut/musc (1hr)	3.9	8.2

Reference 54

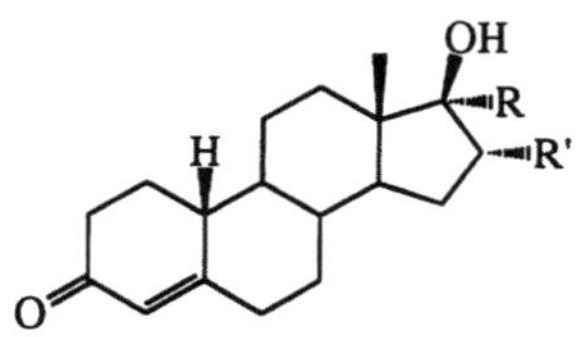

R	R'	RBA (PgR)
H	I	2.6
$CHI{=}CH_2$	H	2.0
(E)$CH_2{=}CH_2I$	H	25
(Z)$CH_2{=}CH_2I$	H	58

References 55, 56
Relative to R5020=100%

Androgens Labeled With Halogens

The work involving androgens for radiolabeling has been less forthcoming compared to the work with estrogens. The proposed difficulty in producing a labeled androgen receptor ligand is that the AR has a more specific binding region which discriminates to a much greater extent than the ER. For this reason, ligand structural requirements are much more stringent and substitutions which do not greatly affect an estrogen's ability to bind to the ER remove affinity of the corresponding androgen for its receptor. For example, a 16α-iodo substituent has been attached to estradiol without adverse effects on affinity or stability [35,58], while the analogous dihydrotestosterone derivative lacks any affinity for the AR [59].

Recent developments in preparing fluorine-18 and carbon-11 labeled derivatives are promising since the products should retain many of the characteristics of the parent compounds. A number of fluorine-labeled androgens have recently been synthesized and evaluated both *in vitro* and *in vivo*. [60-63] One of these labeled androgens, 16β-[^{18}F]fluoro-5α-dihydrotestosterone [61,62], is currently in preliminary clinical trials for evaluation of its ability as an imaging agent for prostate carcinoma in humans. Again, the behavior of the ligands in rats and primates has varied considerably from what was expected, presumably due to the action of SHBG.

Although a great many iodinated androgens have been synthesized, only a fraction have been measured for binding affinity, and even fewer found to be worthy of evaluation *in vivo*. A summary of halogenated androgens is found in Tables 5 and 6. Those that have been evaluated *in vivo* were found to either lack sufficient target specificity or to be unstable.

Table 5. Halogenated Testosterone, Nortestosterone, and Mibolerone Derivatives.

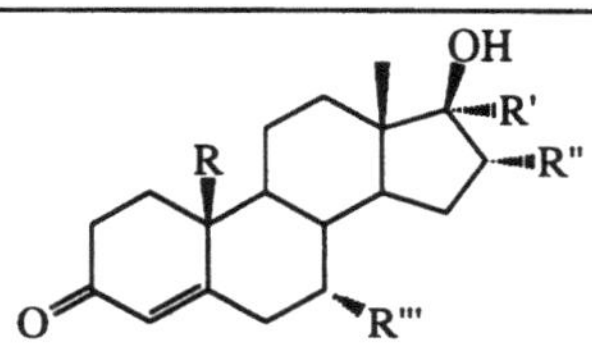

R	R'	R''	R'''	RBA (AR,0°)	RBA (PgR,0°)	%ID/g (vP,1hr)	vP/NT (4hr)	Ref.
CH_3	(Z)CH=CHI	H	H	7.2	4.2			[64]
CH_3	(E)CH=CHI	H	H	18.6	0.7			[64]
CH_3	(Z)CH=CHI	H	CH_3	12.7	2.6			[64]
CH_3	(E)CH=CHI	H	CH_3	14.3	0.7			[64]
H	(Z)CH=CHI	H	H	25.0	92.7	0.35	0.88[a]	[64]
H	(E)CH=CHI	H	H	26.4	9.1	0.16	1.84[a]	[64]
H	(Z)CH=CHI	H	CH_3	32.9	64.5	0.40	1.25[a]	[64]
H	(E)CH=CHI	H	CH_3	15.9	3.3	0.24	1.57[a]	[64]
H	(E)CH=CHI	H	CH_3	2.9 (rat) 73 (human)	20			[65]
CH_3	H	β-^{18}F	H	2.1	–	0.566	21.12[b]	[60,61]
H	CH_3	β-^{18}F	CH_3	30.8	3.0	36.5	21.9[b]	[60,61]
H	H	β-^{18}F	CH_3	36.5	1.6	0.572	14.70[b]	[60,61]
H	H	α-^{18}F	CH_3	21.9	5.7	0.527	35.00[b]	[60,61]
$\Delta^{8,10}$	$CH_2{}^{18}F$	H	H	18.8	10.5	1.128	5.95[b]	[61]
H	$CH_2{}^{18}F$	H	CH_3	53.2	43.7	0.969	13.25[b]	[62]

[a]NT=non-target, includes muscle, spleen, lung
[b]NT=muscle
All AR RBAs are relative to R1881; all PgR RBAs are relative to R5020. $\Delta^{8,10}$ indicates the presence of a double bond between C8 and C9, and between C10 and C11 in the B,C ring systems.

Table 6. Halogenated Dihydrotestosterone Derivatives

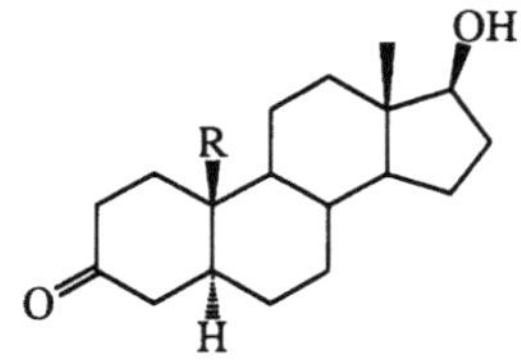

R	Label	RBA (AR,0°)	RBA (PgR,0°)	%ID/g (vP,1hr)	vP/musc (4hr)	Ref.
CH_3	7α-I	74.0 (rat)[a]	1.12 (rat)[a]			[66]
		74.4 (human)[a]	0.239 (human)[a]			
CH_3	17α-CH=CHI	7.0 (human)	0.1 (human)			[65]
		2.9 (rat)				
CH_3	16β-^{18}F	42.7	0.12	0.432	24.87	[60,61]
CH_3	11β-^{18}F	53.1	0.22	0.486	19.715	[63]
H	11β-^{18}F	75.3	0.72	0.284	2.919	[63]

[a]Measured at 4°C

A recently synthesized iodo compound, 7α–iodo-5α-dihydrotestosterone (7α-IDHT), has been shown to have high affinity for the androgen receptor, but has not yet been evaluated *in vivo*. [66] This compound has an exceptionally high relative binding affinity (RBA) of 74 relative to R1881 for the AR, which will hopefully indicate its promise as an *in vivo* radiotracer for imaging of the AR.

Carbon-11 Labeling of Androgens

Two reports of C-11 androgens have been published. The first reported synthesis of C-11 labeled 17α-methyltestosterone produced low specific activity steroid (1-5Ci/mmole). [48] An improvement in the synthesis by using a different starting material and reaction conditions greatly improved the specific activity (1-2Ci/mmole). [67] It does not appear however that the product was evaluated either *in vitro* or *in vivo*.

Metal Radionuclides as Steroid Labels

DiZio and coworkers [68] explored the tolerance of the progesterone receptor to ligands containing a bulky bisamino-bisthiol (BAT, N_2S_2) complex at various positions on the molecule. They found that several positions could tolerate sizeable substituents. (Figure 2.) Out of four systems studied, only the 11β-substituted conjugate showed reasonable affinity for the receptor. These compounds, analogs of the antiprogestin RU 486,have been labeled with technetium-99, technetium-99m and rhenium-186 [69]. The products contain stereoisomers and of these a syn pair and two individual diastereomers have been isolated. In competitive binding studies, the syn pair had an affinity for the progestin receptor that was 161% that of progesterone while the individual anti diastereomers had affinities of 300% and 45% that of progesterone (Table 7). The technetium-99m compounds have been studied in a rat model and show specific receptor mediated uptake in the rat uterus. However, there is also high uptake in nontarget tissue due to the high lipophilicity of these metal complexes which would prevent acceptable imaging.

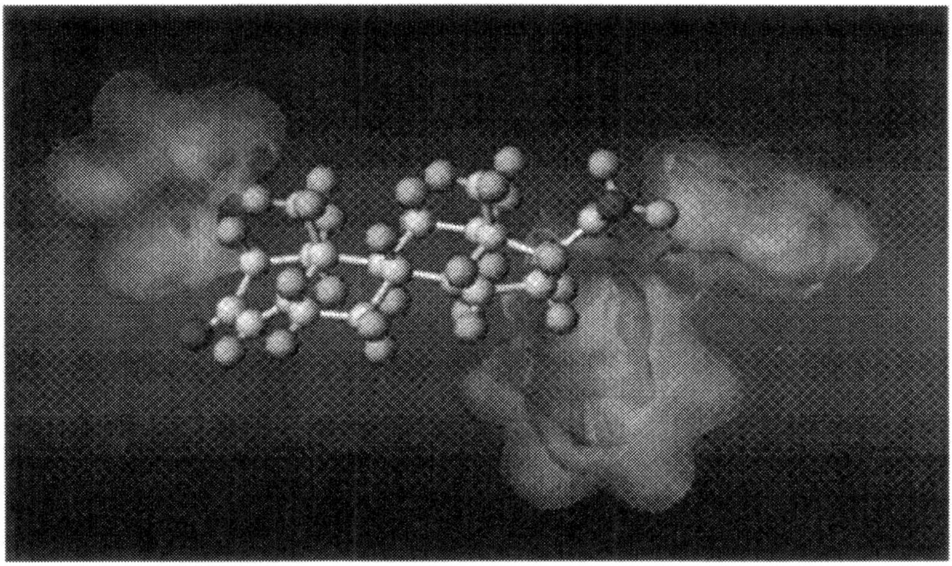

Figure 2. Model of Substitution Sites on Progesterone Which Retain Affinity

To reduce the lipophilicity, three metal conjugates of a progestin-monoamine-monoamide (MAMA') bisthiol chelate system have been studied. [70] Although these conjugates are structurally similar to the BAT conjugates discussed above, the octanol/water partition coefficient is almost two orders of magnitude less indicating a decrease in lipophilicity. These agents also bind to the receptor with an affinity greater than that of progesterone itself (Table 7). Specific uptake in the uterus is again observed, and blocking by coadministration of a PgR ligand reduces uterine uptake by approximately 60%. Even with the less lipophilic MAMA' compounds, high nonspecific binding is still observed. However, both of these studies suggest that high affinity compounds labeled with technetium can be prepared

Table 7. Chelated Metal-Labeled Ligands for the Progesterone Receptor

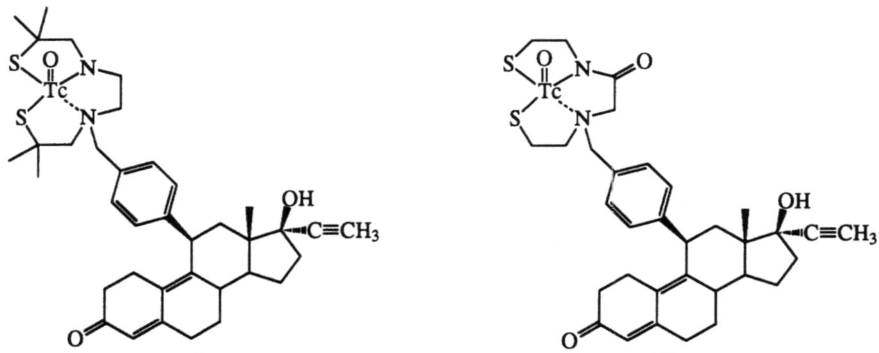

I II

	I	II
RBA [log Po/w]	47 [6.3]	35 [5.3]
%ID/g (Ut,1hr)	1.0	0.75
Ut/musc (1hr)	1.3	1.3
Reference	[67,68]	[70]

RBA is expressed relative to R5020

Chi and coworkers investigated the possibility of preparing complexes of rhenium and technetium which incorporate the metal directly into the structure of the steroid [71]. The B,C ring system of the steroid is replaced by an N_2S_2 complex of oxorhenium or oxotechnetium to generate a metal complex system with a size and shape similar to that of a steroid. A molecular mechanics model of such a steroid is shown in Figure 3. The dimensions between the 2- and 17-hydroxy groups are within 0.15Å of that of the hydroxy groups in a steroid. Several complexes have been synthesized and the radiochemistry and stereochemistry verified by spectroscopic methods. The biodistributions of some of these compounds have been carried out, and the complexes appear to be relatively stable in blood. [71] This integrated synthetic approach [72] is a novel way to prepare receptor based ligands containing technetium-99m.

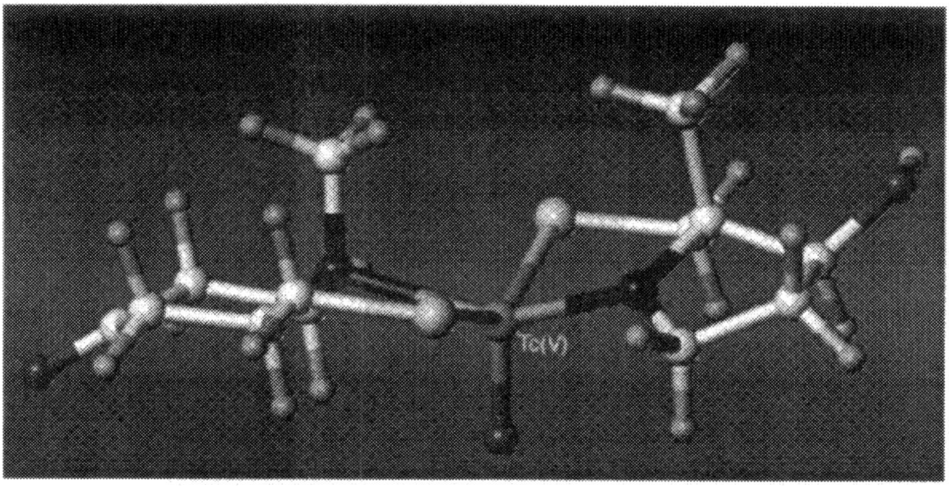

Figure 3. Molecular Mechanics Model of an Integrated Tc(V) N_2S_2 Steroid Complex

Another approach to labeling steroids with metals is through organometallic structures (Table 8). Jaouen, et al., have reported the synthesis of a number of steroids in which transition metals are joined to the steroids through a tricarbonylarene, tricarbonylcyclopentadienyl, or similar organometallic linkage. [73,74] In these structures, the metal is firmly held by the organometallic linkage and the overall structure is non-polar. There are significant problems in preparing these agents at high specific activity and the preliminary radiolabeling studies [75] that have been reported were presumably carried out at very low specific activity.

Table 8. Organometallic Ligands for the Estrogen Receptor

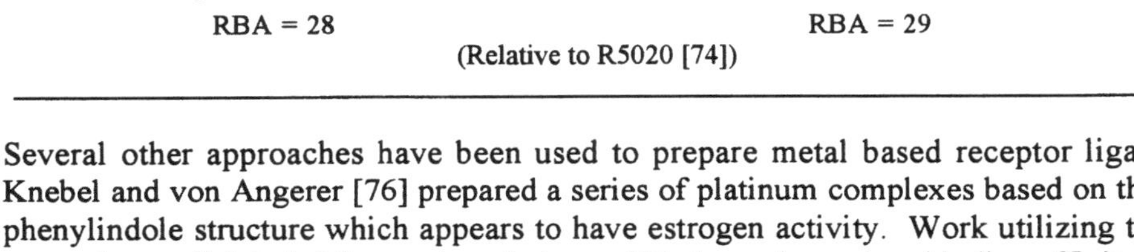

RBA = 28 RBA = 29

(Relative to R5020 [74])

Several other approaches have been used to prepare metal based receptor ligands. Knebel and von Angerer [76] prepared a series of platinum complexes based on the 2-phenylindole structure which appears to have estrogen activity. Work utilizing these agents in a radiolabeled form using platinum-191 showed very low binding affinity and no evidence of selective uptake by estrogen target tissue. [77]

To date, no metal based steroid has been prepared with characteristics suitable for studies in humans. The approaches outlined above, however, give promise that such agents can be designed in the near future.

Steroid Receptor Based Imaging Agents in Humans

The first estrogen receptor based image of a tumor was obtained in 1982 using 16α-[^{77}Br]-bromo-estradiol. [78] The image quality was poor due to the nuclear characteristics of bromine-77. Two iodinated estrogens have been used in clinical imaging studies. 16a-[^{123}I]Iodoestradiol has been studied at several centers.

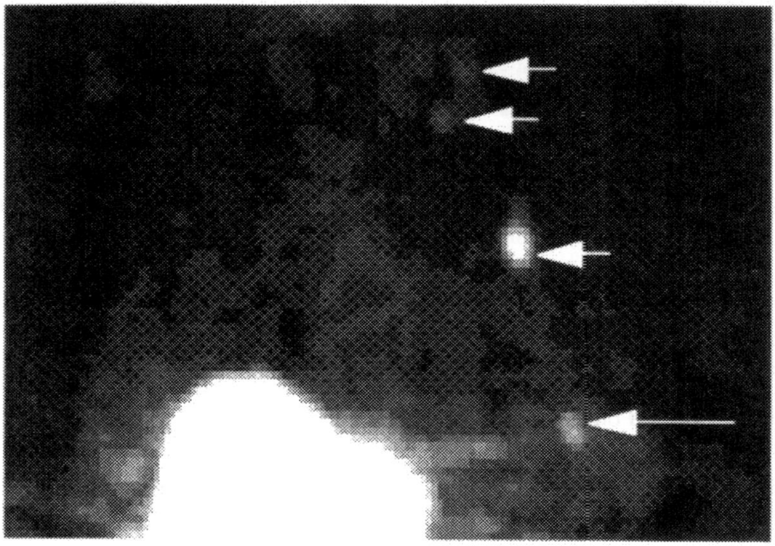

Figure 4. PET image (anterior view) obtained using FES in a patient with small estrogen receptor positive primary breast cancer (long arrow) with axillary and suraclavicular lymph node disease (small arrows).

Preston [79] and others [80] have reported that this agent imaged primary metastatic tumors and a reasonable correlation between tumor uptake and receptor levels was observed. Several studies [81] have confirmed these findings and demonstrate that this agent can be used to identify estrogen receptor positive tumors. A second agent, 11β-methoxy-17α-[^{123}I]iodoestradiol, has also been studied, but appears to be less specific and less sensitive in imaging tumors compared to 16α-[^{123}I]iodoestradiol. [82]

Extensive studies have been carried out using 16α-[^{18}F]fluoroestradiol (FES). Both primary and metastatic tumors have been imaged [83] and the effect of the antiestrogen tamoxifen on uptake has been studied. [84] An example of an image obtained using

FES in an ER positive patient is shown in Figure 4. The correlation between the uptake of FES and patient response to hormone and chemotherapy has also been investigated. [85] In this report, comparison studies using FES and 2-fluoro-2-deoxyglucose (FDG) demonstrate that there is no direct relationship between tumor metabolism (measured by FDG uptake) and the ER mediated uptake of FES. However, further analysis showed that it may be possible to predict response to antiestrogen treatment of ER positive tumors by monitoring changes in glucose metabolism. In a preliminary study [86] it has been shown that metabolism increases following the initiation of antiestrogen therapy, which means that increases in FDG uptake may indicate a positive response to therapy. A combination of metabolic and receptor based agents may be beneficial in evaluating the effectiveness of hormonal therapy early in treatment.

A relatively new consideration in designing radiolabeled ligands for steroid hormone receptors is the binding affinity of the ligand to sex hormone binding globulin (SHBG). It was initially assumed by most investigators that a high affinity for SHBG would decrease effectiveness. According to the free-hormone hypothesis only the free unbound steroid is available for uptake by the steroid receptors, so high affinity for a plasma protein would be undesirable [87]. However, a number of studies using various steroid derivatives has begun to cast doubts on this theory. It appears as though affinity for SHBG may in fact increase the binding of steroids for their receptors, although whether this is due to increased stability in plasma as the steroid-SHBG complex, increased circulation time (slower blood clearance), directed delivery of the complex to the target site, or some other mechanism is unknown. A number of ligands for each of the receptor systems have demonstrated potential after evaluation in rats, but vastly different distributions when studied in primates and vice versa - compounds which did not appear to be as promising after use in rats gave better results in primates. A possible explanation is that the uptake is altered due to the lack of native SHBG in mature rats and its presence in primates in quite significant quantities.

SHBG has been implicated in a number of surprising results. A limited patient study was performed with 11β-methoxy-17α-ethynyl-16β-[^{18}F]fluoroestradiol (FMOX), another promising fluorinated estrogen. [88] Although this agent had very high receptor binding affinity and showed superior target tissue selectivity in the rat compared to FES, in humans it has proven to be a very poor imaging agent. FMOX has a lower affinity for SHBG than does FES and this difference could account for the contradictory behavior. This protein may also cause the differences in behavior of the two iodinated estrogens discussed above. Similarly, a high affinity PgR ligand, 16α-ethyl-21-[^{18}F]fluoro-19-norprogesterone (FENP), showed high selectivity in rats but fell short of expectations when studied in humans. [89] The uptake of FENP in breast tumors was too low to provide imaging of tumors, but had appeared to be quite promising in rat biodistribution studies. Based upon considerations of serum protein binding effects, new agents are currently being investigated for human studies.

Conclusions

The discovery of steroids and their receptors was a major milestone in the initial stages of modern cancer therapy and imaging. Over the last few decades the use of radiolabeled steroid hormones has proven itself to be one of the most effective ways to predict responsiveness to therapy, estimate survival and prognosis, and to localize and stage both primary and metastatic carcinomas. The future in this ever expanding field looks bright as new and more effective agents are developed, leading to new insights into the physiology and development of cancer.

Acknowledgements

The authors wish to thank David Reichert for producing the excellent molecular modeling images, and Timothy J. McCarthy for the formatting of the FES tumor image. The authors' research is supported by the United States Department of Energy and National Institutes of Health.

References

1. Beatson GT. On the treatment of inoperable cases of carcinoma of the mamma: Suggestions for a new method of treatment with illustrative cases. Lancet 1896; 2:104-107.
2. Dodds EC, Golberg L, Lawson W, Robinson R. Oestrogenic activity of certain synthetic compounds. Nature (London) 1938; 141:247-248.
3. Dodds EC, Lawson W, Noble RL. Biological effects of the synthetic oestrogenic substance 4:4'-dihydroxy-a:b-diethylstilbene. Lancet 1938; 1:1389-1391.
4. Mueller GC. Estrogen receptors--Highlights of their history, properties, and actions. In: Jordan VC, ed. Estrogen/Antiestrogen Action and Breast Cancer Therapy. Madison, Wisconsin: The University of Wisconsin Press, 1986: 3-17.
5. Jensen EV, Jacobsen HI. Fate of steroid estrogens in target tissues. In: Pincus G, Vollmer EP, eds. Biological Activities of Steroids in Relation to Cancer. New York: Academic Press, 1960:161-178.
6. Noteboom WD, Gorski J. Stereospecific binding of estrogens in the rat uterus. Arch Biochem Biophys 1965; 111:559-568.
7. King RJB, Gordon J. The localization of [6,7-^{3}H]oestradiol-17β in rat uterus. J Endocr 1966; 34:431-437.
8. Stumpf WE. Subcellular distribution of ^{3}H-estradiol in rat uterus by quantitative autoradiography: A comparison between ^{3}H-estradiol and ^{3}H-norethynodrel. Endocrinology 1968; 83:777-782.
9. Toft D, Gorksi J. A receptor molecule for estrogens: Isolation from the rat uterus and preliminary characterization. Proc Nat Acad Sci 1966; 55:1574-1581.
10. Harper MJK, Walpole AL. Contrasting endocrine activities of *cis* and *trans* isomers in a series of substituted triphenylethylenes. Nature (London) 1966; 212:87.
11. Herrmann W, Wyss R, Riondel A, Philibert D, Teutsch G, Sakiz E, Baulieu EE. The effects of an antiprogesterone steroid in women: Interruption of the menstrual cycle and early pregnancy. C R Seances Acad Sci Ser D 1982; 294:933-938.
12. Philibert D, Deraedt R, Tournemine C, Mary I, Teutsch G. RU 38486 -- A potent antiprogesterone. Int Congr Horm Steroids, 6th Jerusalem 1982: Abstract 204.
13. Healy DL, Baulieu EE, Hodgen GD. Induction of menstruation by an antiprogesterone steroid (RU 486) in primates: Site of action, dose-response relationships and hormonal effects. Fertil Steril 1983; 40:253-257.

14. Sadler SE, Bower MA, Maller JL. Studies of a plasma membrane steroid receptor in Xenopus laevis oocytes using the synthetic progestin RU486. J Steroid Biochem 1985; 22:419-426.
15. Jensen EV, Jacobson HI, Smith S, Kyser K, DeSombre ER. Estrogen receptors and breast cancer responce to adrenalectomy. In: Hall TC, ed. Prediction of Response to Cancer Therapy. Cancer Institute Monograph 34, 1971: 55-70.
16. Maass H, Engel B, Hohmeister H, Lehmann F, Trams G. Estrogen receptors in human breast cancer tissue. Amer J Ob Gyn 1972; 113:377-382.
17. Engelsman E, Persijn JP, Korsten CB, Cleton FJ. Oestrogen receptors in human breast cancer tissue and response to endocrine therapy. British Medical Journal 1973; 2:750-752.
18. Leung BS, Fletcher WS, Lindell TD, Wood DC, Krippaehne WW. Predictability of response to endocrine ablation in advanced breast carcinoma. Arch Surg 1973; 106:515-519.
19. Savlov ED, Wittliff JL, Hilf R, Hall TC. Correlations of certain biochemical properties of breast cancer and response to therapy: A preliminary report. Cancer 1974; 33:303-309.
20. McGuire WL, Carbone PP, Vollmer EP, eds. Estrogen Receptors in Human Breast Cancer. New York: Raven Press, 1975.
21. LeMaistre CF, McGuire WL. Progesterone receptor determinations: A refinement of predictive tests for hormone dependency of breast cancer. In: Jordan VC, ed. Estrogen/Antiestrogen Action and Breast Cancer Therapy. Madison, Wisconsin: The University of Wisconsin Press, 1986: 341-354.
21. Barrack ER, Tindall DJ, A critical evaluation of the use of androgen receptor assays to predict the androgen responsiveness of prostatic cancer. Progr Clin Biol Res 1987; 239:155-187.
22. Ekman P, Dahlberg E, Gustaffson JÅ, Högberg B, Pousette A, Snochowski M. Present and future clinical value of steroid receptor assays in human prostatic carcinoma. In: Iacobelli S, ed. Hormones and Cancer. New York: Raven Press, 1980: 361-370.
23. Katzenellenbogen JA. The development of gamma-emitting hormone analogs as imaging agents for receptor-positive tumors. Progr Clin Biol Res 1981; 75B:313-327.
24. Concolina G, Maroechi A, Margiotta G, et al. Steroid receptors and hormone responsiveness of human prostatic carcinoma. The Prostate 1982; 3:475-482.
25. Diamond DA, Barrack ER. The relationship of androgen receptor level to androgen responsiveness in the Dunning R3327 rat prostate tumor sublines. J Urol 1984; 132:821-827.
26. Ekman P, Snochowski M, Dahlberg E, Gustaffson JÅ. Steroid receptors in metastatic carcinoma of the human prostate. Eur J Cancer 1979; 15:257-262.
27. Ekman P, Snochowski M, Zetterberg A, Högberg B, Gustaffson JÅ. Steroid receptor content in human prostatic carcinoma and response to endocrine therapy. Cancer 1979; 44:1173-1181.
28. Pertschuk LP, Rosenthal HE, Macchia RJ, et al. Correlation of histochemical and biochemical analysis of androgen binding in prostatic cancer: Relation to therapeutic response. Cancer 1982; 49:984-993.
29. Mobbs BG, Johnson IF. Basal and estrogen-stimulated hormone receptor profiles in four R3327 prostatic carcinoma sublines in relation to histopathology and androgen sensitivity. Cancer Res 1988; 48:3077-3083.
30. Müntzing J, Kirdani RY, Murphy GP, Sandberg AA. A rat prostatic adenocarcinoma as a model for the human disease. Invest Urol 1979; 17:37-41.
31. Trapma J, Stalpers CR, van der Korput JAGM, Kuiper GGJM, Brinkmann AO. The androgen receptor: Functional structure and expression in transplanted human prostate tumors and prostate cell lines. J Steroid Biochem Molec Biol 1990; 37:837-842.
32. Sade MV, Barrack ER. Image analysis of androgen receptor immunostaining in metastatic prostate cancer: Heterogeneity as a predictor of response to hormonal therapy. Cancer 1993; 71:2574-2580.
33. Blankenstein MA, Bolt-de Vries J, van Aubel OG, van Steenbrugge GJ. Hormone receptors in human prostate cancer. Scan J Urol Nephrol 1988; 107:39-45.
34. Cummins CH, Radiolabeled steroidal estrogens in cancer research. Steroids 1993; 58:245-259.
35. Hochberg RB. Iodine-125-labeled estradiol: A gamma-emitting analog of estradiol that binds to the estrogen receptor. Science 1979; 205:1138-1140.
36. Zielinski JE, Larner JM, Hoffer PB, Hochberg RB. The synthesis of 11β-methoxy-16α-[^{123}I]iodoestradiol and its interaction with the estrogen receptor in vivo and in vitro. J Nucl Med 1989; 30:209-215.

37. Ali H, Rousseau J, van Lier JE. 7α-Methyl- and 11β-ethoxy-substitution of [^{125}I]-16α-iodoestradiol: Estrogen receptor-mediated target tissue uptake. J Med Chem 1993;36:264-271.
38. McElvany KD, Katzenellenbogen JA, Shafer KE, Seigel BA, Senderoff SG, Welch MJ. 16α-[^{77}Br]bromoestradiol: Dosimetry and preliminary clinical studies. J Nucl Med 1982; 23:425-430.
39. Ali H, Rousseau J, Ghaffari MA, van Lier JE. Synthesis, receptor binding, and tissue distribution of (17α,20E)- and (17α,20Z)-21-[^{125}I]iodo-19-norpregna-1,3,5(10),20-tetraene-3,17-diol. J Med Chem 1988; 31:1946-1950.
40. Hanson RN, Franke LA. Preparation and evaluation of 17α-[^{125}I]iodovinyl-11β-methoxyestradiol as a highly selective radioligand for tissues containing estrogen receptors: Concise communication. J Nucl Med. 1980; 25:998-1002.
41. Jagoda EM, Gibson RE, Goodgold H, et al. [I-125] 17α-Iodovinyl 11β-methoxyestradiol: In vivo and in vitro properties of a high-affinity estrogen-receptor radiopharmaceutical. J Nucl Med 1985; 25:472-477.
42. Hanson RN, Franke LA, Kaplan ML. Synthesis and evaluation of (17α,20E)-21-[^{125}I]iodo-11-substituted-19-norpregna-1,3,5(10),20-tetraene-3,17β-diols: The influence of 11-stereochemistry on tissue distribution of radioiodinated estrogens. Nucl Med Biol (Int J Radiat Appl Instrum Part B) 1989; 16:3-9.
43. DeSombre ER, Pribish J, Hughes A. Comparison of the distribution of radioiodinated di-and tri-hydroxyphenylethylene estrogens in the immature female rat. Nucl Med Biol 1995; 33:679-687.
44. Hanson RN, El-Wakil H, Murphy F. Synthesis and evaluation of ^{82}Br and ^{77}Br labeled (17α,20E)-21-bromo-19-norpregna-1,3,5(10),20-tetraene-3,17β-diol. J.Lab.Comp.Radiopharm. 1989;27:615-627
45. Katzenellenbogen JA, Heiman DF, Carlson KE, Lloyd JE. In vivo and in vitro steroid receptor assays in the design of estrogen radiopharmaceuticals. In: Eckelman WC, ed. Receptor-Binding Radiotracers. Vol 1. Boca Raton, Florida: CRC Press, Inc., 1982: 93-126.
46. Katzenellenbogen JA, Heiman DF, Senderoff SG, et al. Estrogen receptor-based agents for imaging breast tumors: Binding selectivity as a basis for design and optimization. In: Morcos N, Lambrecht RM, eds. Applications of Nuclear and Radiochemistry. New York: Pergamon Press, 1982:311-323.
47. Katzenellenbogen JA. The pharmacology of steroid radiopharmaceuticals: Specific and non-specific binging and uptake selectivity. In: Nunn AD, ed. Radiopharmaceuticals: Chemistry and Pharmacology. New York: Marcel Drekker, Inc., 1992: 297-331.
48. Reiffers S, Vaalberg W, Wiegman T, Wynberg H, Woldring MG. Carbon-11 labeled methyllithium as a methyl donating agent: The addition to 17-keto steroids. Int J Appl Radiat Isot 1980; 31:535-359.
49. Dence CS, Napolitano E, Katzenellenbogen JA, Welch MJ. Carbon-11 labeled estrogens as potential imaging agents for breast tumors. Nucl Med Biol 1996: (in press).
50. Pomper MG, Katzenellenbogen JA, Welch MJ, Brodack JW, Mathias CJ. 21-[^{18}F]Fluoro-16α-ethyl-19-norprogesterone: Synthesis and target tissue selective uptake of a progestin receptor based radiotracer for positron emission tomography. J Med Chem 1988; 31:1360-1363.
51. Verhagen A, Elsinga PH, de Groot TJ, et al. A fluorine-18 labeled progestin as an imaging agent for progestin receptor positive tumors with positron emission tomography. Cancer Res 1991; 51:1930-1933.
52. Verhagen A, Luurtsema G, Pesser JW, et al. Preclinical evaluation of a positron emitting progestin ([^{18}F]fluoro-16α-methyl-19-norprogesterone) for imaging progesterone receptor positive tumors with positron emission tomography. Cancer Lett 1991; 59:125-132.
53. Kochanny MJ, VanBrocklin HF, Kym PR, et al. Fluorine-18-labeled progestin ketals: Synthesis and target tissue uptake selectivity of potential imaging agents for receptor-positive breast tumors. J Med Chem 1993; 36:1120-1127.
54. Buckman BO, Bonasera TA, Kirschbaum KS, Welch MJ, Katzenellenbogen JA. Fluorine-18 labeled progestin 16α,17α-dioxolanes: Development of high-affinity ligands for the progesterone receptor with high in vivo target site selectivity. J Med Chem 1995; 38:328-337.
55. Salman M, Stotter PL, Chamness GC. ^{125}I-Ligand for progesterone receptor: 17α–(6'-iodohex-1'ynyl)-19-nortestosterone. J Steroid Biochem 1989; 33:25-31.

56. Hochberg RB, Hoyte RM, Rosner W. E-17α-(2-[^{125}I]iodovinyl)-19-nortestosterone: The synthesis of a gamma emitting ligand for the progesterone receptor. Endocrinology 1985; 117:2550-2552.
57. Hoyte RM, Rosner W, Johnson IS, Zielinski J, Hochberg RB. Synthesis and evaluation of potential radioligands for the progesterone receptor. J Med Chem 1985; 28:1695-1699.
58. Hochberg RB, Rosner W. Interaction of 16α-[^{125}I]iodoestradiol with estrogen receptors and other steroid-binding proteins. Proc Natn Acad Sci USA 1980; 77:328-332.
59. Hoyte RM, Rosner W, Hochberg RB. Synthesis of 16α-[^{125}I]iodo-5α-dihydro-testosterone and evaluation of its affinity for the androgen receptor. J Steroid Biochem 1982; 16:621-628.
60. Liu A, Carlson KE, Katzenellenbogen JA. Synthesis of high affinity fluorine-substitued ligands for the androgen receptor. Potential agents for imaging prostatic cancer by positron emission tomography. J Med Chem 1992; 35:2113-2129.
61. Liu A, Dence CS, Welch MJ, Katzenellenbogen JA. Fluorine-18-labeled androgens: Radiochemical synthesis and tissue distribution studies on six fluorine substituted androgens, potential imaging agents for prostatic cancer. J Nucl Med 1992; 33:724-734.
62. Liu A, Katzenellenbogen JA, VanBrocklin HF, Mathias CJ, Welch MJ. 20-[^{18}F]Fluoromibolerone, a positron-emitting radiotracer for androgen receptors: Synthesis and tissue distribution studies. J Nucl Med 1991; 32:81-88.
63. Choe YS, Lidström PJ, Chi DY, Bonasera TA, Welch MJ, Katzenellenbogen JA. Synthesis of 11β-[^{18}F]fluoro-5a-dihydrotestosterone and 11β-[^{18}F]fluoro-19-nor-5α-dihydro-testosterone: Preparation via halofluorination-reduction, receptor binding, and tissue distribution. J Med Chem 1994; 38:816-825.
64. Ali H, Rousseau J, van Lier JE. Synthesis of (17α,20E/Z)iodovinyl testosterone and 19-nortestosterone derivatives as potential radioligands for androgen and progesterone receptors. J Steroid Biochem Molec Biol 1994; 49:15-29.
65. Salman M, Chamness GC. A potential radioiodinated ligand for androgen receptor: 7α-Methyl-17α-(2'-(E)-iodovinyl)-19-nortestosterone. J Med Chem 1991; 34:1019-1024.
66. Hoyte RM, Borderon K, Bryson K, Allen R, Hochberg RB, Brown TJ. Synthesis and evaluation of 7α-iodo-5α-dihydrotestosterone as a potential radioligand for androgen receptor. J Med Chem 1994; 37:1224-1230.
67. Berger G, Maziere M, Prenant C, Sastre J, Comar D. Synthesis of high specific activity ^{11}C-17α-methyltestosterone. Int J Appl Radiat Isot 1981; 32:811-815.
68. DiZio JP, Fiaschi R, Davison A, Katzenellenbogen JA. Progestin-rhenium complexes: Metal-labeled steroids with high receptor binding affinity, potential receptor-director agents for diagnostic imaging or therapy. Bioconjugate Chem 1991; 2:353-366.
69. DiZio JP, Anderson CJ, Davison A, et al. Technetium- and rhenium-labeled progestins: Synthesis, receptor binding and in vivo distribution of an 11β-substituted progestin labeled with technetium-99 and rhenium-186. J Nucl Med 1992; 33:558-569.
70. O'Neil JP, Carlson KE, Anderson CJ, Welch MJ, Katzenellenbogen JA. Progestin radiopharmaceuticals labeled with technetium and rhenium. Synthesis, binding affinity, and in vivo distribution of a new progestin N_2S_2-metal conjugate. Bioconjugate Chem 1994; 5:182-193.
71. Chi DY, O'Neil JP, Anderson CJ, Welch MJ, Katzenellenbogen JA. Homodimeric and heterodimeric bis(amino thiol) oxometal complexes with rhenium(V) and technetium(V). Control of heterodimeric complex formation and an approach to metal complexes that mimic steroid hormones. J Med Chem 1994; 37:928-937.
72. Hom RK, Chi DY, Katzenellenbogen JA. Heterodimeric bis(amino thiol) complexes of oxorhenium(V) that mimic the structure of steroid hormones. Synthesis and stereochemical issues. J Org Chem (in press).
73. Jaouen G, Vessieres A, Butler IS. Bioorganometallic chemistry: A future direction for transition metal organometallic chemistry. Acc Chem Res 1993; 26:361-369.
74. Top S, El Hafa H, Vessieres A, et al. Rhenium carbonyl complexes of β-estradiol derivatives with high affinity for the estradiol receptor: An approach to selective organometallic radiopharmaceuticals. J Am Chem Soc 1995; 117.8372-8380.
75. Wenzel M, Klinge C. Tc-99m markierte östradiol-derivate synthese, organverteilung und tumor-affinität J Label Comp Radiopharm 1994; 34:981-987

76. Knebel NG, von Angerer E. 2-Phenylindole linked (2-aminoalkylpyridine)-dichloro-platinum(II): Complexes with a selective action on estrogen receptor positive mammary tumors. J Med Chem 1991; 34:2145-2152.
77. DiZio JP, Carlson KE, Bannochie CJ, Welch MJ, von Angerer E, Katzenellenbogen JA. Estrogen platinum-diamine complexes: Preparation of a non-steroidal estrogen platinum-diamine complex labeled with platinum-191 and a study of its binding to the estrogen receptor in vitro and its tissue distribution in vivo. J Steroid Biochem Molec Biol 1992; 42:363-373.
78. McElvany KD, Katzenellenbogen JA, Shafer KE, Siegel BA, Senderoff SG, Welch MJ. 16α-[^{77}Br]bromoestradiol: Dosimetry and preliminary clinical studies. J Nucl Med 1982; 23:425-430.
79. Preston DF, Spicer JA, Baranczuk RA, et al. Clinical results of breast cancer detection by imageable estradiol (I-123 E2) J Nucl Med 1990; 31:937-938.
80. Schober O, Scheidhauer K, Jackisch C, et al. Breast cancer imaging with radioiodinated oestradiol. Lancet 1990; 335:1522.
81. Kenady DE, Pavlik EJ, Nelson K, et al. Images of estrogen-receptor-positive breast tumors produced by estradiol labeled with iodine-123 at 16α. Arch Surg 1993; 25:1212-1221.
82. Ribeiro-Barras MJ, Foulon C, Baulieu JL, et al. Estrogen receptor imaging with 17α-[^{123}I]iodovinyl-11β-methoxyestradiol (MIVE$_2$)—Part II. Preliminary results in patients with breast carcinoma. Nucl Med Biol 1992; 19:263-267.
83. Mintun MA, Welch MJ, Siegel BA, et al. Breast cancer: PET imaging of estrogen receptors. Radiology 1988; 169:45-48.
84. McGuire AH, Dehdashti F, Siegel BA, et al. Positron tomographic assessment of 16α-[^{18}F]fluoro-17β-estradiol uptake in metastatic breast carcinoma. J Nucl Med 1991; 32:1526-1531.
85. Dehdashti F, Mortimer JE, Siegel BA, et al. Positron tomographic assessment of estrogen receptors in breast cancer: Comparison with FDG-PET and in vitro receptor assays. J Nucl Med 1995; 36:1766-1774.
86. Flanagan FL, Dehdashti F, Mortimer JE, Siegel BA, Jonson S, Welch MJ. PET assessment of response to tamoxifen therapy in patients with metastatic breast cancer. J Nucl Med (in press).
87. Mendel CM. The free hormone hypothesis: A physiologically based mathematical model. Endocr Rev 1989; 10:232-274.
88. Dehdashti F. Unpublished data.
89. Dehdashti F, McGuire AH, Van Brocklin HF, et al. Assessment of 21-[^{18}F]fluoro-16α-ethyl-19-norprogesterone as a positron-emitting radiopharmaceutical for the detection of progestin receptors in human breast carcinomas. J Nucl Med 1991; 32:1531-1537.

LABELLING OLIGONUCLEOTIDES WITH IMAGABLE RADIONUCLIDES

Donald J. Hnatowich

Introduction

Oligonucleotides are relatively short polymers of either ribonucleic (RNA) or deoxyribonucleic (DNA) acids joined in a linear fashion through their phosphate-sugar backbone. In the single-stranded oligonucleotide, the nucleotides within are arranged in space in such a manner that their bases are uniquely positioned to bind via hydrogen bonds to complementary bases on a second single-stranded oligonucleotide. One of the purine bases will bind with a pyrimidine base, adenine with thymidine (or uracil in RNA) and guanine with cytosine. The process by which a double-stranded oligonucleotide is formed by the "zippering" of two complementary single-stranded oligonucleotides by Watson-Crick base pairing can be termed hybridization [1]. It is this property of hybridization, unique to RNA and DNA (if artificial oligomers are excluded), which is likely to render in the near future radiolabeled oligonucleotides useful as radiopharmaceuticals.

Radiolabeling with beta-emitting radionuclides

Although the focus of this chapter is oligonucleotides labeled with imagable (i.e. gamma-emitting) radionuclides for in vivo studies, some brief comments may be useful regarding those methods which have become standard in molecular biology for radiolabeling oligonucleotides with beta-emitters, usually for in vitro uses. Radiolabeling may be illustrated as in figure 1 by the structure of the deoxynucleotide adenosine triphosphate (dATP). This and the other deoxynucleotides of DNA and the nucleotides of RNA may be radiolabeled in a variety of ways prior to their incorporation into an oligonucleotide. In particular, a stable phosphate atom may be replaced in either the alpha, beta or gamma position with ^{33}P or, more commonly, ^{32}P [2]. In the special case of a phosphorothioate DNA in which one of the non-bonding oxygen atoms in the phosphate backbone of phosphodiester DNA is replaced with a sulphur atom [3], the non-radioactive sulphur atom may be replaced with ^{35}S. Once radiolabeled, the nucleotides may be incorporated into an oligonucleotide during its synthesis.

S. J. Mather (ed.), Current Directions in Radiopharmaceutical Research and Development, 157–168.

Because of the ready availability of preformed oligonucleotides, such as those now provided by many commercial suppliers, methods of radiolabeling after synthesis are much more useful. Enzymes are commercially available which permit the incorporation of a ^{32}P in the 5' or 3' end of a single-stranded oligonucleotide. Figure 1 also diagramatically illustrates the labelling of an oligonucleotide (in this example, consisting of the nucleotides cytosine and guanine in which the phosphate groups are represented by lower case p's). When radiolabeled in the alpha position, one or more dATP nucleotides (in this example) may be added to the 3' end of the single-stranded oligonucleotide using the enzyme terminal deoxynucleotidyl transferase. It is also possible to radiolabel on the opposite 5' end by first treating the oligonucleotide with alkaline phosphatase. The terminal phosphorus atom on the 5' end may thus be removed and replaced with a hydroxyl group. Using a polynucleotide kinase, the dephosphorylated oligonucleotide may then be labeled with radiophosphorus by adding dATP (in this example) labeled with a radiophosphorus atom in the gamma position [2].

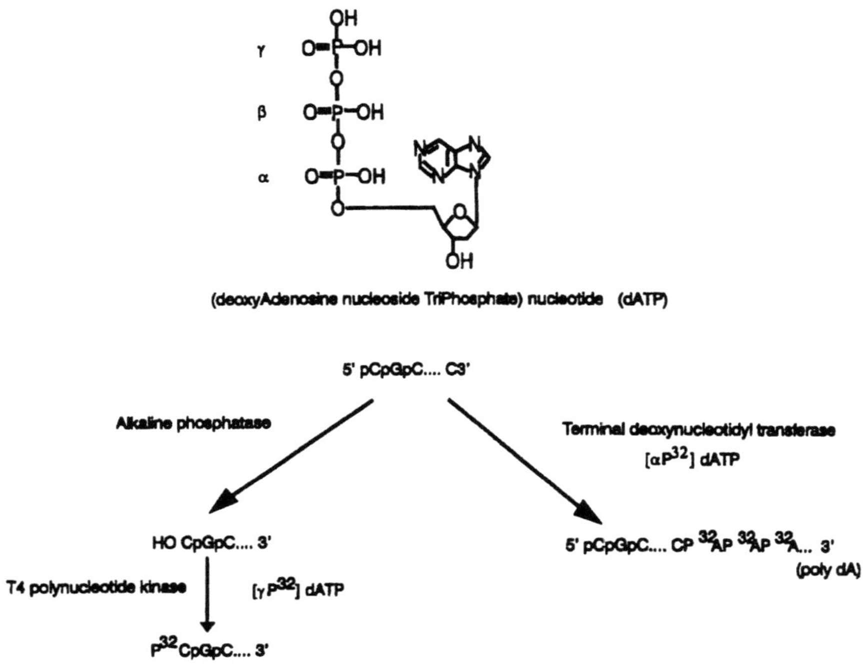

Figure 1.Chemical structure of deoxyadenosinetriphosphate (dATP) nucleotide (top). Diagrammatic representation of DNA end labelling showing only three bases (CGC) and their phosphate groups (represented by "p"). Labelling on the 3' end with terminal deoxynucleotidyl transferase and on the 5' end with alkaline phosphatase and T4 polynucleotide kinase. Adapted from ref. (3).

Radiolabeling with Radioiodine

As useful as these, and other, labelling method may be for molecular biology investigations, they are of little value for in vivo radioimaging purposes since they are usually used to attach beta-emitting radionuclides. Of more interest to the nuclear medicine research community are methods which attach imagable gamma emitters. The earliest method of radiolabeling with gamma-ray emitting radioisotopes was reported in 1971 for iodine-125 (^{125}I) and iodine-131 (^{131}I) [4]. Using thallic ion as a mild oxidising agent, cytosine bases may be labeled with radioiodine under non-denaturing conditions to generate 5-iodocytosine. In this fashion, one or more of the cytosine bases may be radiolabeled in a preformed single- or double-stranded oligonucleotide.

More recently, Dewanjee and his colleagues described a novel method of radiolabeling with ^{125}I in which p-methoxyphenyl isothiocyanate was first conjugated to an amine-linked oligonucleotide and then radiolabeled on the phenol ring with ^{125}I using iodogen. Alternatively, the phenol group in p-methoxyphenyl isothiocyanate could be radioiodinated before conjugation [5].

Radiolabeling of oligonucleotides by chelation would be advantageous for a variety of reasons having to do with convenience and with the superior imaging properties of some of the chelatable metallic radionuclides. Accordingly, Dewanjee and his colleagues [6] and Hnatowich et al [7], have labeled oligonucleotides using "bifunctional" chelators (i.e. moieties capable of both conjugating to the carrier and retaining the radionuclide by chelation) which have been applied successfully for many years to radiolabel proteins and peptides. Thus far, only single stranded oligonucleotides, and only those derivatised on one end with a primary amine, have been radiolabeled in this way.

Radiolabeling with ^{111}In

The first report describing the radiolabeling of oligonucleotides with ^{111}In was that of Dewanjee et al. [6]. A 15-base single stranded DNA was synthesised to include a primary amine on one end attached by a six-carbon spacer. An isothiocyanate derivative of DTPA was synthesised according to published procedures and was coupled to the amine on the DNA. Optimal conditions for coupling were determined to be a ten-fold molar excess of bifunctional chelator to DNA and a 24 hr. incubation period at 45°C. Radiolabeling was achieved in 0.1 M sodium acetate buffer, pH 5.0, to which ^{111}In was added as the acetate complex. After pH adjustment to 6.5 (found to be optimum for chelation), the labeled DNA was purified from unbound radiolabel by open column gel filtration. Labelling efficiency was 45-60% Successful labelling was confirmed by size exclusion HPLC in which the radiolabel showed the same retention time as the oligonucleotide. Maximum specific activity was about 50 uCi/ug.

A similar study was performed more recently in this laboratory using, in place of the isothiocyanate derivative, the commercially available cyclic anhydride of DTPA [7]. A 22-base single stranded DNA was synthesised with a primary amine attached on one end via a six-member methylene carbon spacer and with a biotin group attached to the other end. Conjugation was achieved at a large (>2000-fold) molar excess of the bifunctional chelator over DNA to minimise crosslinking through the multifunctional anhydride. After 30 min. at room temperature, the conjugated DNA solution was adjusted to pH 3.5 and the DNA was purified by anion exchange chromatography using gradient elution. The DTPA-conjugated and purified DNA was radiolabeled with ^{111}In acetate at pH 6. Labelling efficiencies were often 100% and specific activities of 100 uCi/ug were achieved.

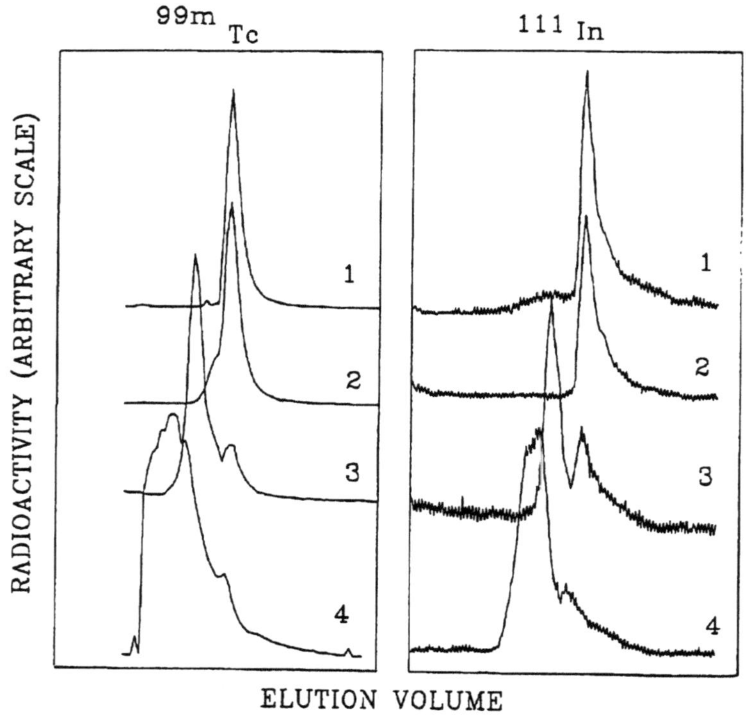

Figure 2.Radiochromatograms obtained by size exclusion HPLC of ^{111}In-labeled (right column) and ^{99m}Tc-labeled (left column) DNA in saline (trace 1), in saline containing biotin saturated streptavidin (trace 2), in saline containing streptavidin (trace 3) and in saline containing complementary DNA bound to streptavidin (trace 4). Taken from ref. (7) with permission.

The radiolabeling of DNA was confirmed using the complementary DNA (i.e., with a base sequence complementary to that of the radiolabeled DNA) derivatised with biotin on one end. Figure 2 presents on the right, size exclusion HPLC radiochromatographic profiles of ^{111}In-labeled DNA in saline (trace 1). No change in the profile is apparent after the addition of biotin-saturated streptavidin (trace 2), demonstrating that the radiolabeled DNA does not bind non-specifically to this protein. A shift to higher molecular weight (i.e. smaller elution volumes) is evident after the addition of streptavidin to the biotinylated DNA (trace 3) and is the result of biotin binding of the DNA to streptavidin. Finally, the addition of streptavidin to which the complementary DNA has been bound results in a much larger shift to higher molecular weight (trace 4) as binding occurs by both biotin binding and hybridization. It is obvious that these shifts to higher molecular weight could only occur if the radiolabel was attached to DNA.

Stability studies in 37°C serum showed a 14% loss of the label from DNA (immobilised on beads) in 24 hrs.

Radiolabeling with ^{99m}Tc using SHNH

In the field of diagnostic imaging, the radiolabel of choice is almost always ^{99m}Tc. It may be assumed that this radioisotope will be the label of choice for most oligonucleotide imaging applications as well, particularly since relatively short single stranded oligonucleotides usually have a biological half lives more consistent with the physical half life of ^{99m}Tc (6 hrs.) rather than that of the longer-lived radioisotopes such as ^{111}In (67 hrs.), ^{125}I (25 days) or ^{131}I (8 days).

As described above, DTPA has been used to attach ^{111}In to oligonucleotides [6,7]. This chelator has also been used to radiolabel DNA with ^{99m}Tc [8]. However, some time ago we were able to show that DTPA is a poor chelator for ^{99m}Tc [9]. A better choice may therefore be the 6-hydrazinonicotinate (SHNH, "hynic") chelator which was first developed as a method of radiolabeling antibodies with ^{99m}Tc [10] and has been shown to provide a stable chelate [11]. The N-hydroxysuccinimide (NHS) ester of SHNH has been synthesised to facilitate conjugation [10]. We have investigated the NHS-SHNH bifunctional chelator for the labelling of oligonucleotides [7]. The identical amine-derivatised single stranded DNA used in the above-described ^{111}In study was again used in this investigation. The NHS-SHNH was dissolved in DMF and was added dropwise to the DNA in a stirred solution buffered to about pH 8.5. The SHNH was added at a 1 : 1 molar ratio and the solution was incubated at room temperature for 1 hr. before purification by open column gel filtration chromatography.

The SHNH-conjugated DNA was radiolabeled with ^{99m}Tc by transchelation from labeled tricine. The tricine was prepared in a pH 7.0 buffer and was mixed with stannous ion immediately before adding to a neutral solution of the DNA and pertechnetate. After 10 min. at room temperature, the labeled DNA was purified by column chromatography. Labelling efficiencies varied between 30-60% and typical specific activities were about 50 uCi/ug. Confirmation that the DNA was radiolabeled was obtained by size exclusion HPLC analysis. As shown on the left in fig. 2, shifts in the radioactivity profiles identical to that observed with ^{111}In (and which provided proof that the ^{111}In label was on the DNA) were seen with ^{99m}Tc.

Stability studies in 37°C serum showed a 4% loss of ^{99m}Tc from DNA (immobilised on beads) in 24 hrs.

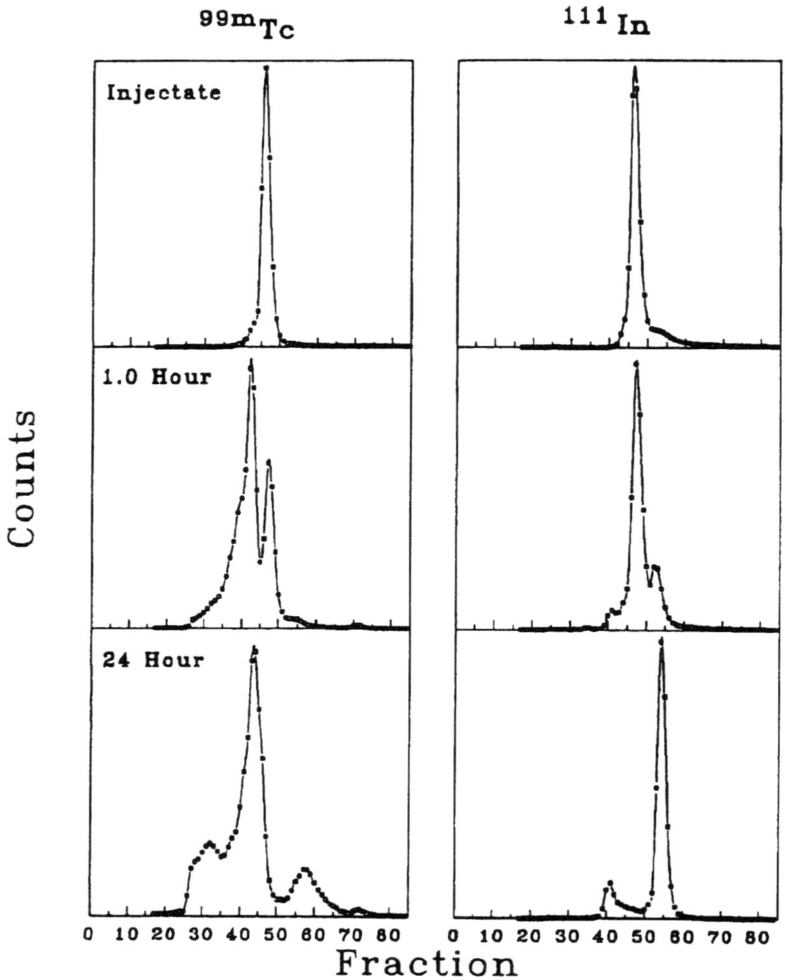

Figure 3. Size exclusion HPLC radiochromatograms of serum incubates of ^{99m}Tc labeled DNA (left column) and ^{111}In (right column) showing the profiles before (top panels) and after 1 hr. (middle panels) and 24 hrs. (bottom panels) of incubation in 37°C fresh human serum. Taken from ref. (7) with permission.

The stability of the label during serum incubation was investigated for both the ^{99m}Tc and ^{111}In labeled DNAs. Each was incubated in fresh human serum at 37°C and samples were removed periodically for size-exclusion HPLC analysis. As shown in figure 3. in the right panel, in the ^{111}In case, a lower molecular weight peak appeared after only 1 hr. of incubation and became the predominant labeled species at 24 hrs. The natural phosphodiester DNAs, particularly the single stranded DNAs used in this investigation, are known to be rapidly digested by nucleases in serum. The lower molecular weight peaks are apparently due to smaller chains of DNA still labeled with ^{111}In and are the result of nuclease digestion. However, in the case of ^{99m}Tc, shown on the left in the figure, instead of low molecular weight peaks, a high molecular weight peak appeared. Further investigations revealed that this peak was due to serum protein binding of the intact oligonucleotide, which occurred in the ^{99m}Tc case only, and was associated with the SHNH chelate [7].

Although serum protein binding obviously interfered with nuclease attack of ^{99m}Tc-SHNH-DNA (as shown by the absence of lower molecular weight peaks in fig. 3), and therefore could be viewed as advantageous, we have subsequently observed that this affinity for serum (and tissue) proteins seriously interferes with hybridization. Accordingly, we have searched for an alternative chelator for labelling oligonucleotides with ^{99m}Tc.

Radiolabeling with ^{99m}Tc using MAG3

The N-[N-[N-[(benzoylthio)acetyl]glycyl]glycyl]glycine (MAG3) chelator of ^{99m}Tc was originally developed as an alternative to radiolabeled hippuran for renal function studies [12]. This N_3S chelator is protected against disulphide-bond formation by a benzoyl group which is removed by heating at 100°C for 10 min during labelling. The MAG3 chelator has also been used to radiolabel antibodies with ^{99m}Tc [13] and radiorhenium [14]. However, past use of the chelator for protein labelling has been limited since the benzoyl leaving group requires extreme alkaline pH or boiling temperatures for sulphur deprotection. Accordingly, the chelator is usually radiolabeled prior to conjugation (i.e. preconjugation labelling) to carriers such as proteins or polypeptides which cannot withstand harsh conditions. Preconjugation labelling can be a complex procedure with multiple intermediate purification steps.

Recently, we developed the alternative synthesis of MAG3 which is illustrated in fig. 4 [15]. The salient features are: 1) that the synthesis can be performed simply in two steps; 2) that the end product is an NHS-ester to facilitate conjugation of the chelator to amines; and 3) that the sulphur atom is protected by an acetyl group in place of the benzoyl group. One result of this [15] and two additional studies from this laboratory [16,17] is that acetyl protection greatly simplifies the synthesis and use of MAG3. The acetyl protection of NHS-MAG3 and MAG3-conjugated amines is stable, apparently indefinitely, to storage even at room temperature yet the acetyl group will dissociate during standard radiolabeling procedures. Once radiolabeled, the serum stability of ^{99m}Tc when incubated on MAG3-conjugated antibodies was essentially identical to ^{99m}Tc on SHNH-conjugated antibodies (16). The stability to cysteine challenge was more favourable for SHNH vs. MAG3, particularly at higher cysteine molar ratios [16].

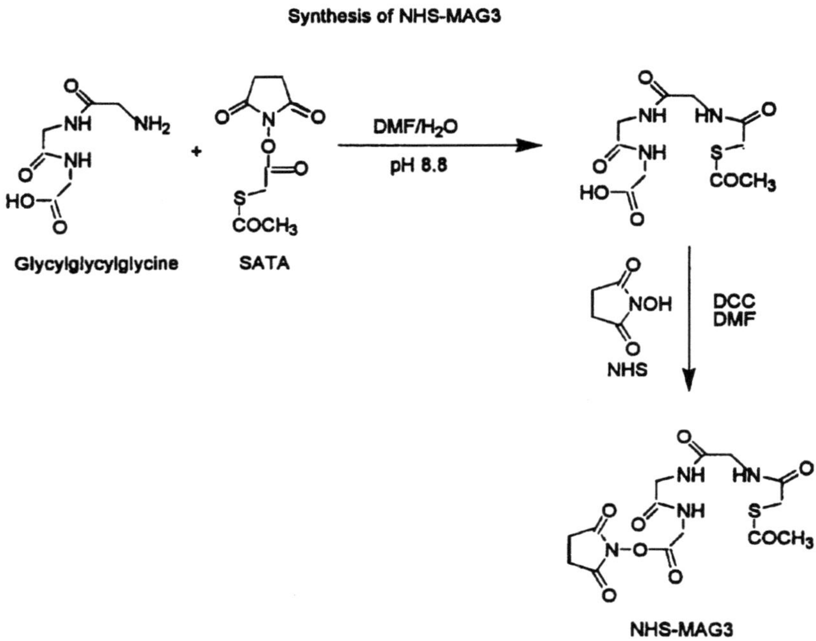

Figure 4. The synthesis of acetyl-protected NHS-MAG3.

We have used the acetyl-protected NHS-MAG3 bifunctional chelator to radiolabel DNA [15]. The same 22-base amine-derivatised phosphodiester DNA was again used and was conjugated by adding dropwise a DMF solution of NHS-MAG3 into a stirred solution of the DNA buffered in bicarbonate to pH 8.5. The molar ratio at conjugation was about 20 : 1 MAG3 to DNA. After 15 min. at room temperature, the solution was purified on an open gel filtration column into pH 5.2 ammonium acetate buffer.

The conjugated DNA was radiolabeled by transchelation using tartrate. The tartrate was added to a solution of the DNA and ^{99m}Tc-pertechnetate buffered at pH 7.6. Radiolabeling was accomplished by the addition of a fresh stannous ion solution. After 15 min. at room temperature, the labeled DNA was purified on an open gel filtration column into pH 5.2 ammonium acetate buffer. Specific activities of up to 70 uCi/ug were achieved. Control labellings with unconjugated DNA showed 0-2% binding under identical conditions.

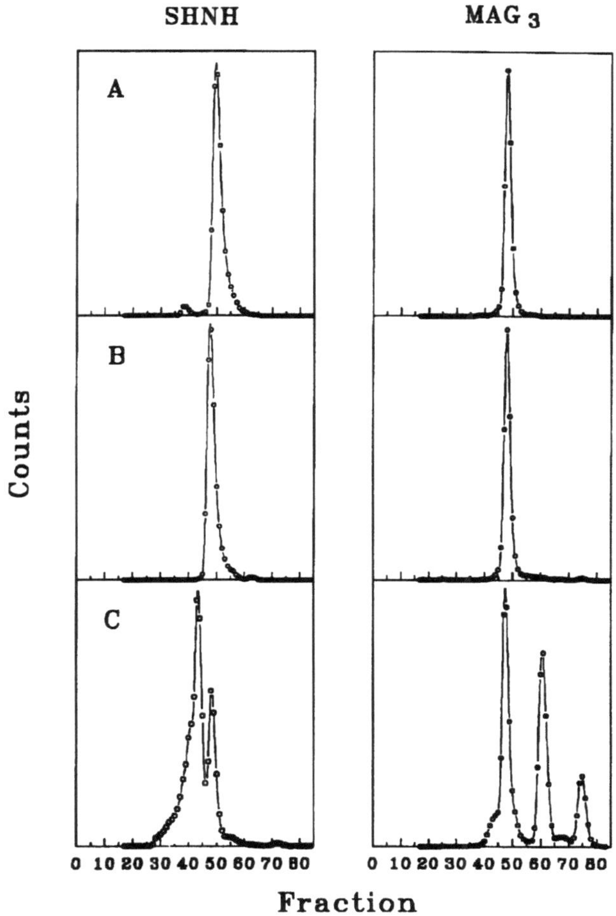

Figure 5. Radiochromatograms obtained by size exclusion HPLC analysis of SHNH-coupled DNA (left column) and MAG3-coupled DNA (right column) after labelling with 99mTc and showing the profiles in saline (panels A), in saline with a large molar excess of cysteine (panels B) and after 1 hr. of incubation in 37°C serum (panels C). Taken from ref. (15).

Figure 5 presents size exclusion HPLC radiochromatograms of the same DNA radiolabeled with ^{99m}Tc via MAG3 (right column) and SHNH (left column). The radiochromatograms are essentially independent of the chelator when analysed in saline solution (row A) and in a cysteine solution (row B). Major differences are, however, readily apparent when analysed from a serum incubate (row C). Whereas a shift to higher molecular weight is again evident in the SHNH case and is due to serum protein binding, in the MAG3 case, no such shift occurs to signify the absence of significant serum protein binding. Lowed molecular weight peaks are present which signify nuclease digestion as in the earlier study with ^{111}In.

Conclusions

To judge from a recent symposium on radiopharmaceutical chemistry, interest in radiolabeled oligonucleotides is increasing [18]. Among the radioisotopes considered therein for oligonucleotide labelling were carbon-11, fluorine-18, yttrium-90, iodine-123 and iodine-124. Whereas certain of these, and other, radionuclides may be of value under specialised circumstances (e.g., positron-emitters used in connection with positron detection devices and beta-emitters for therapy), most likely it will be the chelatable metallic radionuclides (for convenience of labelling) emitting gamma rays (for use with existing gamma cameras) which will be most often used in future in vivo studies with radiolabeled oligonucleotides. Of the two commonly used radionuclides with these properties, ^{99m}Tc will almost certainly be the more popular for reasons of cost, availability and decay properties. The longer physical half life of ^{111}In may be advantageous in certain situation (e.g., slow cell membrane transport kinetics), however the shorter half life of ^{99m}Tc is a better match with the rapid in vivo clearance kinetics of the short oligonucleotides now being considered [19].

Of the two methods which have been considered for radiolabeling amine derivatised single stranded oligonucleotides with ^{99m}Tc (i.e. via SHNH or MAG3), this laboratory prefers MAG3 to avoid difficulties due to the affinity of the SHNH chelate for serum proteins. In our hands, the MAG3 method has been successful by most measures. With acetyl protection, the NHS-MAG3 is not difficult to synthesis and, being stable to long-term storage, may be safely shipped to different laboratories. Amine conjugation is via familiar NHS technology and, once conjugated, the MAG3-DNA may be safely stored. Radiolabeling efficiencies and specific activities are adequate and the label does not bind to serum proteins. In related studies, we have shown greater instability of ^{99m}Tc to cysteine transchelation when labeled to antibodies via MAG3 vs. SHNH although in the same study, only a few important differences were seen in the biodistributions in normal mice [16].

If acetyl-protected MAG3 can be used to radiolabel oligonucleotides with ^{99m}Tc as suggested, then the focus may confidently shift to a discussion of which class of oligonucleotide to use in vivo. This laboratory has judged both the phosphodiester and phosphorothioate DNAs to be unsuitable for different reasons[19]. We have recently begun an investigation of peptide nucleic acid (PNA) oligomers for in vivo imaging studies [17]. Figure 6 presents a whole body anterior/posterior image of one mouse injected 2 hrs earlier with a ^{99m}Tc-MAG3 labeled 15-base single stranded PNA. The mouse has been injected subcutaneously in the left thigh with beads containing the complementary PNA and in the right thigh with beads without PNA. Apart from radioactivity in the liver, kidney and bladder, uptake only in the left thigh is evident. This demonstration of in vivo hybridization shows that with the proper radiolabel and the proper oligomer class, it will be possible to use oligomers as potential radiopharmaceuticals.

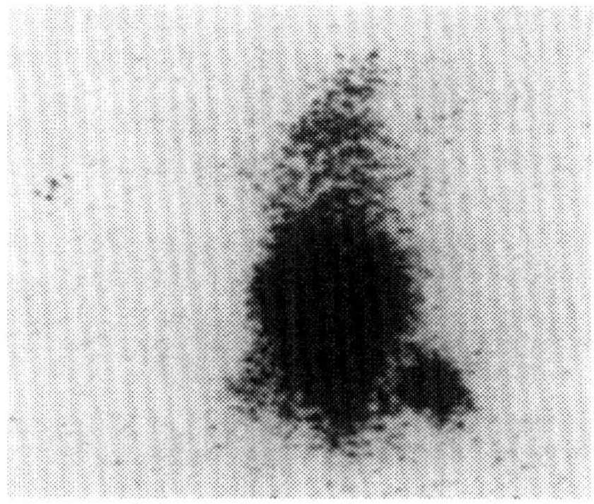

Figure 6. Whole body anterior/posterior images of one mouse injected 2 hrs earlier with a ^{99m}Tc-MAG3 labeled 15-base single stranded PNA. The mouse has beads containing the complementary PNA in the left thigh (on the right in the image) and beads without PNA in the right thigh.

Acknowledgements

This work was supported in part by DE-FG02-93ER61656 from the U.S. Department of Energy and by CA59785 from the U. S. National Cancer Institute.

References

1. Watson JD, Gilman M, Witkowski J, Zoller M. Recombinant DNA. Scientific American Books, W.H. Freedman and Co., New York. 1992, Second Edition.
2. Sambrook J., Fritsch E.F., Maniatis T. Molecular Cloning, (2nd edition) Vol. 2. Cold Spring Harbor Lab Press, New York, 1989, pp 11.23-11.28.
3. Goodchild J. Conjugates of oligonucleotides and modified oligonucleotides: a review of their synthesis and properties. Bioconj. Chem. 1: 165-187, 1990.
4. Commerford S.L. Iodination of nucleic acids in vitro. Biochemistry 10: 1993-1999; 1971.
5. Dewanjee M.H., Glafouripour, A.K., Werner R.K. et al. Development of sensitive radioiodinated anti-sense oligonucleotide probes by conjugation techniques. Bioconj Chem 2: 195-200; 1991.
6. Dewanjee M.K., Ghafouripour A.K., Kapakvanjwala M., Dewanjee S, Serafini AN, Lopez DM, Sfakinakis GN. Noninvasive imaging of c-myc oncogene messenger RNA with indium-111-antisense probes in a mammary tumor-bearing mouse model. J Nucl Med 35: 1054-1063, 1994.
7 Hnatowich D.J., Winnard P. Jr., Virzi F., et al. Labeling deoxyribonucleic acid oligonucleotides with 99mTc. J Nucl Med 36: 2306-2314; 1995.
8. Dewanjee MK., Ghalfouripour AK., Subramanian M., et al. Labeling antisense deoxyoligoonucleotide with Tc-99m and hybridization with c-myc oncogene mRNA in P388 leukemic cells. J Lab Compd Radiopharm 35: 40-42; 1994 (Abstract).
9. Childs R.L., Hnatowich D.J. Optimum conditions for labeling of DTPA-coupled antibodies with techneitum-99m. J Nucl Med 26: 293-299; 1985.

10. Abrams M.J., Juweid M., tenKate C.I., et al. Technetium-99m-human polyclonal IgG radiolabeled via the hydrazino nicotinamide derivative for imaging focal sites of infection in rats. J Nucl Med 31: 2022-2028, 1990.
11. Hnatowich D.J., Mardirossian G., Ruscowski M. et al. Directly and indirectly technetium-99m-labeled antibodies-a comparison of in vitro and animal in vivo properties. J Nucl Med 34; 109-119, 1993.
12. Fritzberg AR., Kasina S., Eshima D., Johnson D.L. Synthesis and biological evaluation of technetium-99m MAG_3 as a hippuran replacement. J Nucl Med 27: 111-116; 1986.
13. Fritzberg A.R., Berninger R.W., Hadley S.W. et al. Approaches to radiolabeling of antibodies for diagnosis and therapy of cancer. Pharmaceutical Res. 5: 325-334; 1988.
14. Goldrosen MH., Biddle WC., Pancook S. et al. Biodistribution, pharmacokinetics, and imaging studies with ^{186}Re-labeled NR-LU-10 whole antibody in LS174T colonic tumor-bearing mice. Cancer Res. 50: 7973-7978; 1990.
15. Winnard P. Jr., Rusckowski M, Mardirossian G, Hnatowich DJ, A simplifed synthesis of MAG_3-coupled oligonucleotides for technetium-99m labeling. Bioconj Chem (Submitted).
16 Lei K., Rusckowski M., Chang F., Qu T., Mardirossian G., Hnatowich DJ. Technetium-99m antibodies labeled with MAG_3 and SHNH-an in vitro and animal in vivo comparison. (Submitted).
17. Mardirossian G., Rusckowski M., Chang F., Qu T., Lei K., Egholm M*. Hnatowich DJ. In vitro hybridization of technetium-99m labeled peptide nucleic acid (PNA). (Submitted).
18. Multiple contributions. Eleventh international symposium on radiopharmaceutical chemistry. J Lab Compd Radiopharm 1995: 38; 324-352. (Abstracts).
19. Hnatowich DJ, Mardirossian G, Fogarasi M, et al. Comparative Properties of a technetium-99m-labeled single-stranded natural DNA and a phosphorothioate derivative in vitro and in vivo. Pharm Exp Therap 276: 326-334;1996.

RADIOLIGAND BINDING ASSAYS: THEORY AND PRACTICE

Anthony P. Davenport and Fraser D. Russell

Introduction

Transmitters and hormones generate signals in target cells by interacting with a signal transducing protein or receptor. Receptors may be located in the cytosol, allowing for example, steroid and thyroid hormones to control gene transcription. However, the largest family comprises G-protein linked seven transmembrane spanning receptors located in the plasma membrane. In addition to the endogenous transmitter or hormone, selective drugs are continuously being developed that act via receptors or discrete recognition sites. Drugs may mimic the action of the endogenous transmitter by binding to a receptor to induce a biological response such as muscle contraction and therefore function as an agonist. At the other end of the spectrum, competitive antagonists bind to receptors without inducing a functional response themselves but block the action of an agonist or endogenous transmitter. It is difficult to differentiate between agonists and antagonists in a binding assay and both classes of compounds will therefore be referred to as ligands.

During the 1960s, ligands were first radiolabelled to high specific activity which allowed receptors that are usually expressed in comparatively low densities to be characterised in vitro. More recently, ligands for positron or single photon emission tomography have been developed for in vivo imaging of human receptors. Unlabelled ligands require a radioactive isotope to be incorporated into the molecule. In a few cases, the ligand may already contain a group that is suitable for incorporating or substituting a radioactive isotope. Alternatively, the ligand has to be structurally modified to provide a suitable site for radiolabelling. In both cases, it is not always predictable that the selectivity and specificity of an unlabelled ligand will be retained following labelling.

The aim of this review is to discuss how new radiolabelled ligands can be characterised using human membrane bound receptors derived from preparations of surgical samples. The development of a radiolabelled ligand that is selective for endothelin ET_A receptors

S. J. Mather (ed.), Current Directions in Radiopharmaceutical Research and Development, 169–179.

will be used as an example [1-3]. For more detailed discussion of the techniques see reviews [4-8].

Why use radioligand binding to characterise receptors interaction?

When injected in vivo, radiolabelled ligands are initially limited by the rate of diffusion of the compound to the tissue expressing the target receptors. At close range a variety of forces of different magnitude (including ionic, hydrogen and Van der Waal) will be established between a ligand and its receptor to form a reversible complex. Under physiological conditions, these forces are made and broken rapidly. Specificity results from the complimentary surfaces of the ligand and receptor and it is this interaction that can be quantified in vitro using ligand binding assays. Ligands can be selective for a target receptor over a certain range of concentrations but at higher doses may interact with other receptor types. The interaction between ligands and receptors can be quantified in ligand binding assays. Two important parameters can be calculated: the affinity of a ligand for a receptor, the K_D, and the maximum density of receptors, the Bmax.

The K_D (units M) is the equilibrium dissociation constant and is a measure of the strength of interaction of a ligand to its receptor. By definition, the K_D is the concentration of ligand that will occupy 50% of the receptors. A ligand binding with a K_D of 1 nM or less is generally considered to have a high affinity for its receptor whereas ligands binding with a K_D of 1 uM have low affinity. The K_D can be used to calculate the concentration of a radiolabelled ligand needed to occupy a desired proportion of receptors. The fraction of receptors is equal to L/K_D+L, where L in the free ligand concentration. For example, a radioligand with a K_D of 0.2 nM would occupy 9% of the receptors at a concentration of 0.02 nM.

Bmax is the maximum density of receptors. This is usually corrected using the amount of protein present in the binding assay and expressed as amount of ligand bound/mg protein (e.g. 50 pmol/mg protein). The determination of the maximum density of receptors in a particular tissue is unique to ligand binding.

Desirable properties of radioligands

Ideally, candidate ligands for radiolabelling should have the following desirable properties:

i) High affinity (K_D of 1 nM or less) to favour specific over non-specific binding.
ii) Low non-specific binding.
iii) High specific activity to detect low receptor densities.
iv) Receptor specificity.

In addition, the following may be important for radioligands that are to be used as radiopharmaceuticals for the in vivo imaging of receptors:

i) The permeability of the blood-brain barrier to the radioligand.
ii) Low rate of metabolism.
iii) Low toxicity.

Ligand binding assays

SATURATION BINDING

Receptor affinity and density can be readily determined by saturation analysis. In this assay a number of tissue preparation are commonly used: partially purified plasma membrane fractions from tissue homogenates, cells transfected with cloned receptors, freshly isolated or cultured cells. Alternatively, freshly frozen tissue sections (usually 5-30 um thick) are cut on a microtome and mounted on microscope slides. The latter method has the advantage that radioactivity can be determined in the whole section by wiping the tissue from the slide or by apposing to radiation sensitive film for autoradiography.

Two strategies are commonly adopted for this experiment: i) the amount of radioligand added is increased while maintaining a constant specific activity of the radioligand or ii) a constant concentration of radioligand is used and the specific activity of the radioligand is decreased by the addition of unlabelled ligand. The first strategy is illustrated using [^{125}I]-PD151242, an endothelin ET_A selective ligand, in slide mounted tissue sections of human heart [1-3]. Endothelin-1 is an endogenous peptide that has two major actions in the human cardiovascular system: it is a powerful constrictor of blood vessels and potent inotropic agent by a direct action on endothelin receptors in the heart. We have previously shown that both endothelin receptor sub-types, ET_A and ET_B are present in left ventricle in a ratio of about 60% ETA: 40 ET_B% [9], allowing ligands to be characterised against both receptors in the same tissue.

In saturation assays, the concentration chosen for a new ligand must be determined empirically. However, as an initial starting point sections are labelled with radioligand concentrations that are selected to span a range at least an order of magnitude above and below the K_D of the unlabelled compound, if this is known. Non-specific binding is determined at each concentration of [^{125}I]-PD151242 by co-incubation of sections with a 1000 fold excess of unlabelled ligand over the K_D. The sections are incubated for a defined period of time at a constant temperature in order to ensure equilibrium conditions; these conditions will have been determined previously in association experiments (see below). For [^{125}I]-PD151242 a 2h incubation at 23°C is sufficient to reach equilibrium [3]. Equilibrium is rapidly broken by washing to separate bound from free ligand and conditions for this should be examined to find an optimal compromise between retention of bound label and a high percentage of specific binding. Sections are wiped from the slide and the amount of radioactivity bound to the tissue is measured. For homogenates, separation of the bound from the free ligand can be achieved by rapid filtration of the incubation mixture through a filter or by centrifugation.

GRAPHICAL ANALYSIS

An example of a saturation isotherm for the binding of [^{125}I]-PD151242 to human heart is shown in Figure 1. The total, specific and non-specific binding has been plotted against increasing concentrations of the radiolabelled ligand. Non-specific binding occurs because the ligand may also bind to other proteins and lipids. This is linear and not saturable.

The amount of specific binding observed where the isotherm plateaus is an approximation of the Bmax. An estimate of the K_D can also be derived from the concentration of [^{125}I]- PD151242 that labels half of the target receptors (50% of the Bmax). However, a better estimate can be achieved by linearising the data using a Scatchard plot (Figure 1B). Here the ratio of bound and free radioligand (B/F) is plotted on the ordinate against the amount of bound radioligand (B) on the abscissa. The slope of the line through the points is equal to the negative reciprocal of the K_D and the intercept of the line with the abscissa is an estimate of Bmax. This latter parameter is generally standardised against a suitable reference that allows a direct comparison of receptor density in different tissues and in different studies. Protein content of the tissue homogenate or slide mounted section is commonly used as the reference and is readily measured spectrophotometrically.

A linear Scatchard plot indicates that the radioligand binds with a single affinity. Under certain circumstances the Scatchard plot yields a concave line indicating that the ligand binds to multiple populations of sites with differing affinities for the radioligand or alternatively negative co-operativity. A curvi-linear convex line may indicate positive co-operativity. The Hill plot of log (Bound/Bmax-Bound) versus log [Free] is used to interpret these possible anomalous binding interactions (Figure 1C). The Hill coefficient (the slope of the line through the points) will be approximately one when the ligand binds to a single population of sites or when the ligand is binding to multiple populations of sites with similar affinity for the radioligand. A value less than one may indicate either negative co-operativity or multiple populations of binding sites with differing affinities for the radioligand.

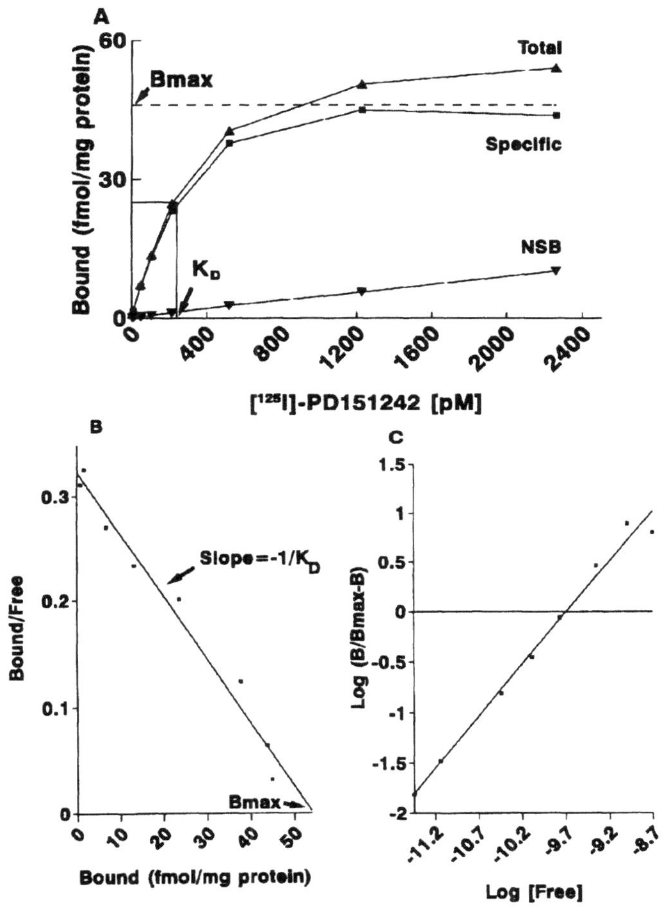

Figure 1A: Saturation isotherm for the binding of increasing concentrations [^{125}I]-PD151242 to cryostat sections of human heart. The amount of radioactivity bound to the tissue, measured in DPM by gamma counting, has been converted to fmol of [^{125}I]-PD151242 per mg of protein present in the incubation mixture. Non-specific binding (NSB) was subtracted from the total to give the amount of specific binding. An approximate value for the Bmax can be estimated from the ordinate and a K_D from the abscissa. 1B: Scatchard transformation of the data from 1A. The slope of the line is equal to the negative reciprocal of the K_D (approximately 0.3 nM) and the intercept of the line with the abscissa is an estimate of Bmax (approximately 55 fmol/mg protein). These values were then used as initial estimates in the computer programme LIGAND which used non-linear curve fitting to calculate the final binding parameters for [^{125}I]-PD151242; K_D=0.24 nM, Bmax=50.6 fmol/mg protein. IC: Hill plot of the data from 1A. The slope of the line = the Hill coefficient (nH). For [^{125}I]-PD15242, nH=1.03, indicating that the radioligand was binding with a single affinity to receptors within the heart tissue.

NON-LINEAR CURVE FITTING PROGRAMMES

In practice non-linear iterative curve fitting programmes are used to calculate final estimates of the binding parameters [1-3,9,10-12]. Non-linear regression analysis utilises equations that can define curves. KELL (Biosoft, Cambridge, UK. and Ferguson, MO, USA.) contains EBDA (Equilibrium Binding Data Analysis) and LIGAND [10,11] programmes. EBDA performs the preliminary analysis of both saturation and competition binding experiments, converting radioactivity in DPM into molar concentrations of ligand. Hill slopes are calculated and a Scatchard transformation is used to provide initial estimates of K_D and Bmax. LIGAND uses the files created by EBDA together with initial estimates of the binding parameters to fit the data to a specified model of the radioligand binding, which may be to one, two or more sites. A weighted non-linear curve fitting routine is iteratively refined to provide more accurate estimates of the K_D and Bmax values than those obtained with linear transformations.

A runs test is used to determine whether the data points differ significantly from the fitted curve. A good fit will have points randomly distributed around the fitted line whereas a run of consecutive points appearing either above or below the fitted line, may provide evidence for a significant lack of fit. In a saturation assays over a limited concentration range, many radioligands will bind with a single affinity, and a one sit fit is an appropriate model. However, curvilinear Scatchard plots displayed in the EBDA results (or a significant departure of the data from the fitted curve in the runs test) may suggest that the ligand is binding with different affinities to more than one population of receptors and a two (or possibly three site) fit should be tested, compared with a one site model. This can be tested using LIGAND by fitting a two site model and the programme calculates an F value, taking into account the improvement in the goodness of fit that accompanies an increase in the number of parameters to be fitted in the two site model compared with a one site fit. The programme will indicate which of the two models is statistically the better fit.

BINDING KINETICS

One of the first objectives in any binding study is to ensure that binding equilibrium is reached (Figure 2). The time taken for a radioligand to reach equilibrium (defined as 97% or more of the ligand bound [6] is equivalent to 5 times the $t_{1/2}$ for association (5.($\log_e$(2)/Kobs)), where Kobs is the effective or observed association rate constant. The time to reach equilibrium is dependent on temperature and the concentration of the radioligand, particularly when the concentration used in the incubation mixture to label the receptors is higher than the K_D. Kinetic experiments determine the time course of ligand association and dissociation. In association studies sections are labelled with a fixed concentration of radioligand for increasing time periods. Non-specific binding defined at each time point using a high concentration of unlabelled ligand. The plot of $\ln(B_{eq}/(B_{eq}-B_t))$ against time, where B_{eq} is the amount of ligand bound at equilibrium and B_t is the amount of ligand bound at time t, should yield a straight line through the points with slope equal to Kobs.

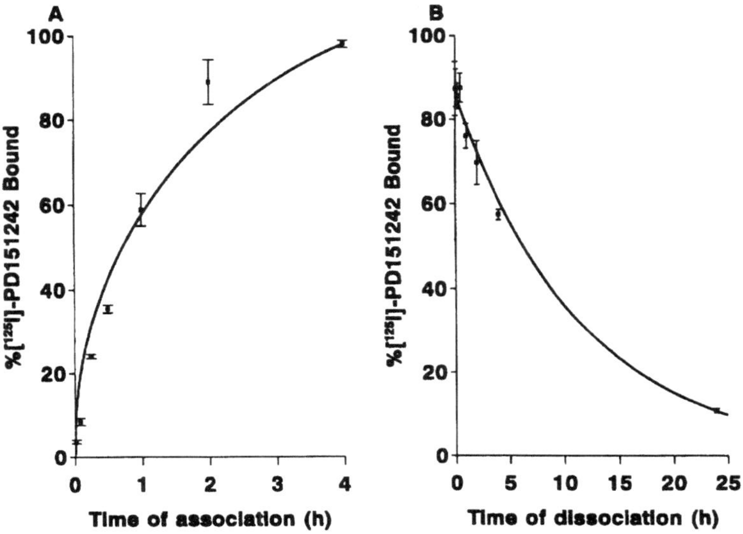

Figure 2A: An example of an association curve for 0.7nM [125I]-PD151242 binding to sections of heart muscle at 23°C. The curve plateaus after two h, indicating that equilibrium has been reached for this ligand. The calculated observed association rate constant (Kobs) was 0.0172 min-1. 3B: Time course for the dissociation of [125I]-PD151242 initiated by washing the sections in a large volume of buffer. The calculated dissociation rate constant (K-1) was 0.00144 min-1 [3].

When equilibrium is reached, dissociation of the radioligand from the receptors is achieved either by incubation of tissue sections with a high concentration of unlabelled competitor or by infinite dilution of the labelled sections by immersion in a large volume of buffer. The plot of $\ln(B_t/B_0)$ against time, where B_0 is binding at time 0, should be linear with the slope equal to the dissociation rate constant (K_{-1}, K_{21} or K_{off}). The association (K_1, K_{12} or K_{on}) and dissociation rate constants are described by the following relationship: K_1=(Kobs-K_{-1})/[L], where [L] is the concentration of free ligand. Kinetic experiments provide additional means of calculating the equilibrium dissociation constant, K_D=K_{-1}/K_1, and this should approximate that determined by saturation analysis (see above). A number of packages (for example, KINETIC in the KELL suite of programmes) are available for the non-linear curve fitting of kinetic data.

COMPETITION BINDING

Having determined the K_D of a radiolabelled ligand for a target receptor in a saturation assay, this information can be used to determine the ability of other unlabelled compounds, tested over a much wider concentration range (typically 10 pM-100 uM), to compete binding of a fixed concentration of the labelled ligand. Competition binding experiments can also be used to determine the selectivity (if any) of a particular ligand for receptor sub-types and thus allow determination of the density and proportion of each sub-type in the tissue. Competition curves are obtained by plotting specific binding as a percentage of total binding (binding in the absence of competitor) against the log concentration of the competing ligand. In Figure 3, [^{125}I]-ET-1 has been used to label all of the endothelin receptors in heart tissue, since the peptide has equal affinity for both the ET_A and ET_B sub-type. A steep competition curve is usually indicative of binding to a single population of receptors. However, increasing concentrations of unlabelled PD151242 inhibited the binding [125I]-ET-1 biphasically. A shallow curve or a curve with clear inflection points (as shown in Figure 3) is indicative of multiple populations of binding sites. The partial F-test and the runs test can again be used to differentiate single and multiple populations of binding sites. In this case, a two site fit was preferred, consistent with PD151242 binding with high affinity to the ET_A site but low, micromolar affinity to the ET_B receptors, giving about 15000 fold selectivity for the ET_A receptor.

The plot of log (%B/(100-%B)) against log [L*], where %B is the percentage of radioligand bound and [L*] is the concentration of the competing ligand, gives a line through the points with slope equal to the pseudo Hill coefficient. This approximates unity for a one site fit and is less than unity if negative co-operativity is indicated or if two or more populations of receptors with differing affinities for the competing ligand are present. However, binding constants for multiple receptor populations is difficult to determine accurately by graphical means. EBDA uses an equation that allows interpretation of a heterogeneous population of binding sites and provides estimates of the pseudo Hill coefficient and receptor affinity. LIGAND is then used to test for one, two or more binding sites as described for the analysis of saturation data.

What are the limitations of ligand binding assays?

Binding parameters may be altered by many factors including the type and ionic strength of buffer, presence of divalent ions and temperature. No standard conditions have emerged for binding assays and these parameters may have to be optimised during the development of a new radioligand. Binding assays are frequently carried under non-physiological conditions, for example to minimise degradation of the ligand. Whilst binding assays can be used to estimate the affinities of radioligands binding to human receptors in vitro, factors such as metabolism need to be considered in order to extrapolate the results to the use of radiopharmaceuticals that are to be used in vivo.

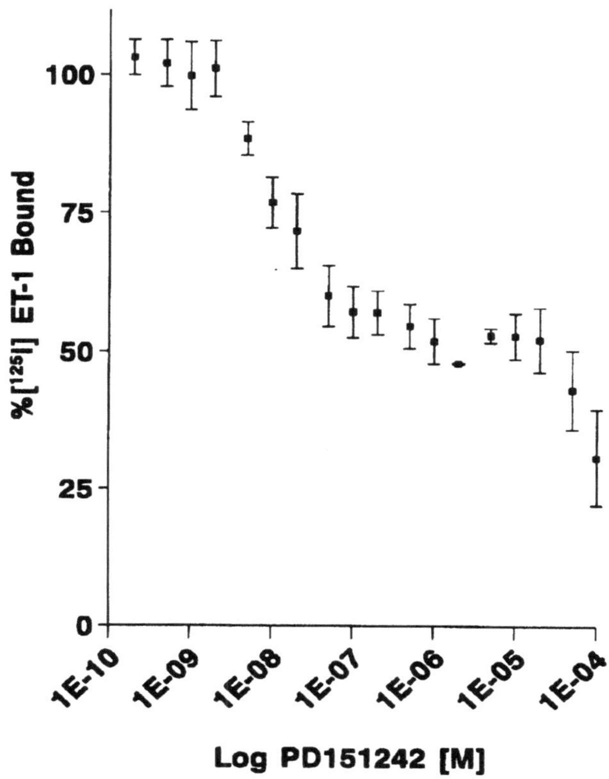

Figure 3: An example of a competition binding curve. Inhibition of 0.1 nM [125I]-ET-1 binding by increasing concentrations of unlabelled PD151242 to sections of human heart. Over the concentration range tested, PD151242 competed in a biphasic manner and a two site fit was preferred to a one site or three site model using LIGAND. The high affinity site corresponded to the endothelin ET_A receptor (K_D=7.2+2.8 nM), the low affinity site to the ET_B receptor, K_D=104+23 uM. Each value represents the mean+s.e.m. of three individuals.

Autoradiography

A detailed discussion of microautoradiography is included elsewhere in this volume. Autoradiography can be used to visualise the localisation of receptors in discrete regions of tissue and to confirm that the radioligand binds to cells that would be expected to express the target receptor. The principle of the technique is that the spatial distribution of radiolabelled ligands can be detected by the blackening of radiation sensitive film apposed directly to the section containing radiolabelled tissue. Slide mounted tissue sections are used. Sections are pre-incubated in buffer, labelled with the radioligand in the absence or presence of selective competing ligands, washed in buffer, dipped in water to remove buffer salts, and dried rapidly under a stream of cool dry air. The K_D (determined by saturation analysis) is used to calculate the concentration of the radioligand required to label a fixed proportion of receptors in the tissue. Using a concentration calculated to label 10% of the receptors results in a high ratio of total to NSB. At the end of the assay, sections are apposed to radiation sensitive film for macro-autoradiography and exposed in the dark for a period that will be determined by the type of isotope used, the density of binding sites in the tissue section and by the tissue section thickness. The films are then developed, fixed and viewed. When higher resolution is required, sections can be apposed to coverslips coated in nuclear emulsion. Developed silver grains represent the location of the bound radioligand in the underlying tissue when viewed using a microscope equipped with darkfield illumination. A number of useful derivations of the standard labelling procedure have been developed, for example computer assisted quantitative autoradiography and high resolution electron microscopic localisation of receptors.

Conclusion

The effect of radiolabelling a ligand is not always predictable. However, the selectivity and specificity of structurally novel radiolabelled ligands such as [^{125}I]-PD151242 can be tested in vitro using saturation and competition binding assays. Non-linear curve fitting programmes are recommended to test for the most appropriate model to be fitted to the data and to calculate accurate final binding parameters.

Acknowledgements

Supported by grants from the British Heart Foundation, Royal Society, BBSRC, Isaac Newton Trust and Glaxo Group Research.

Selected references

1. Davenport AP, Kuc RE, Fitzgerald F, Maguire JJ, Berryman K, Doherty AM. [125I]-PD151242: a selective radioligand for human ETA receptors. Brit J Pharmacol 1994;111:4-6.
2. Davenport AP, O'Reilly G, Kuc RE. Endothelin ETA and ETB mRNA and receptors expressed by smooth muscle in the human vasculature: majority of the ETA sub-type. Brit J Pharmacol 1995;114:1110-1116.
3. Peter MG, Davenport AP. Selectivity of [125I]-PD151242 for the human, rat and porcine endothelin ETA receptors in the heart. Brit J Pharmacol 1995;114,297-302.
4. Bylund DB, Yamamura HI. Methods in receptor Binding. In: Yamamura HI, Enna SJ, Kuhar MJ, editors. Methods in Neurotransmitter Receptor analysis. New York;Raven Press, 1990;1-35.
5. Davenport AP, Beresford IJM, Hall MD, Hill RG, Hughes J. Quantitative autoradiography. In editors van Leeuwen FW, Buijs RM, Pool, CW, Pach, O. Molecular Neuroanatomy. Elsevier;Amsterdam.1988;121-145.
6. Hulme EC, Birdsall NJM. Strategy and tactics in receptor binding studies. In:Hulme EC, editor. Receptor-ligand interactions.Oxford;IRL Press, 1992;63-176.

7. Hulme EC, Buckley NJ. Receptor preparations for binding studies. In:Hulme EC, editor. Receptor-ligand interactions. Oxford;IRL Press, 1992;177-212.
8. Jones CR, Molenaar P, Summers RJ. New Views of human cardiac B-adrenoceptors, J Mol Cell Cardiol 1989:21;519-535.
9. Molenaar P, O'Reilly G, Sharkey A, Kuc RE, Harding DP, Plumpton C, Gresham GA, Davenport AP. Characterization and localization of endothelin receptor sub-types in the human atrioventricular conducting system and myocardium. Circ Res 1993;72:526-538
10. Munson PJ, Rodbard D. LIGAND: a versatile computerized approach for characterization of ligand bonding systems. Anal Biochem 1980;107;220-239.
11. Munson PJ. LIGAND: a computerized analysis of ligand binding data. Methods Enzymol 1983;92;543-576.
12. Unnersall JR. Computer-assisted analysis of binding data. In: Yamamura HI, Enna SJ, Kuhar MJ, editors. Methods in Neurotransmitter Receptor analysis. New York;Raven Press, 1990;37-68.

MOLECULAR MODELLING - AN INTRODUCTION

David Barlow

Introduction

Computer-aided molecular modelling was once viewed as a rather specialised enterprise undertaken predominantly by protein crystallographers, but over the last ten years or so has become a key component in all research concerned with the relationships between molecular structure and function. The computing systems used not only provide the ideal means for storing, visualising and manipulating molecular structures, but also facilitate quantitative analyses and predictions of their properties and interactions. The following sections provide a general overview of the basic requirements and common methodologies involved in molecular modelling, including practical considerations and limitations of the various methods, together with specific illustrations of their utility as research tools. For further information the reader can consult Newman and Sproul for a comprehensive treatise on the principles and practice of interactive computer graphics [1]; Barrat & Mackay [2] for an account of some of the mathematics involved in molecular geometric measurements; and Clark [3] for detailed discussions of the methods employed in computational chemistry.

Generation of Models

DATA REQUIRED

The first requirement in molecular modelling is to obtain a computer model for the molecule of interest. The standard internal description of a molecule's structure takes the form of a list of the labels, coordinates and (covalent bond) connectivities for its constituent atoms. For some applications, e.g. molecular mechanics calculations, it is also necessary to provide and store details about the type of each atom, e.g. sp3, sp2 carbon, etc, and for work involving protein modelling it is also common to provide a separate summary of the protein's amino acid sequence. These data can be generated automatically if the modelling package incorporates model-building routines (vide infra), but will otherwise be entered manually (from the literature) or by accessing an appropriate structural database. Intelligent interfaces cogniscent of the file formats for

S. J. Mather (ed.), Current Directions in Radiopharmaceutical Research and Development, 181–199.

the major databases are now standard in molecular modelling packages. The databases most commonly used are the Cambridge Crystal Data File [4] and the Brookhaven Protein Databank [5] (which also holds coordinates for a number of nucleic acids and polysaccharides). Other structure descriptors may include the van der Waal's' radii and point charges of the atoms in the molecule, and the crystal lattice type and associated unit cell parameters.

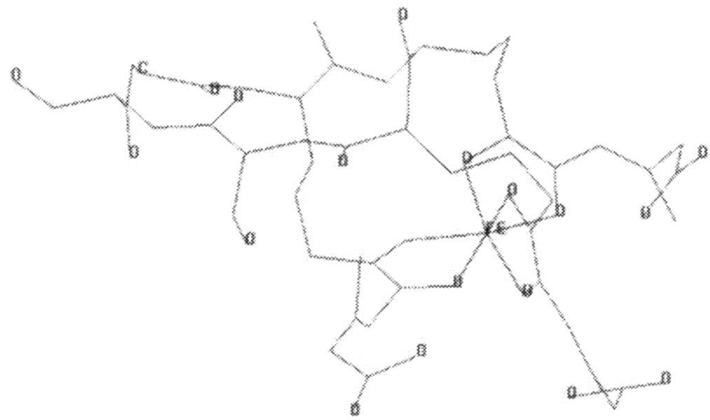

a)

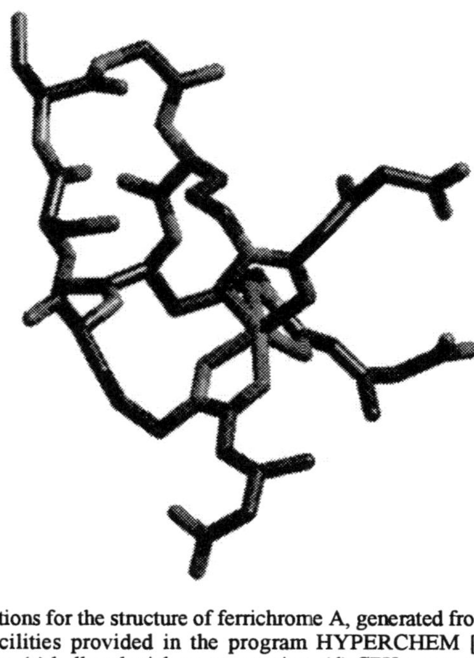

b)

Figure 1. Computer graphics representations for the structure of ferrichrome A, generated from the data of van der Helm et al. [6] using the facilities provided in the program HYPERCHEM [7]. (a) stick representation, (b) 'tubes' representation, (c) ball and stick representation, (d) CPK representation. Note that in (a)-(c) the hydrogen atoms have been omitted for the sake of clarity.

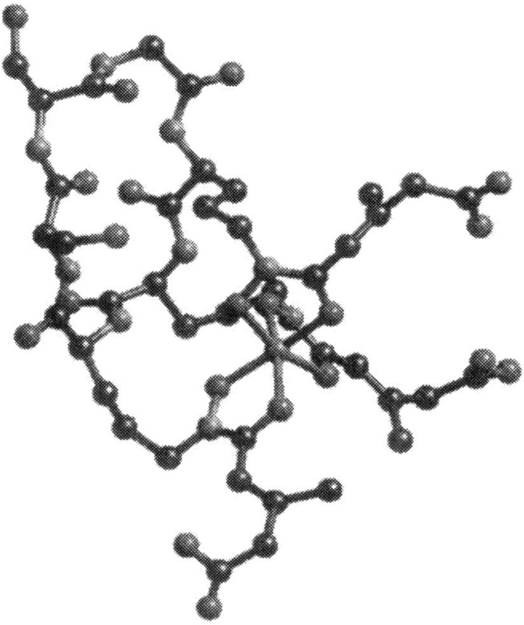

c)

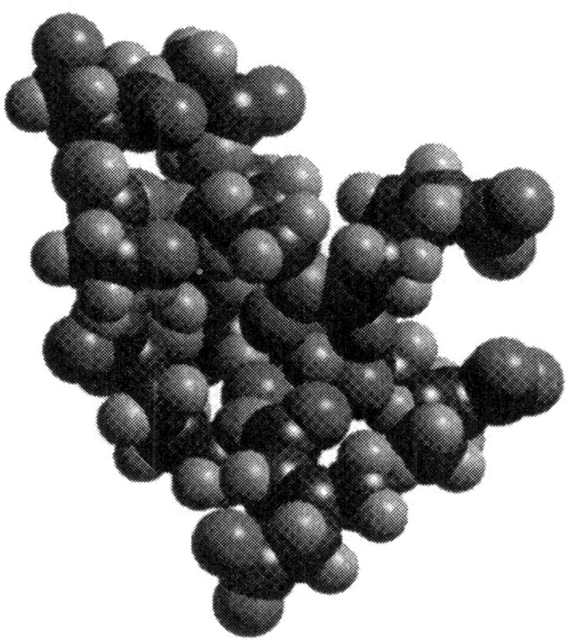

d)

For all geometric measurements on a molecule's structure, and also for the purposes of its computer graphics display and manipulation, the positions of its constituent atoms must be expressed as orthogonal (or Cartesian) coordinates, meaning simply that their spatial arrangements will be measured (usually in units of Ångstroms) relative to some arbitrary origin in a reference frame provided by three mutually perpendicular (x, y and z) coordinate axes. In the structure databases, however, the positions of the atoms in a molecule may instead be specified by fractional coordinates, so that their positions in space are mapped with reference to coordinate axes that have a geometry dictated by the molecule's unit cell. In order to convert the fractional coordinates into orthogonal coordinates it is necessary to perform an appropriate matrix transformation using the unit cell parameters, a, b, c, a, b and g.

STRUCTURE REPRESENTATION

A variety of different forms of representation are used in the computer graphics display of molecular structure. At the simplest level, the molecule will be displayed as an array of points representing its atoms (with positions determined by the atom coordinates) joined by lines (or 'tubes') indicating their covalent bonding. The resulting models are relatively uncluttered, similar in appearance to Dreiding models (see Figure 1a,b) and they can be rotated and translated interactively even when the molecules contains several thousand atoms. As a slight variation on this theme, the molecule might also be displayed as a 'ball-and-stick' structure (Figure 1c).

These 'skeletal' types of models are ideal for analyses of the conformations and interatomic interactions of molecules, but suffer the major disadvantage that they make no attempt to represent the volumes of atoms, and so give the misleading impression that molecules are quite open structures. In order to allow for a better appreciation of molecular volumes and surfaces (an important requirement when modelling the structures of intermolecular complexes), it is preferable to use some form of space-filling model. For this purpose each atom is commonly treated as a hard sphere, with a radius given by its van der Waal's radius. Each atom can then be considered as a solid object, intersecting the spheres of its bonding partners, and obscuring those of the atoms which it hides from the viewer. In this instance, the finished product is a realistic (albeit opaque) CPK-like model, which with many programs nowadays will be further enhanced by simulating the effects of light and shade (Figure 1d). As an alternative, however, the space-filling properties may be conveyed in a much more transparent manner using a 'dot surface' representation (Figure 2). Here the molecular envelope is visualised as spherical clouds of dots, the positions of which are calculated using the concept of atomic accessible area [8].

More simplified forms of structure representation have also been devised [9], specifically for use in studying complex macromolecules like proteins and nucleic acids (see Figure 3). This 'cartoon' style of representation is particularly valuable for eliminating extraneous detail present in full-atom models of these molecules, so that specific aspects of structure can be highlighted such as the spatial arrangements of secondary structures or the basic framework of an enzyme's active site.

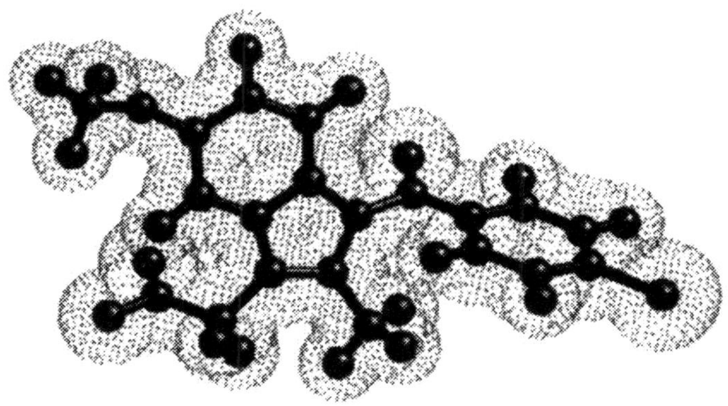

Figure 2. Computer graphics display obtained using the program HYPERCHEM [7] showing the 3-dimensional structure of the drug indomethacin, overlaid with a 'dot surface' representation of its van der Waal's surface.

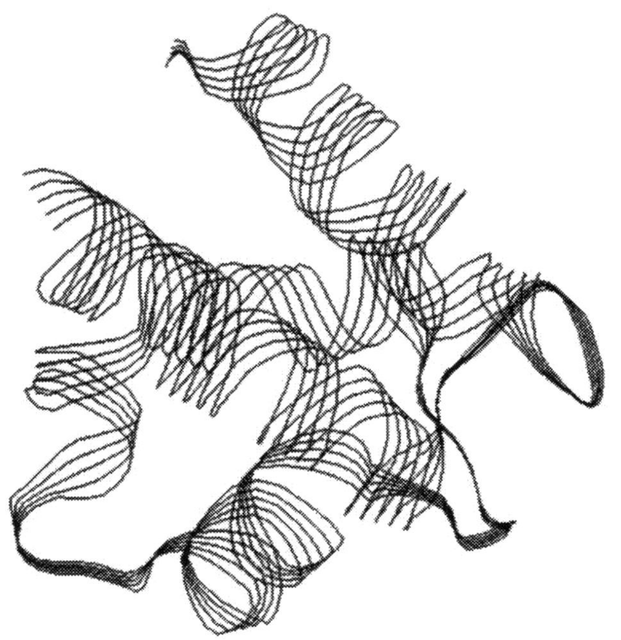

Figure 3. A 'ribbon' model illustrating the polypeptide main chain folding in the vitamin-D dependent calcium binding protein from bovine intestine [10], rendered using the program RASMOL [11].

Model Building

In the absence of any crystallographic data on the 3-dimensional structure of a molecule, computer modelling programs will often allow for the required atomic coordinates to be generated automatically. The user simply supplies the details of the atom types and their connectivities, and then the coordinates are calculated using a dictionary of 'standard' bond lengths and bond angles. At the most basic level, the model is constructed atom by atom. Each new atom added might be picked from a menu of atom types, and its bonding partner(s) in the nascent structure identified using a light pen or mouse controlled cursor. In some programs, the model can be entered simply as a free-hand, 2-dimensional 'sketch', and then a 'clean-up' tool used to convert this to a 3-dimensional chemical structure.

Since the atom-by-atom approach to model-building becomes protracted and tedious in the case of large and/or polymeric molecules, there is usually an added convenience provided by the modelling programs which allows for construction using common molecular 'building blocks', e.g., amino acids, organic bases, heterocyclic rings, etc. These building blocks are joined together merely by specifying which atoms in the structures are to be removed and replaced by a covalent bond. Modifications to the structures are then made either by deleting unwanted substituents or adding new substituents in place of hydrogen atoms. In order to speed the process of producing a fully saturated molecule, some programs also have the option to allow for a global addition of hydrogen atoms to satisfy all unfilled valencies.

Interactive Molecular Graphics

Programs that allow the interactive manipulation of molecular models are complex and sometimes machine-specific. They range from the relatively basic microcomputer-based packages like ALCHEMY [12] and NEMESIS [13], to those like INSIGHT [14] and SYBYL [15] that require more sophisticated hardware. Some of the programs like CEREUS [16] and CHEM-X [17], have a modular construction, which not only provides the versatility required to support a range of graphics devices but also facilitates expansion of the systems to cover new developments in modelling techniques. (From a practical point of view, it also means that a user can purchase only those elements of the complete package that they require or can afford!)

The basic functions supported by molecular graphics programs are summarised in Table 1. They include the facilities for inspecting the displayed models from different viewpoints and at different magnifications, and for carrying out interactive structural modifications. These and any other features supported are normally 'picked' from a fixed or 'pull down' menu of commands displayed on the computer graphics screen, using a cursor controlled by a mouse or light pen and tablet. With programs that cater for the simultaneous display of multiple molecular structures, there will be the option to manipulate each of the displayed structures independently. This allows the study of intermolecular interactions, enabling, for example, the 'docking' of substrates and inhibitors into an enzyme's active site.

Table 1. Molecular graphics structure manipulation functions

Function	Purpose
Rotation & Translation	Global movement of the molecule along and around the x, y and z axes
Pan & Zoom	Global scaling of the molecule for viewing close-up or at a distance
Slab	Alter the depth of field for the displayed structure
Rock	Continuously rotate the displayed molecule about the vertical axis, backwards and forwards through 30°
Torsion	Calculate and/or interactively alter the values of single bond torsion angles
Fragment	Identify a molecule or part of a molecule to be moved independently of the remainder of the structure(s)
Fit	Perform a least-squares fit of one structure on to another

In order to simulate the rotation and translation of the computer graphics models (at the same creating the illusion of 3-dimensionality), the atomic coordinates of the molecules are transformed by various matrix operations. Control of the rotations and translations is achieved via some peripheral device such as a joystick, tracker ball or mouse. When the molecular models are 'stationary', the impression of 3-dimensions is preserved by the use of depth-cueing and perspective techniques, so that those atoms and bonds which are furthest from the viewer are drawn more diffusely and to a smaller scale than those that are closer.

As an alternative means to obtain 3-dimensionality, the displayed figures may be drawn in 'stereo'. This requires that two views of the molecule(s) are displayed on the computer graphics screen, one rotated 6 degrees with respect to the other. If the two models are superposed and displayed simultaneously, one coloured red and the other green, a single 3-dimensional object is perceived by viewing through spectacles fitted with red/green filters. In a more sophisticated system (developed at Leeds University) the two images flash on and off the screen in rapid alternation; the user in this case wears spectacles fitted with liquid crystal lenses, which are made alternately transparent and opaque, so that each eye sees only the corresponding graphics image [18].

Structure Analysis

SIMPLE GEOMETRIC PROPERTIES

The tools necessary for performing simple geometric analyses of molecular structures are routinely provided within the multi-purpose graphics programs designed for interactive modelling. All of the programs offer the same basic set of facilities but differ in the range of additional features they provide. These differences reflect the fact that some programs are written specifically to aid in analyses of macromolecules, whilst others are more general or else are tailored for use with small or medium sized organic molecules.

The basic functions provided will generally allow for calculations of interatomic distances, bond angles, dihedral angles and real or pseudo-bond torsion angles. Among the further features provided there may be routines for obtaining the least-squares plane through a set of atoms, the absolute configuration at chiral centres, molecular volumes or molecular and/or accessible surface areas.

Simple stand-alone programs can also provide the means to calculate properties such as the extent of steric congestion around a given atom centre [19], and the dimensions of an ellipsoid having the same inertial properties as a molecule [20].

STRUCTURE COMPARISONS

In a great many modelling applications it is necessary to make both qualitative and quantitative comparisons of molecular conformations. This is particularly valuable, for example, when modelling the structures of homologous proteins, and when correlating the structures and activities of drugs acting at a common receptor. For most purposes the problem is reduced to one of superposing the atomic coordinates of the molecules and evaluating the 'fit' between them. The least-squares routines for performing these operations are available in purpose-built programs [21] and are also included in some of the general molecular graphics packages. The researcher simply identifies which atoms in the molecules are to be considered equivalent, and then uses a least-squares facility to fit the structures so that the sum of the squared distances between these atom pairs is minimised. The conformations of the molecules are normally fixed during the fitting procedure, in which case their superpositioning is achieved simply by carrying out rigid body rotations and translations of one molecule on to the other (Figure 4). With some algorithms, however [22], the fit of the molecules may be further optimised by allowing systematic variations in single bond torsion angles, and in this event the user is required to enter an upper limit for the (energy) 'penalty' incurred as a result of the conformational changes. In addition to the standard least-squares methods for molecular superpositioning, it is also possible to obtain the required fit using quaternion transformations [23], and this has the advantage that particular atom pairs can be identified as more important than others in the fitting process, so that the final superposition obtained is 'weighted' in their favour.

When performing molecular superpositions it is advantageous to do so using interactive graphics facilities because the equivalent atoms can then be more conveniently selected by means of a graphics cursor, and because the structures can first be manipulated manually, so that the user can experiment with different molecular overlaps (a feature which is especially useful when dealing with 'distantly related' molecules, where the choice of atoms for equivalencing may not be immediately obvious).

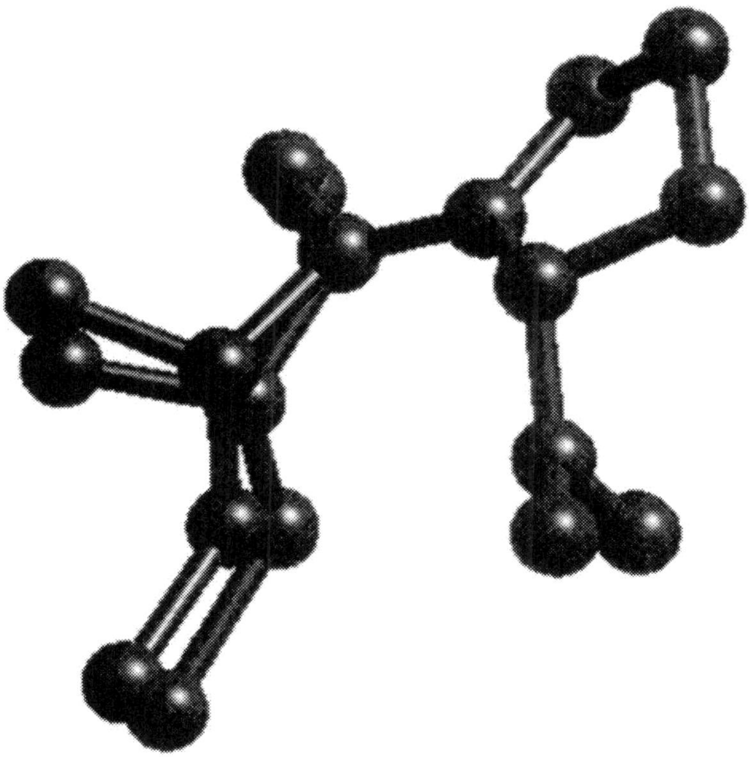

Figure 4. Computer graphics superpositioning of two conformers of the drug captopril, performed according to ref. 23, and visualised using HYPERCHEM [7].

Computational Chemistry

With nearly all modelling applications there will be an inherent subjectivity involved whenever the structures, properties or interactions of molecules are determined purely by manual or visual means. In addition of course there may be pertinent information required which just cannot be obtained by simple inspection or geometric analysis. For example, we may wish to know the relative stability of a particular conformation of a molecule, the distribution of its electron density, or the free energy change involved when it binds different ligands. As a means to obtaining solutions to these types of problems, we must have recourse to computational chemistry, and carry out some form of molecular mechanics and/or quantum mechanics calculation(s).

MOLECULAR MECHANICS

With molecular mechanics calculations we can obtain estimates of molecular and intermolecular potential energies. The total potential energy of the system is calculated as the sum of the energies associated with the different kinds of interatomic interaction. The interactions considered can be broadly grouped as those between bonded atoms and those between non-bonded atoms. The terms for bonded atom interactions essentially measure the 'strain' within the covalent structure of the molecule(s), and include terms for bond stretching, bond angle deformation and torsional (or bond twisting) deformation. The non-bonded atom interactions include those due to van der Waal's forces and electrostatic or charge-charge interactions. The total molecular (or intermolecular) potential energy ($\mathbf{E}_{total}$) is obtained as:

$$\mathbf{E}_{total} = \sum\mathbf{E}_{stretch} + \sum\mathbf{E}_{bend} + \sum\mathbf{E}_{torsion} + \sum\mathbf{E}_{vdw} + \sum\mathbf{E}_{charge}$$

where $\sum$ indicates a summation of the different energies over all atoms and bonds within the molecule(s) under investigation. For the bond stretching term, the atoms are considered as masses proportional to their atomic masses and the bonds between them are treated as mechanical springs. The deformation of each bond is considered to obey Hooke's law, with the square of the deformation and the associated strain energy related by a force constant, $k_{stretch}$:

$$\mathbf{E}_{stretch} = \mathbf{k}_{stretch}(\mathbf{d}_{obs} - \mathbf{d}_{ideal})^2$$

where $\mathbf{d}_{obs}$ and $\mathbf{d}_{ideal}$ are respectively, the calculated and ideal bond lengths. The values of $\mathbf{k}_{stretch}$ and $\mathbf{d}_{ideal}$ are different for different types of bonds (-C=C-, -C-H etc.), and are determined from analyses of small molecule crystallographic data ($\mathbf{d}_{ideal}$) and the observed modes of infrared or Raman spectroscopic bond vibrations ($\mathbf{k}_{stretch}$). Similar kinds of terms are used for evaluating the strain associated with bond angle and torsion angle deformations:

$$\mathbf{E}_{bend} = \mathbf{k}_{bend}(\mathbf{q}_{obs} - \mathbf{q}_{ideal})^2$$

$$\mathbf{E}_{torsion} = \mathbf{k}_{torsion}[1 + \cos(n\varphi - \gamma)]/2$$

with $\mathbf{k}_i$ in each case being the force constant for the deformation, the *obs* and *ideal* subscripts respectively denoting the calculated and ideal bond angles (θ), φ the observed torsion angle, n the torsion angle Fourier periodicity, and γ the corresponding phase shift.

The non-bonded interaction terms are considered for all pairs of atoms in the system investigated, with the exception of those considered in the evaluation of the bonded interactions (because the bonded interactions are calculated taking the relevant non-bonded interactions into account). The relative importance of the non-bonded interaction energies is strongly dependent upon the separations of the atoms involved, being highly significant at short range, and much less significant at long range. The charge-charge (or Coulombic) energy is evaluated as:

$$\mathbf{E}_{charge} = \theta_i\theta_j / \varepsilon r_{ij}$$

where θ_i and θ_j are the electronic charges on atoms i and j, r_{ij} is their distance of separation, and ε is the effective dielectric constant of the intervening medium. The van der Waal's interactions can be calculated using several different equations, but the Lennard-Jones potential function is perhaps the most common:

$$\mathbf{E}_{vdw} = \zeta\,[(\mathbf{d}_{min} / \mathbf{d}_{ij})^{12} - 2(\mathbf{d}_{min} / \mathbf{d}_{ij})^{6}]$$

Here, $\mathbf{d}_{ij}$ is the distance of separation of the atoms i and j and $\mathbf{d}_{min}$ is their distance of separation at the minimum energy, ζ. The first term in the expression represents the repulsive component of the interaction, which becomes dominant when the atoms approach so close to one another that their electron clouds start to overlap. The second term represents the attractive component of the interaction and measures the force arising through transient dipole-induced dipole interactions.

Other non-bonded interaction terms which might form part of the potential energy calculations include those dealing specifically with hydrogen bonding groups, and those intended to provide an estimate for the contribution to stability gained through changes in solvent entropy. In regard to this latter point, it is important to note that a great many of the reported molecular mechanics calculations are performed in the absence of solvent (that is, in vacuo), and so tend to overestimate the potential energy because of the undue weight given to electrostatic interactions. Facilities are now available, however, which will allow for the system of interest to be immersed in a 'bath' of water molecules, so that the dielectric shielding of the charge-charge interactions is handled in a more realistic fashion.

The complete set of equations used in describing the various interatomic interactions, together with the associated force constants and ideal parameter values, is commonly referred to as a *force field*. The use of such a force field for calculating molecular or intermolecular potential energies is nowadays quite painless and the results are obtained relatively quickly. Using a fairly modest desktop personal computer, the potential energy for a molecule involving less than 100 atoms will usually be evaluated within just a few seconds. It is not advisable to use such low level hardware when dealing with macromolecules like proteins, however, and for these molecules (where the numbers of atoms will generally run into the thousands) it is preferable to perform the calculations on some form of workstation incorporating RISC chip architecture.

The molecular mechanics calculations have their basis in 'classical' models of atomic and molecular structure, and so provide a relatively quick and reliable means to quantitate, for example, the relative stabilities of different conformations of a given molecule, or the relative energies involved in different modes of ligand binding to a 'receptor' structure. With some of the more recent sophistications, it is even possible now to compute changes in free energy - evaluating the ΔG associated with a particular process, therefore, and not just the ΔH. It is important to note, however, that the form of the force field employed in any molecular mechanics calculation must be appropriate for the molecule under study. That is to say, the force constants, ideal bond lengths and ideal bond angles etc., are usually optimised for use with a restricted subset of molecules (proteins, saccharides etc.), and will not necessarily give sensible results when used in calculations made for molecules not included within this subset. Some of the more widely used force fields include MM2/MM+ [24], COSMIC [25], AMBER [26] and CHARMM [27]; the former are good general-purpose force fields, whilst that latter two are intended primarily for simulations involving proteins and nucleic acids.

The most significant disadvantage of the molecular mechanics calculations is the fact that they are only concerned with the atomic nuclei in a molecule and so they cannot be used to provide information about its electronic properties. In order to obtain this type of detail it is necessary to perform quantum mechanical calculations.

QUANTUM MECHANICS

With the aid of quantum mechanical (QM) calculations it is possible to determine the distribution of electron density in a molecule, and from this then to derive a great many other properties of interest. The QM calculations are much more complex than the molecular mechanics calculations and in consequence require far greater computing time and resources. The calculations involve the use of molecular orbital theory to find solutions to the Schrödinger wave equation. In order to make the calculations tractable, the required solutions are sought following two simplifying approximations. The first of these is the Born-Oppenheimer approximation, in which the atomic nuclei are regarded as stationary, because of the fact that their masses are around 1800 times lighter, and their movements thus that much slower, than those of their orbiting electrons. The second is the Hartree-Fock approximation, in which the interaction of each electron with all other electrons in the system is subsumed within a single 'effective field' term. Even with these simplifications, however, the solutions to the wave equations cannot be determined in an exact, analytic fashion, and so the further step is taken to obtain the solutions using an iterative numeric procedure. The most rigorous and thus most reliable of these numeric procedures will treat each electron within the system explicitly and take account of its interaction with every other electron and proton present. These methods (often referred to as ab initio methods) are provided for in programs such as the GAUSSIAN programs [28]. Note, however, that they are highly costly in terms of computer resources and are entirely prohibitive for molecules involving 100 or more atoms. If the molecule of interest is larger than this, therefore (or if the only computer available is just not up to it!) it is necessary instead to use one of the semi-empirical QM procedures. These procedures are about 1000 times faster than the ab initio methods, and they achieve this improved performance by simplifying or approximating particular atomic orbital interactions (using estimates based upon empirical findings). In the most commonly used semi-empirical procedures, CNDO [29] and MNDO [30], the simplifying assumptions made involve varying degrees of simplification in the treatment of electron orbital overlaps. A more recent, and more accurate semi-empirical method is provided by AM1 [30].

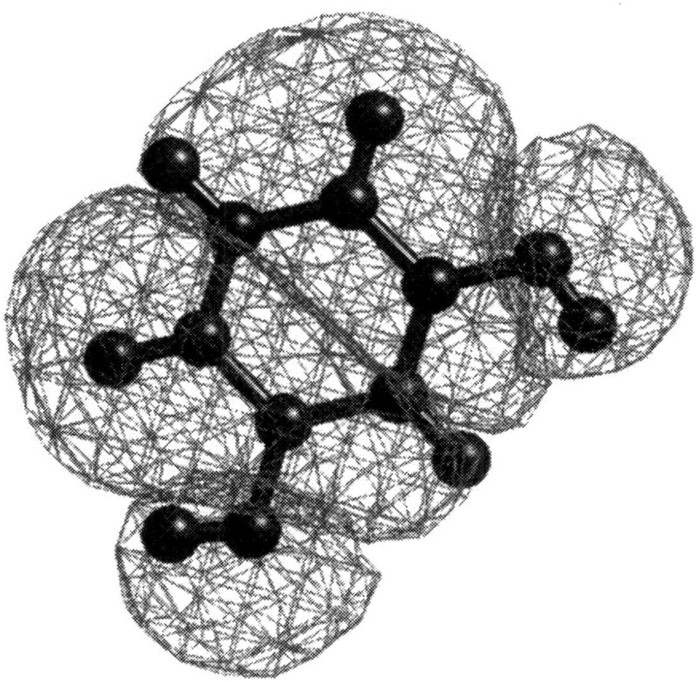

Figure 5. Computer graphics display of the 3-dimensional structure of resorcinol, together with its highest occupied molecular orbital (HOMO). The display and necessary QM calculations were performed using HYPERCHEM [7], with the frontier orbitals modelled using the semi-empirical method, AM1 [30].

Most frequently the QM modelling methods are used to provide a set of atomic point charges for use in quantitating the contribution made by electrostatic interactions in force field calculations. In addition they are employed as a means to determine the electrostatic fields surrounding molecules, providing a guide to experimenters concerned with complementarity in intermolecular complexes. The molecular orbitals themselves also have utility, in enabling the identification of sites of reactivity within a molecule. The two specific orbitals of interest in this context are the highest occupied molecular orbital (or HOMO) and the lowest unoccupied molecular orbital (or LUMO). The HOMO is the highest energy orbital occupied by an electron, and its shape and location reveal the site of the most reactive electron in a molecule. The LUMO is the lowest energy orbital which is not occupied by an electron, and it is this orbital which will be filled when an extra electron adds to the molecule. Knowledge of these two (frontier) orbitals for molecules (see Figure 5) can give insights into their relative susceptibilities towards nucleophilic and electrophilic attack and allow predictions to be made about their likely mechanisms of reaction.

In choosing between ab initio and semi-empirical calculations, most users will generally opt for the latter, simply because life is too short to do otherwise. It should be noted, however, that the extra accuracy of the ab initio calculations may not be warranted in any case, and that perfectly satisfactory 'working models' can be obtained with the semi-empirical methods. The choice between the various flavours of semi-empirical calculations may be more difficult to make, and in this instance the user should pay heed to the kinds of problems that each is able to cope with. Extended Hückel calculations [31], for example, do not include any explicit treatment of the electron-electron interactions within a molecule, and so are particularly ill-suited for systems involving π-bonds, although they are perfectly adequate in qualitative applications of QM calculations, such as frontier orbital estimates of chemical reactivity. The CNDO calculations, although generally better than the Extended Hückel calculations, are completely incapable of dealing with systems where electron spin is important. In compensation, however, the CNDO method allows mixed mode calculations, which means that defined parts of the system under investigation can be treated using classical mechanics, whilst the remainder of the system is treated in QM fashion. MNDO provides some improvement over CNDO, particularly in the treatment of polar compounds, but still has limitations; it is not very good in its treatment of hydrogen bonds, sterically crowded molecules or four membered ring systems. AM1 will tend to give better results on the whole (being much better for molecules with hydrogen bonds) but MNDO has the edge in dealing with fluorine- and phosphorus-containing molecules.

Structure Refinement by Energy Minimisation

As a means to optimise the geometry of a molecular model (to 'iron out' the imperfections in 'hand-built' structures) it is common practice to use the technique of potential energy minimisation. This involves using a molecular mechanics force field to calculate the potential energy of the system, and some form of iterative procedure which will transform it stepwise to a state of lower potential energy. At each iteration the conformation of the molecule(s) may be altered through rotations about single bond torsion angles, with the interatomic bond lengths and bond angles all kept fixed.

Optimisations of this kind are speedily performed but are unlikely to yield a structure corresponding to the 'true' energy minimum (because small changes in bond lengths and/or bond angles may very often serve to alleviate some of the strain associated with unfavourable non-bonded atom interactions). For more reliable results, therefore, the iteration process is better performed using a stepwise refinement of the individual atom positions. The termination criteria employed in the refinement process will generally involve a continuation of the iterations until the computed potential energy or its gradient (that is, its difference from one iteration to the next) reaches some user-specified limit. The number of iterations required to achieve these convergence criteria will depend upon the size and complexity of the system studied, and its conformation at the start of the minimisation process. It will also be a function of the mathematical procedure employed to achieve the refinement.

During the course of the iteration process, a variety of different algorithms may be used to direct the structure towards a potential energy minimum. Methods such as the steepest descent method are quick to take a poor structure to the general vicinity of a potential minimum, but may tend to 'hunt' around the minimum when they get close to it. Other methods like the Newton-Raphson method are quite a bit slower but solid and dependable. The best general-purpose compromise is provided by the so-called conjugate gradient methods (for example, the Fletcher-Reeves and Polak-Ribiere algorithms). For a good general discussion of the various optimisation algorithms the reader may refer to Bunday [32].
The computing time required to energy minimise a molecular model will obviously depend on the size of the system under study, the nature of the hardware used, and also on the type of force field and optimisation algorithm employed. Table 2 shows some representative statistics for the calculations performed on an average-sized molecule (a peptide with 50 atoms) using several different computing platforms.

Table 2. Potential energy minimisation times for Thyrotropin releasing hormone

Hardware	Force field	Minimisation time (for 100 iterations)
386 SX 25MHz PC	Cosmic [25]	186 seconds
486 DX2 66MHz PC	Cosmic	60 seconds
SG Indigo	Amber [26]	30 seconds
SG Iris 4D 35 GT	Amber	20 seconds

As with the QM modelling, it pays to give some thought to the purpose of carrying out the energy, and then to judge the level of treatment most appropriate. Thus, if the only reason for performing the refinement is to regularise the bonded geometry of a model, it will certainly not be necessary to include solvent in the calculations, and probably also unnecessary to worry too much about the electrostatic interactions. The choice of convergence criteria will often be rather arbitrary and, in addition to monitoring the change in potential energy during the minimisation, it is a good idea also to visualise the structure at various intervals, so that when the changes to the atomic coordinates become visibly imperceptible, the user can intervene to avoid superfluous calculations. Note too, that at the end of the minimisation it is best to check the final molecular geometry 'by hand', because there is no guarantee that the minimiser will have done its job properly, particularly if the starting structure was very poor.

Molecular Dynamics

As a means of studying the *dynamic* behaviour of one or more molecules, it is only necessary to determine the forces experienced by their component atoms (which can be achieved using force field calculations) and then to solve Newton's equations of motion to obtain the trajectories of the atoms as a function of time [33]. For each atom i, the differential equation which must be solved is:

$$-\delta V_i / \delta r_i = m_i (\delta^2 r_i / \delta t_i^2)$$

where r_i is its position vector (that is, the set of its Cartesian coordinates), m_i is its mass, V_i is the potential energy resulting from its interaction with all other atoms in the system, and t is time. The solution to the equation is evaluated numerically using a Taylor series expansion:

$$r_{(t + \Delta t)} = r_{(t)} + \Delta t (\delta r / \delta t) + \Delta t^2 (\delta^2 r / \delta t^2) / 2 + \ldots\ldots$$

We thus need to know the position (r), velocity ($\delta r / \delta t$) and acceleration ($\delta^2 r / \delta t^2$) of each atom i at time t, and we can then work out its new position a short time later (at time, $t + \Delta t$).

In order to perform these molecular dynamics (or MD) calculations successfully, it is important to ensure that the time step, Δt, is sufficiently small that we can properly model the fastest vibrating atoms in the structure. Given that the fastest moving atoms are hydrogen atoms, which, in C-H bonds are known to vibrate with a frequency of 10^{-14} s, it is apparent that we must use time steps of about 10^{-15}s (i.e., one femtosecond). Since the motions of the heavy atoms in the molecule will occur on a picosecond (ps) time scale (that is, 10^{-12} s) the complete dynamics simulation must be run for at least 10ps, and ideally for several 100ps. It should be noted, however, that the MD simulations will generally take quite some time to calculate (particularly if the molecule has several hundred atoms) and so the 10ps runs are more common than the longer simulations. As a result of this limitation, full MD simulations which are run at normal temperatures cannot be used to probe dynamic events which occur on second or even millisecond time scales. This means that they cannot be used for studying protein folding or unfolding, nor can they be used to follow the dynamic exchange of surfactant molecules between micelles and solution.

At each iteration of an MD simulation, the atomic coordinates of the molecule(s) will normally be saved to a disk file so that, on completion of all the calculations, the movements of its atoms over time can be 'replayed' on the computer graphics screen in the form of a movie. From a study of such a movie it is possible to visualise the extent of a molecule's conformational freedom, and to judge the importance of specific interatomic interactions in maintaining its structure.

CONFORMATIONAL SEARCHING

When seeking to find the global potential energy minimum for a molecule, or when endeavouring to obtain a population of its conformers all of which have low energy, the MD procedures can be modified to enable simulated annealing calculations. With this approach the system studied will first be equilibrated at a low temperature of say 300K (so that the atomic velocities are fairly low) and will then be subjected to a period of 'heating' to take it to a much higher temperature. At the higher temperature (typically around 600-1000K) the atoms will have much higher velocities and so in any given time period the molecule can 'visit' a greater range of conformations. Over the period of the high temperature simulation the coordinates of the molecule(s) studied will be stored at regular intervals. Each of these conformers can then be subjected to a separate MD simulation in which the temperature of the system is slowly returned to its starting level. A subsequent energy minimisation for each of these 'cooled' conformations will then provide the required population of low energy structures, and if the conformer corresponding to the global energy minimum is required the user can simply select the one from this set that has the lowest energy. (Whether or not this conformer actually corresponds to the global energy minimum will of course depend on the efficiency with which the simulated annealing process has allowed the molecule to sample the available conformational space.)

Both the simulated annealing and normal (quenched) MD simulations (and indeed any energy minimisation calculations) can be carried out with certain constraints in force. Such constrained simulations are commonly used in generating one or more molecular models consistent with 2D-1H NMR data, for example, where the constraints applied take the form of lower and upper bounds for specific interatomic separations determined from the spectroscopic results.

Conclusions

The foregoing discussions will hopefully have conveyed that computational chemistry and molecular graphics techniques provide invaluable tools for all aspects of chemical and biochemical research. The computer programs required are nowadays made very easy to use, and the necessary hardware is readily available and affordable. Users are no longer required to be card-carrying members of the computer literati, therefore, merely scientists who have an interest in pursuing interpretations of their experimental data at the molecular level.

References

1. Newman WM, Sproul DF. Principles of interactive computer graphics. New York: McGraw-Hill, 1979.
2. Barrat AN, Mackay AL, editors. Spatial structures and the microcomputer. Basingstoke: Macmillan, 1987.
3. Clark T. A handbook of computational chemistry. New York: Wiley, 1985.
4. Allen FH, Bellard SH, Brice MD, Cartwright BA, Doubleway A, Higgs H, Hummelink T, Hummelink-Peters BG, Kennard O, Motherwell WDS, Rodgers JA, Watson DA. The Cambridge crystallographic data centre: computer-based search, retrieval, analysis and display of information Acta Crystallogr 1978;35:2331-9.
5. Bernstein FC, Koetzle TF, Williams GJB, Meyer Jr EF, Brice MD, Rodgers JR, Kennard O, Shimanouchi T, Tasumi M. The protein data bank: a computer-based archival file for macromolecular structures. J Mol Biol 1977;112:535-42.
6. van der Helm D, Baker JR, Loghry RA, Ekstrand JD. Structures of alumichrome A and ferrichrome A at low temperature. Acta Cryst Sect B 1981;37:323-30.
7. HYPERCHEM, distributed by Hypercube, Inc., 419 Phillips Street, Waterloo, Ontario N2L 3X2.
8. Richards FM. Areas, volumes, packing and protein structure. Ann Rev Biophys Bioeng 1977;6:151-176.
9. Richardson JS. Anatomy and taxonomy of protein structure. Adv Protein Chem 1981;34:167-339.
10. Szbenyi DME, Obendorf SK, Moffat K. Structure of vitamin D-dependent calcium binding protein from bovine intestine. Nature 1981;294:327-32.
11. Sayle RA, Milner-White EJ. Rasmol - biomolecular graphics for all. TIBS 1995;20:374-6.
12. ALCHEMY, distributed by Evans & Sutherland / Tripos, Parkers House, 46 Regent Street, Cambridge CB2 1DB.
13. NEMESIS, distributed by Oxford Molecular Ltd., South Parks Road, Oxford OX1 3UB.
14. INSIGHT, developed by Hagler A, Agouron Institute, University of California, San Diego; distributed by Biosym Technologies Inc, Suite 101, 9605 Scranton Road, San Diego, California.
15. SYBYL, developed by Marshall G, University of Washington, St Louis, Missouri.
16. CEREUS, distributed by Molecular Simulations Inc, 9685 Scranton Road, San Diego, California.
17. CHEM-X, developed by Davies K, University of Cambridge; distributed by Chemical Design Ltd, Unit 12, 7 West Way, Oxford OX2 0JB.
18. Leeds Liquid crystal 3-D viewer, Millenium, Steveange, Herts SG1 4QX.
19. Wipke WP, Gund P. A conformation-dependent measure of steric environment. J Am Chem Soc 1974;96:299-300.
20. Taylor WR, Thornton JM, Turnell WG. An ellipsoid approximation of protein shape. J Mol Graphics 1983;1:30-9.
21. Cory M, Bentley J. MATCHMOL, an interactive computer graphics procedure for superposition of molecular models. J Mol Graphics 1984;2:39-42.
22. Lejeune J, Michel AG, Vercauteren DP. Interactive flexible molecular fitting program to be integrated into computer-adied molecular modelling systems. J Mol Graphics 1986;4:194-99.
23. Mackay AL. Quaternion transformation of molecular orientation. Acta Crystallogr Sect A 1984;40:165-166.
24. Allinger NL. Conformational analysis. 130. MM2. A hydrocarbon force field utilizing V1 and V2 torsional terms. J Am Chem Soc 1977;99:8127-37.
25. Vinter JG, Davis A, Saunders MR. Strategic approaches to drug design. I. An integrated software framework for molecular modelling. J Comp Aided Mol Design 1987;1:31-51.
26. Weiner SJ, Kollman PA, Nguyen DT, Case DA. An all atom force field for simulations of proteins and nucleic acids. J Comp Chem 1986;7:230-252.

27. Brooks BR, Bruccoleri RE, Olafson BD, States DJ, Swaminathan S, Karplus M. CHARMM: a program for macromolecular energy minimization and dynamics calculations. J Comp Chem 1983;4:187-217.
28. Binkley JS, Whiteside RA, Raghavachari K, Seeger R, DeFrees DJ, Schlegel HB, Frisch MJ, Pople JA, Kahn LR, GAUSSIAN 82 Release A, Carnegie-Mellon University, Pittsburg, 1982.
29. Pople JA, Beveridge DL. Approximate molecular orbital theory. New York: McGraw-Hill, 1970.
30. Stewart JJP. MOPAC: A semi-empirical molecular orbital program. J Comp Aided Mol Design 1990;4:1-105.
31. Hoffman R. An extended Hückel theory. J Chem Phys 1963;39:1397-1412.
32. Bunday BD. Basic optimisation methods. Baltimore: Edward Arnold, 1984.
33. van Gunsteren WF, Berendsen HJC. Computer simulation of molecular dynamics - methodology, applications and perspectives in chemistry. Ang Chemie 1990;29:992-1023.

COMPUTER MODELLING OF METAL-BASED RADIOPHARMACEUTICALS

Robert D. Hancock

Introduction

The metals of interest in this chapter are primarily Tc, Ga and In, because of their importance in radiopharmaceuticals discussed in other chapters. Metal ions of potential interest such as alkali metals and lanthanides will also be discussed. Molecular Mechanics (MM) is an important aid in molecular design. The use of MM has been greatly facilitated by the availability of user-friendly packages, with menu driven operation, and excellent colour graphics. Most of these packages also make possible wave-mechanical calculations, which are useful in predicting properties such as electronic spectra, and magnetic properties. A selection of computer molecular modelling packages is listed below:

1) CAChe system, CAChe Scientific Inc. P. O. Box 4003, Beaverton, OREGON 97076, USA. (Runs on special Power Mac with enhanced performance).
2) SPARTAN, from Wavefunction, 18401 Von Karman, Suite 370, Irvine CA 92715, USA. (both Silicon Graphics and Power Mac Versions available).
3) SYBYL from TRIPOS Associates, 1699 South Hanley Road, St. Louis, MO, USA. (requires Silicon Graphics or other workstation such as SUN)
4) BIOSYM, from BIOSYM Technologies, Inc.
5) HYPERCHEM, which will run on a 486DX or better PC.
6) ALCHEMY, a simpler package which is very useful, available from TRIPOS. (Both PC and Mac versions available.).

The aim of this chapter will be to show how MM and other theoretical calculations can be used as an aid to ligand design. It is important at the outset to stress that such calculations are an aid to the knowledge, insight and intuition of the researcher, and are not a substitute for these abilities.

S. J. Mather (ed.), Current Directions in Radiopharmaceutical Research and Development, 201–217.

MM modelling of Complexes of Metal ions

In the MM approach[1-5] the bonds and bond angles in the molecule are treated purely mechanically, being described with simple Hooke's Law expressions, as below for bond length deformation:

$$U_B = 1/2K_B(r - r^{\circ})^2 \qquad [1]$$

where U_B is the steric energy of bond length deformation, K_B is the force constant acting to restore the bond length (r) to the ideal bond length (r°), which is the bond length observed in molecules of minimum strain. Other contributions to the steric energy of the molecule are considered, such as torsional contributions (U_f), van der Waal's repulsions (U_{NB}), electrostatic interactions, and hydrogen bonds. The modelling of these contributions in MM is discussed in greater detail elsewhere[1-5]. Of importance later for Tc complexes are torsional contributions, which are given by the expression

$$U_f = V/2[\,1 + S.\cos(n.f)] \qquad [2]$$

In equation 2, V is the torsional barrier to rotation, the periodicity n is the number of minima in energy in a rotation of 360° about the bond, f is the torsional angle, and *S* has a value of +1 when minima occur for staggered systems (e.g. ethane), and -1 when minima occur for eclipsed systems (e.g. ethylene).

Modelling the geometry around metal ions presents some problems, not present for sp^3 hybridised atoms, or atoms of lower coordination number than four. One, which we will call the *labelling problem*, relates to the fact that, in the simplest example of a square planar metal ion, as shown below, some of the donor atoms are *cis* to each other, and require 90° ideal L-M-L bond angles (L = ligand, M = metal), while others are *trans*, and require 180° L-M-L angles. One approach is to define two types of donor atom, which are identical, but form different L-M-L angles with each other. Thus, in square planar $[Cu(NH_3)_4]^{2+}$, for example, the nitrogen donors are labelled N_A and N_B, and N_A-Cu-N_A and N_B-Cu-N_B ideal angles are set to 180°, while N_A-Cu-N_B angles are set to 90°.

For an octahedron, such as in $[Co(NH_3)_6]^{3+}$, three types of donor atom are required (above), and for higher coordination numbers this approach becomes hopelessly complicated. One approach to overcoming this difficulty is not to define L-M-L bond angles around the metal ion, and to let van der Waal's repulsion between the donor atoms generate the geometry. This approach is fairly satisfactory for small metal ions, but for larger metal ions such as octahedral In(III), the approach may fail because the atoms are too far apart to repel each other and maintain regular octahedral geometry.

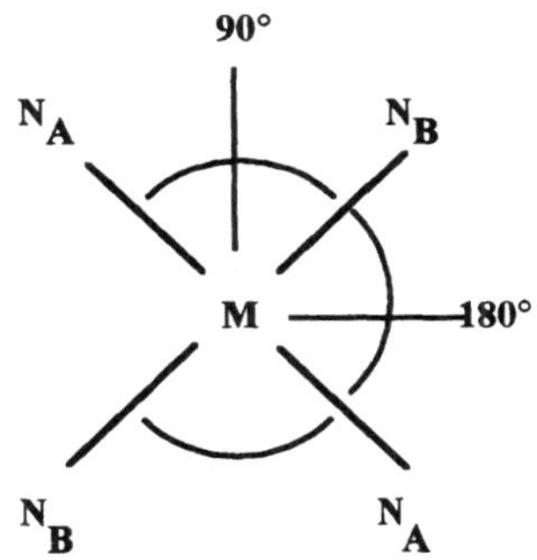

square planar

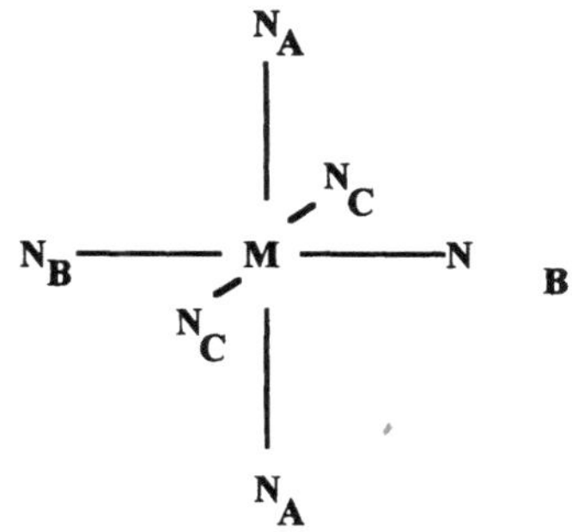

octahedral

Alternatively, the geometry can be generated by electrostatic repulsion between charges on the donor atoms. For coordination numbers above six, the latter two are really the only practical approaches, and are reasonably satisfactory. In SYBYL, the program automatically switches to modelling the geometry around an atom by van der Waal's repulsion when the coordination number is defined in the atom type table to exceed four, although this feature may be overridden if labelling of the donor atoms is required for modelling with defined L-M-L bond angles. A program such as CAChe is able to recognise from the hybridisation specified for a metal ion whether an angle should be 90°, 109.5°, 120° or 180°, and set the ideal L-M-L angle accordingly. A menu containing different hybridisation schemes for metal ions is presented, e.g. dsp^2, dsp^3, or d^2sp^3, and the L-M-L angles are correctly set according to the hybridisation scheme selected. If it is desired to set the force constants for the L-M-L angles to zero, or define a geometry not present in the range of geometries offered, the *s* hybridisation scheme is selected.

Those strategies for representing the resistance of the M-L bond to bond length deformation that use an ideal M-L bond length and associated force constant are usually referred to[1-5] as a 'covalent' representation. An alternative approach is not to define any specific bonds between the metal ion and the ligand, but simply to place negative charges on the donor atoms and allow the attraction between these and the positive charge placed on the metal ion to pull the donor atoms in towards the metal ion. In this approach the donor atoms are prevented from approaching too close to the metal ion by the van der Waal's radii of the donor atoms and the metal ion. The latter approach is usually referred to as the 'ionic' model. One would expect the ionic approach to be appropriate for alkali and alkaline earth metals, and the covalent approach to be more appropriate for most other metal ions. A particular problem with the ionic approach is the estimation of the best charges on the metal ion and donor atoms, to be used in the calculation. A further complication is that these will not be constant, but change as the complex is formed, due to polarisation effects. An advantage of the ionic approach is that coordination number can change during the course of refinement of the structure.

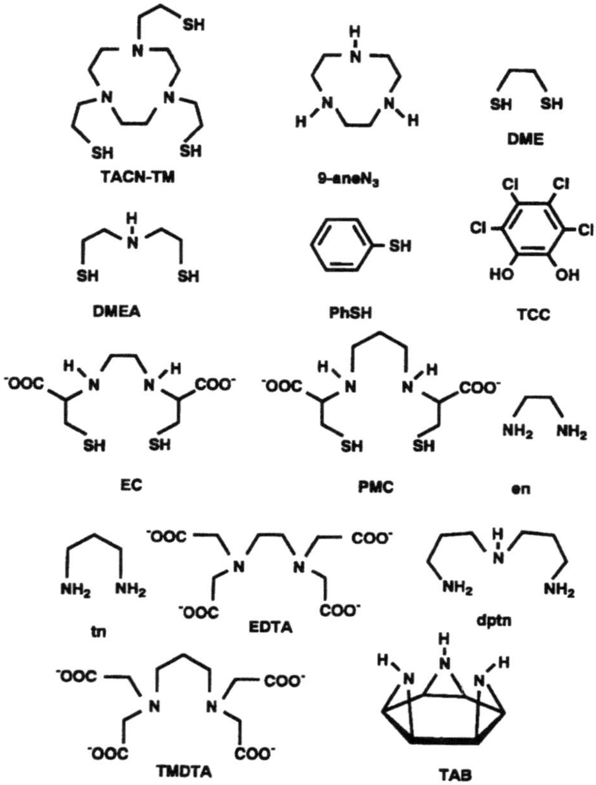

Figure 1. Ligands discussed in this chapter.

DEVELOPMENT OF MM MODELS OF COMPLEXES OF METAL IONS

a) Gallium(III) and Indium(III). In the experience of the present author, the parameters present in commercially available programs for modelling complexes of metal ions are generally not satisfactory for detailed work, and modellers should provide their own parameters for the systems to be studied This arises because of the larger number of oxidation states, spin states, and coordination geometries that are possible for metallic elements, as compared with the limited number adopted by carbon, hydrogen, and other elements commonly found in organic compounds. The literature may be consulted for suitable parameters for metal ions. If these are not available, one can search the Cambridge Crystallographic Data Base for structures containing the metal ion of interest, and of appropriate structure type. Thus, when it was decided[6] to parametrise octahedral complexes of In(III) and Ga(III) with saturated nitrogen, sulphur, and oxygen donors, the Database yielded some six suitable structures for each metal ion. In the case of In(III), this included the structure of the TACN-TM complex[7], (see Fig. 1 for key to ligand abbreviations) which provided a basis for obtaining ideal In-S and In-N bond lengths, and a hydroxy bridged 9-aneN3 complex[8] , which provided In-N and In-O bond lengths. The next step was to model the complexes of In(III), and vary the parameters involving In-L bonds until the agreement between MM generated and crystallographically observed structures was as close as possible. One may write one's own subroutine to carry out the parameter optimisation, although in most cases doing this by hand will yield acceptable results. The parameters in Table 1, developed for In(III) and Ga(III) were used[6] to predict the structures of their complexes with the ligand EC, and subsequent determination[9] of the crystal structures demonstrated good agreement with those predicted[6]. In Figure 2 are shown the MM generated and subsequent crystallographically determined structures of $[In(EC)]^-$. In Table 1 are given parameters which will work satisfactorily with the TAF[10] force field for modelling complexes of In(III) and Ga(III), and, with at most small modification, with the MM2 force field[11].

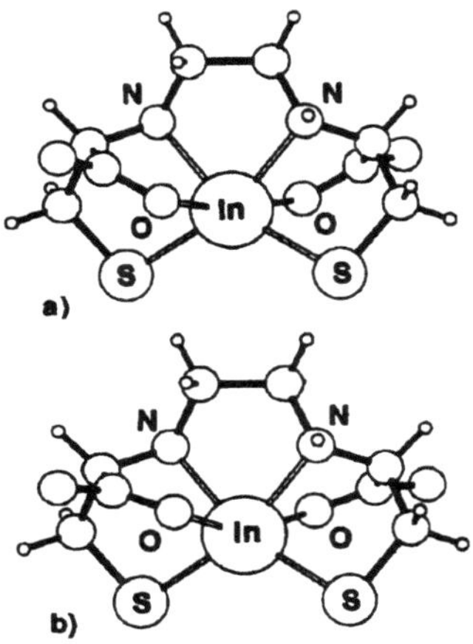

Figure 2. (a) The MM predicted[6], and (b) the structure observed subsequently[9] for the In(III) complex of EC. The structure was generated using the TAFF force field[10] supplemented by parameters shown in Table 1. Redrawn after reference 9.

Table 1. MM parameters for modelling complexes of In(III) and Ga(III)[a].

Bond length deformation parameters.

Bond	strain free length (Å)	force constant ($kcal.mol^{-1}.Å^{-1}$)
In-N	2.38	200
In-S	2.51	100
In-O	2.23	100
Ga-N	2.15	200
Ga-S	2.34	100
Ga-O	2.04	100

Bond angle deformation parameters[b].

Bond angle	strain free angle (deg)	force constant ($kcal.mol^{-1}.deg^{-1}$)
N-In-N	90	0.005
N-In-S	90	0.005
N-In-O	90	0.005
In-N-C	112	0.02
In-O-C	109.5	0.02
S-In-S	90	0.005
O-In-O	90	0.005
O-In-S	90	0.005
In-S-C	97	0.02

[a]For use in conjunction with the TAFF force field present in SYBYL[10], although these parameters should be satisfactory with at most minor modification with the MM2 force field[11]. To convert the units in this table to the other commonly used units, note that 144 kcal.mol^{-1}.Å^{-1} = 1 mdyn..Å^{-1}
[b]The angle constants for Ga(III) are the same as for In(III). Note that all torsional constants in volving Ga and In are set to zero.

b) Complexes containing the Technetium(V) oxo group. This important type of Tc complex presents an interesting problem in MM modelling[12]. The Tc(V) oxo complexes have the oxo group placed on the apex of the Tc, which lies some 0.7Å above the plane created by the other four donor atoms (Figure 3). This aspect of the structural chemistry of these complexes is readily reproduced by defining appropriate ideal O-Tc-L angles. The feature of the Tc(V) oxo complexes that is difficult to reproduce is the fact that, for example (Figure 3), the ethylene bridges in $[TcO(DME)_2]^-$ do not lie symmetrically about the plane formed by the Tc and two S donors, but are displaced above this plane on the side of the complex containing the oxo group. The key to reproducing this feature lies in recognising the proposed[13] role of p-bonding in the Tc-S bond. The need for this contribution becomes apparent when one examines structures such as the [TcO(DMEA)SPh] structure[14] shown in Fig 4. One sees that the O=Tc-S-C torsional angle is close to 90°, and this is typical of structures of Tc(V)=O containing a unidentate thiolate anion. This feature is not reproduced without a torsional barrier to rotation about the Tc-S bond. This barrier is at a minimum when the O=Tc-S-C torsion angle is 90 or 270°. This means that n in equation [2] has a value of 2, and *S* is positive.

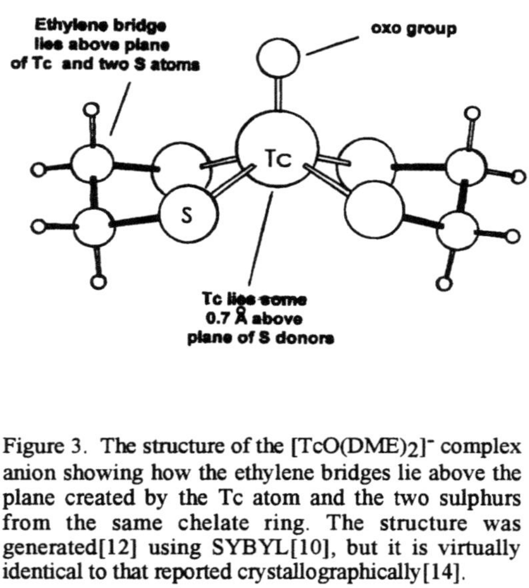

Figure 3. The structure of the $[TcO(DME)_2]^-$ complex anion showing how the ethylene bridges lie above the plane created by the Tc atom and the two sulphurs from the same chelate ring. The structure was generated[12] using SYBYL[10], but it is virtually identical to that reported crystallographically[14].

The same feature is present in the negatively charged N from deprotonated amide groups bonded to Tc, and in phenolic oxygens, where the filled p_z orbital is able to overlap with the empty d_{xz} orbital on Tc, as shown in Fig. 5. The importance of the p-bonding contribution to the structures of Tc(V) oxo complexes is seen in Fig. 6.

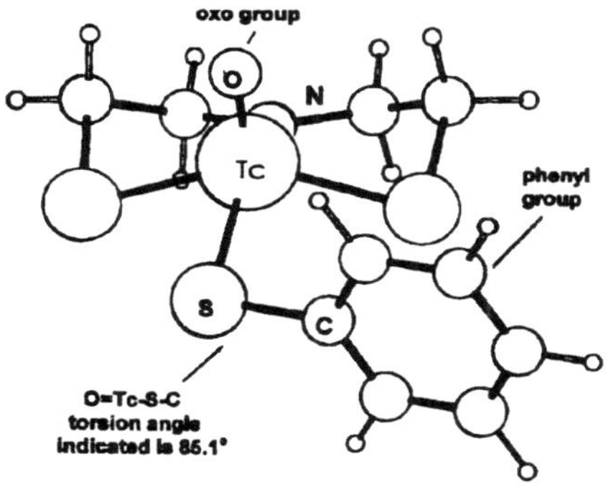

Figure 4. Structure of complex of the Tc(V) oxo group with a monodentate thiolate coordinated to the Tc, showing how the phenyl group of the thiolate is held in the plane of the four donor atoms of Tc by the need to satisfy the energy minimum for the O=Tc-S-C torsion angle at 90°. The structure was generated[12[by MM calculation using SYBYL[10[. If the torsional barrier about the Tc-S bond is reduced to zero, the phenyl group will then rotate out of the plane of the donor atoms to lessen van der Waal's repulsions. A crystal structure showing similar coordination of a thiophenol to Tc(V) can be found in ref. 14.

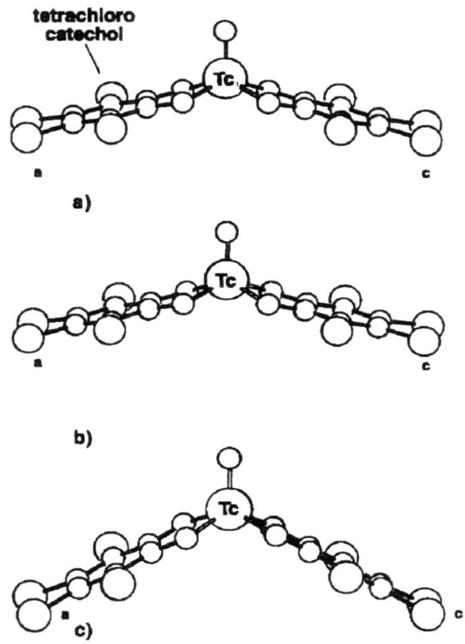

Figure 6. The effect on complex structure[12] of p-bonding in the Tc-O bonds to tetrachlorocatecholate dianion (TCC) . At (a) is shown the structure generated by MM calculation with the barrier to rotation about the Tc-O bond at a value of 3.5 $kcal.mol^{-1}$. At (b) is shown the crystallographically determined structure. At (c) the MM calculation is repeated with the barrier to rotation about the Tc-O bond set to zero. Note that here the tetrachlorocatecholate ligand lies in the same plane as that generated by the Tc and the two oxygen donors from the same catecholate ligand.

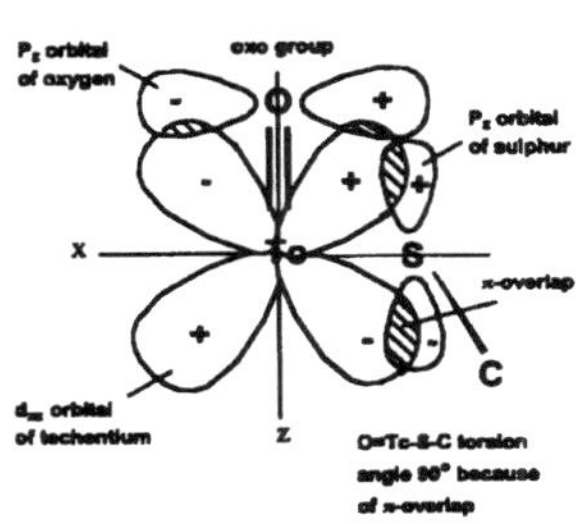

Figure 5. The importance of p-bonding in complexes of the Tc(V) oxo group. Overlap of a p_Z orbital on sulphur with the d_{XZ} orbital of Tc to yield a p-bond. Redrawn after reference 12.

The complex with the two tetrachlorocatechol (TCC) ligands coordinated to Tc(V) is shown generated by MM, first including the torsional contribution in the Tc-O bond, and then without the torsion included. It is seen that only with the O=Tc-O-C torsional barrier included is the subtle folding of the complex across the two oxygens of each ligand, observed in the crystal structure[15], reproduced. It is the attempt to achieve O=Tc-L-C torsion angles of 90° that tilts ligands such as DME or TCC above the plane formed by the Tc and the two donor atoms from the ligand. A further important effect of p-bonding in the Tc-L bond is very considerable bond shortening as compared to ligands where such p-bonding does not occur. Thus, as seen in Table 2, the ideal Tc-N bond lengths to sp^2 hybridised nitrogen in amide bonds is 1.91Å, whereas that to sp^3 hybridised nitrogen is 2.20Å. The sp^2 hybridised nitrogen of pyridines does not appear able to form p-bonds with Tc(V), since the Tc-N bonds here are 2.21Å, This lack of Tc-N bond shortening suggests that the p-electrons of pyridine are too strongly held as part of the aromatic system to be donated to Tc.

Table 2. MM parameters for modelling complexes of Tc(V) oxo complexes[a].

Bond length deformation parameters.

Bond	strain free length (Å)	force constant ($kcal.mol^{-1}.Å^{-1}$)
Tc-N(sp^3)	2.20	100
Tc-N(sp^2, ar)	2.21	200
Tc-S	2.33	100
Tc-O	1.96	200
TcN(sp^2, am)	1.91	200
TcN(sp^2, sat)	1.91	200
Tc=O	1.65	400

Bond angle deformation parameters[b].

Bond angle	strain angle (deg)	free force constant ($kcal.mol^{-1}.deg^{-1}$)
O=Tc-N(sp^2)	117.8	0.008
O=Tc-N(am)	109.1	0.008
O=Tc-N(sp3)	110.0	0.008
O=Tc-S	109.1	0.008
O=Tc-O	108.9	0.008
S-Tc-S(cis)	82.1	0.008
S-Tc-S(trans)	142	0.008
N(sp^2)-Tc-N(sp^3)	90	0.005
Tc-S-C	98	0.008

Torsional Constants.

Torsion angle	Torsional constant, V	Periodicity, n ($kcal.mol^{-1}$)
O=Tc-S-C	3.5	2
O=Tc-N(am)-C	3.5	2

[a]For use in conjunction with the TAFF force field present in SYBYL[10], and also ALCHEMY, although these parameters should be satisfactory with at most minor modification with the MM2 force field[11]. To convert the units in this table to other commonly used units, note that 1 $mdyn.Å^{-1}$ = 144 $kcal.mol^{-1}.Å^{-1}$.

[b]The angle constants for Ga(III) are the same as for Tc(III).

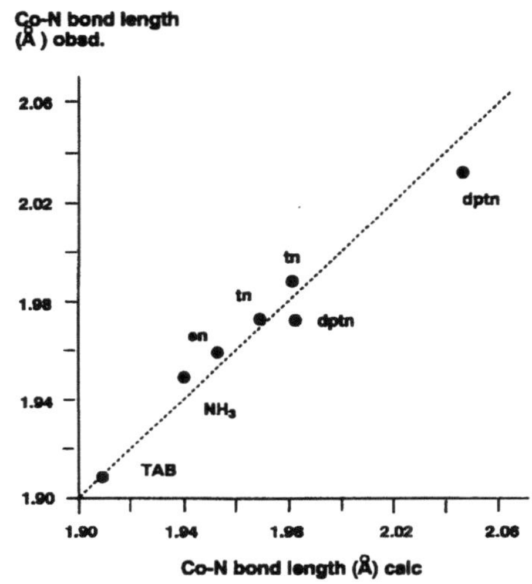

Figure 7. The accuracy of MM calculations on coordination compounds. The Co-N bond lengths observed in crystal structures are plotted against those calculated by MM using the MM2 force field[11] and parameters of the present author similar to those reported previously[2]. For ligand abbreviations, see Fig. 1.

c) Other Complexes of Technetium. Complexes of Tc that one might be interested in modelling[16] include Tc(I), and Tc(III). These are generally octahedral[17] so that they will be well modelled in a simple fashion with a covalent model. Important Tc(I) complexes such as the isocyanide complexes are easily modelled with suitable Tc-C bond lengths and force constants. If no parameters are available in the literature, and only one or two structures of an appropriate type are available, one should simply use a value of the M-L force constant typical of the type of bond under consideration. If the calculations yield some important conclusion, one can simply double and then halve the value of the force constant used to ensure that one's conclusion is not sensitive to the force constant.

Typical constants to use would be 250 kcal.mol^{-1}.Å^{-1} for a very strong and covalent M-L bond such as a bond to carbon, or involving a very covalently bound metal ion such as Co(III), or transition metal ions from the second and third row of the periodic table. Thus, Tc(I) and Tc(III) should be modelled with such force constants until accurate values can be determined. For divalent transition metal ions such as Ni(II) or Cu(II), or for trivalent lanthanides, force constants in the vicinity of 100 kcal.mol^{-1}.Å^{-1} would be satisfactory. For very ionically bound metal ions such as alkali and alkali earth metal ions, should one decide to model these using a 'covalent' representation of the M-L bond, force constants in the vicinity of 50 kcal.mol^{-1}.Å^{-1} would be reasonable. What is needed to pin down accurate values of the M-L force constants is crystal structures where there is considerable distortion of bond lengths and angles due to steric features in the complexes. This is the case with Co(III) and high-spin Ni(II)[2], where many crystal structures are available, many with high degrees of distortion due to steric effects. In Figure 7 is shown a plot of the Co-N bond lengths calculated by MM for complexes of Co(III) with six sp^3 hybridised nitrogen donors, against the Co-N bond lengths observed in the crystal structure. It is seen that the Co-N bond lengths are predicted by MM to an accuracy of about 0.01 Å, with Co-N bond lengths varying over a range of 0.13 Å, which is much larger than the variation in C-C bond length in organic molecules produced by purely steric effects, which is of the order of only 0.02 Å.

USE OF MM CALCULATIONS IN COORDINATION CHEMISTRY

At the simplest level, MM calculations can be used to predict the structures of complexes of interest in the absence of crystallographic information. Thus, the MM calculations[6] on EC complexes of In(III) showed that the alternative conformer with the sulphurs trans to each other was some 5-7 kcal.mol^{-1} higher in energy. In agreement with this, the observed[9] structure has the sulphurs cis to each other as in the conformer predicted by MM to be of lower energy. At a higher level, the MM calculation can be used to explore the effects of structural changes on complexes on the steric strain present in the complex. The steric strain energy, ÂU, of a molecule or complex ion is an unfavourable contribution to its formation. Thus, one can calculate the strain energy change on complex formation, DU, according to

$$\begin{array}{ccccc} M & + & n.L & \xrightarrow{\Delta U} & ML_n \\ U_M & & U_L & & U_{ML} \end{array} \qquad [3]$$

where U_M, U_L, and U_{ML} are the strain energies of the metal aquo ion (if the reaction is occurring in water), the ligand, and the complex, respectively. The value of DU is thus given by $U_{ML} - U_M - n.U_L$. If one is comparing a series of similar ligands with the same metal ion, one can see how DU would be affected by structural changes in the series of ligands, ignoring the value of U_M, which is common to all the complexes. An example of such a calculation might be to decide what the best size of bridge between the two nitrogens on EC might be. Thus, in the ligand PMC this bridge increases from two carbons in EC to three. The energy of the two ligands can be calculated, which using the MM2 force field gives UL as 16.70 kcal.mol^{-1} for the lowest energy conformer found for EC, and 17.35 kcal.mol^{-1} for the lowest energy conformer found for PC. In contrast, the strain energy for $[In(EC)]^-$ is 21.16 kcal.mol^{-1}, while that for $[In(PC)]^-$ is 26.91 kcal.mol^{-1}. Thus, one estimates that DU for the EC complex will be some 5.1 kcal.mol^{-1} more favourable than for the PC complex. This agrees with the experience that five membered chelate rings generally lead to more stable complexes for In(III) than do six membered, as evidenced by $\log K_1 = 24.9$ for[18] the In(III) complex of EDTA (five membered chelate ring involving the two nitrogens) and $\log K_1 = 21.2$ for the TMDTA complex (six membered chelate ring involving the two nitrogens). One similarly finds a scarcity of six membered chelate rings in complexes of the Tc(V) oxo group. Here again, MM calculations show much higher strain energy when the ethylene bridges in a ligand such as L,L-ECD are replaced with trimethylene bridges to give L,L-PCD:

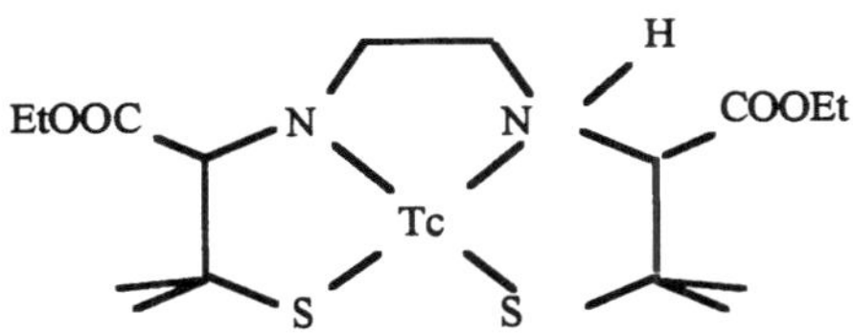

Tc(V)O(L,L-ECD)
U_{ML} = 12.1 kcal.mol^{-1}

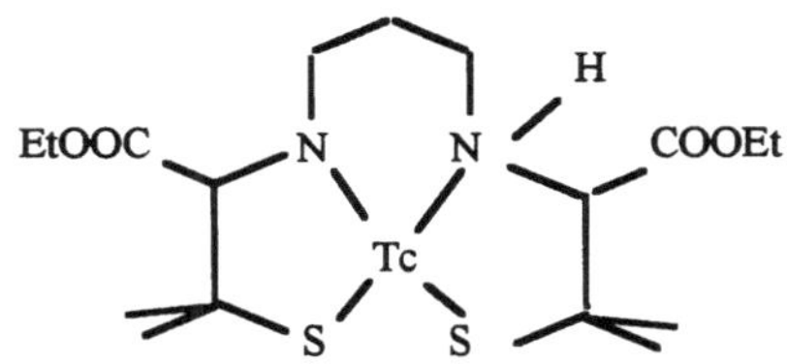

Tc(V)O(L,L-PCD)
U_{ML} = 19.0 kcal.mol^{-1}

Addition of an extra methylene group to free ligands generally raises the strain energy by less than 1 kcal.mol^{-1}, so that one can conclude that the above difference in strain energies reflects the general preference of Tc(V) for five membered chelate rings. The general effects of chelate ring size on metal ion size based selectivity have been discussed[2].

The above complexes raise an interesting point in terms of the presence of C-methyl groups adjacent to the sulphur donors. What effect do such groups have on complex stability? Examination of the literature shows that in general such groups lead to increases in complex stability. A very simple example is provided by comparing NTA with its analogue containing C,C-dimethyl groups:

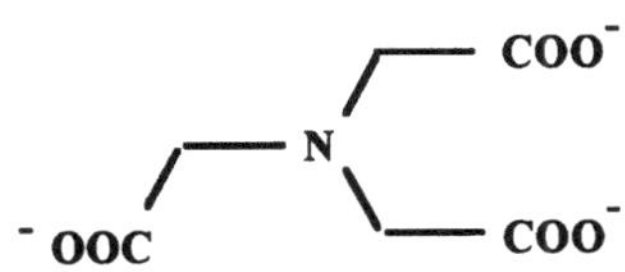

NTA
$\log K_1$[Zn(II)] 10.66
$\log K_1$[Ca(II)] 6.39

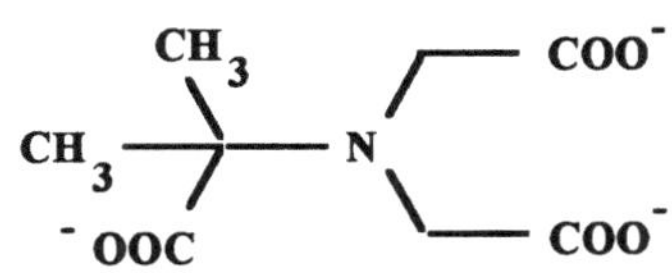

DM-NTA
12.45
8.32

MM calculations can enable us to understand such effects. The above is an example of *preorganisation*, which is one of the most important concepts in chemistry. Preorganisation is a term coined by Cram[19]. A ligand is more preorganised the more nearly it is constrained to be in the conformer required for complex formation. Thus, macrocycles are more preorganised than open chain ligands. The lowest energy conformation for a non-macrocylic ligand will tend to be linear, and energy has to be expended in bending the ligand into a conformer that can coordinate to a metal ion.

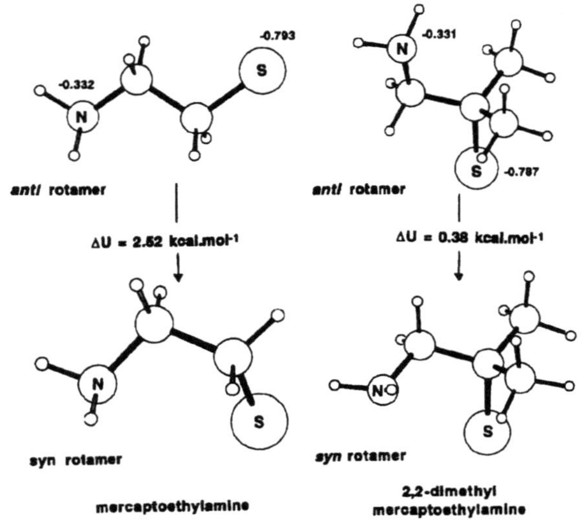

Figure 8. The effect of C-methyl groups on the level of preorganisation of mercaptoethylamine ligands. At left is shown the increase in steric energy caused by passing from the *syn* to the *anti* rotamer, calculated[20] using the SYBYL program, for mercaptoethylamine. This is much larger than the energy for the same transition calculated for 1,1-dimethylmercaptoethylamine

This is illustrated by the simple example[20] of mercaptoethylamine (ME) and 2,2-dimethylmercaptoethylamine (DM-ME) in Fig. 8. For ME, the *anti* rotamer is of lower energy than the *syn* rotamer required for complex formation by some 2.56 kcal.mol^{-1}, and this is an unfavourable contribution to the energy of complex formation. The greater stability of the *anti* rotamer of ME is due to electrostatic and van der Waal's repulsion between the NH_2 and S^- groups of ME. In DM-ME, the *anti* rotamer is destabilised by the presence of the methyl groups, which repel the NH_2 group by van der Waal's interactions. The increase in strain energy for DM-ME in passing from the *anti* to the *syn* rotamer is thus only calculated to be 0.38 kcal.mol^{-1}. This calculation illustrates the origin of the stabilisation observed in complexes where C-methyl groups are present.

Other types of question of interest in ligand design for biomedical applications is the question of coordination number. Will the metal in the proposed complex coordinate a water molecule, and so be much more hydrophilic than expected, or interact with donor groups such as sulphur on cysteines, or imidazole groups, to bind to biomolecules. This type of problem can be addressed at a simple level using MM if one proposes that coordination number in many metal ions is controlled by steric crowding. This would tend to be true for non-transition metal ions, where there is not a strong directionality in the M-L bonds provided by overlap with the d-orbitals, as is true for complexes of transition metal ions. Thus, for In(III), one finds that the EDTA complex is seven coordinate[21], but the complex with TACN-TM is six coordinate[7]. One may carry out a scan of the energy of complexes as a function of metal ion size[2], where the ideal M-L bond length in the calculation is varied over a suitable range. The energy of the complex may then be plotted as a function of M-L bond length. If we carry out a MM calculation on both of these complexes, first with no water molecule present to give six-coordination, and then with a water molecule added to the axial site to give seven-coordination, the scan of energy as a function of metal ion size will indicate[6] where steric crowding will lead to six coordination being favoured over seven coordination. Such scans, for both the In(III) complexes of EDTA and of TACN-TM, are seen in Fig. 9. The scans correctly indicate that for In(III) the EDTA complex should be seven coordinate, while the TACN-TM complex is six coordinate.

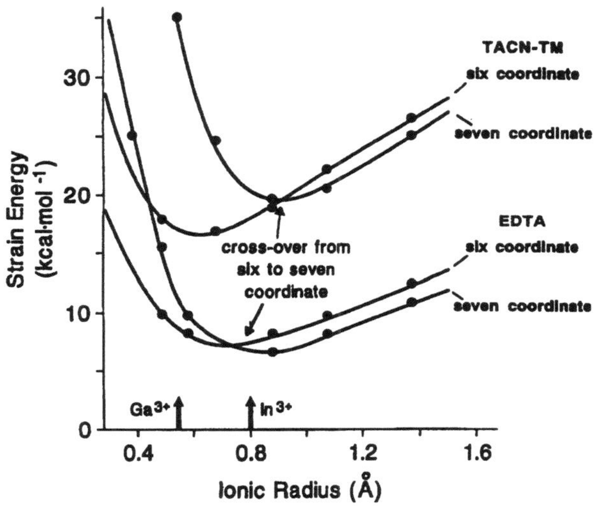

Figure 9. The effect of steric crowding on coordination number. The MM calculation is carried out with the ionic radius varying as shown for six and seven coordinate versions of each complex, with the seventh coordination site occupied by a water molecule. The cross over point indicates where steric crowding becomes serious for the seven coordinate version of the complex. Thus, the In(III) complex with EDTA is seven coordinate, but that with TACN-TM is six-coordinate. Ionic radii (r^+) are related[20] to M-N bond length by r^+ = M-N length + 1.47Å. Redrawn after reference 20.

The MM calculation is particularly suited to examining molecular recognition type of interactions. Katzenellenbogen et al[22]. have synthesised complexes of the Tc(V) oxo group which it is hoped will mimic steroids. In Figure 10 is shown such a Tc(V) complex, compared to a steroid. MM calculations show that the dimensions of the Tc(V) steroid mimic are similar to those of the steroid. However, the question arises of what the charge will be on the Tc(V) oxo oxygen. Will this be sufficiently negative to alter the molecular recognition properties of the Tc(V) steroid mimic that it does not bind to the same sites as the steroid. To answer questions such as this, one needs to turn to MO calculations, which are now readily carried out with many of the commercially available packages mentioned in the introduction.

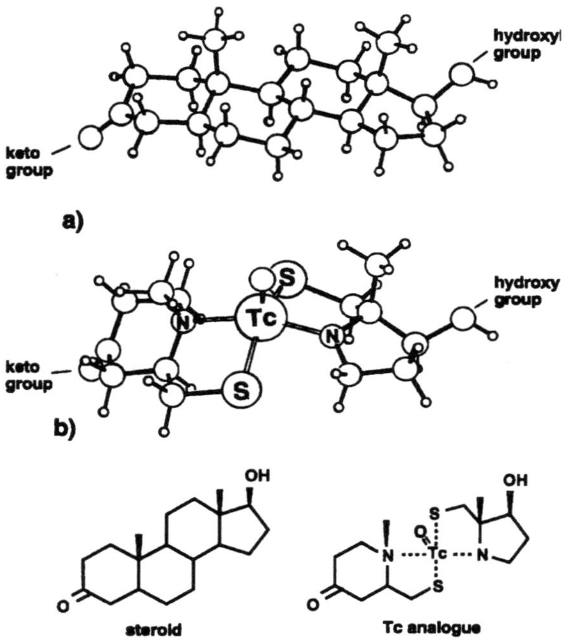

Figure 10. A Tc(V)O based steroid mimic[22]. At (a) is shown the structure of the steroid generated by MM calculation, and at (b) is the MM generated structure of the lowest energy conformer of the Tc(V)O analogue. The dimensions of the Tc(V)O analogue match those of the steroid quite well. The oxygen-oxygen distance from the keto group oxygen to the hydroxyl group oxygen on the steroid is calculated to be 11.10 Å, while the same O--O distance in the Tc(V)O analogue is 11.24 Å. Unpublished work of the present author.

Molecular Orbital Calculations on Complexes of Metal ions

The availability of packages that could be used for Molecular Orbital (MO) calculations on complexes of metal ions, and particularly transition metal ions, was until recently rather limited. Packages such as MOPAC[23,24] were confined to non-transition metals, and even these were limited to some half dozen metals. The program ZINDO[25] has been parametrised for a wide range of metal ions such as the first row of transition metals[25], and the second row of transition metals[26]. ZINDO is thus parametrised for calculations on Tc complexes, but unfortunately not for Ga or In, which, are, however, available in MOPAC[23,24]. ZINDO is a valence electron only program, and as such runs quickly even on a Mac when incorporated into the CAChe system. ZINDO is a useful adjunct to the MM package. Its particular strength is in calculating electronic spectra. The best approach with the latter appears to be to generate the structure using MM, and then use ZINDO to calculate the electronic spectrum from the MM structure. The parameters in ZINDO appear to generate bonds that are too stiff, and so steric effects are not well reproduced, so that MM is a better approach where MM parameters are available. ZINDO also has a tendency, in the experience of the present author, to produce from time to time unrealistic structures, where, for example, atoms become bonded to each other in a way not found in any of the real complexes. One has to experiment with ZINDO with the types of complexes one is interested in, and determine the types of situation where it works well, and where it will fail. ZINDO does fairly well with complexes of Technetium. One can use ZINDO to address the types of problem that are not amenable to solution by MM. Thus, for example, the coordination number of Tc(V) with its covalent and strongly directional bonding, is not controlled by steric crowding, as with In(III), but appears to be controlled more by the p-bonding characteristics of the ligand. Where the ligands coordinated in the plane of the Tc(V) oxo group are weak p-donors, a second oxo group is coordinated to give dioxo complexes[13]. One can thus gain an indication of where this will happen by calculating the energy of the reaction (unpublished work of the present author):

$$Tc(V)OL_4 \quad + \quad 3\,H_2O \quad = \quad TC(V)O_2L_4 \quad + \quad 2\,H_3O^+$$

One is neglecting such things as solvation energies and entropy contributions in such a calculation. One finds, however, that if one carries out the calculation for L as a variety of different ligands, that the results accord well with experience. Thus, for L = NH_3, where p-bonding in the Tc-N bond cannot occur, the reaction is calculated to proceed to the right with a favourable enthalpy change of -188.3 kcal.mol^{-1}. In contrast, for L-L = DME, where strong p-bonding is present in the Tc-S bond, the enthalpy change of the reaction is calculated to be +671 kcal.mol^{-1}. As one experiments with the package, one finds that this type of calculation for Tc(V)O complexes works quite well. ZINDO can also be used to calculate charge distributions on complexes. One is thus able to answer questions such as the size of the charge on the oxo group of Tc(V)O complexes. In Fig. 11 is shown the charge distribution calculated on a Tc(V)O complex similar to that investigated by Katzenellenbogen et al[22]. The figure shows the calculated electron density on the complex, and indicates that the charge density on the oxo group is about the same as that on the keto group present on the complex. This suggests that the complex might have rather different molecular recognition properties from the steroid which it is meant to mimic, where no such region of high charge density is present on the middle of the molecule.

It appears that MO calculations on complexes of metal ions in general, and transition metal ions in particular, are set to become much easier to perform, with better and more extensive parametrisations available. Packages such as SPARTAN are being extended to treat all of the metal ions in the periodic table with greater reliability than ZINDO, and the authors of this package have indicated that they are paying particular attention to the needs of researchers in the biomedical field.

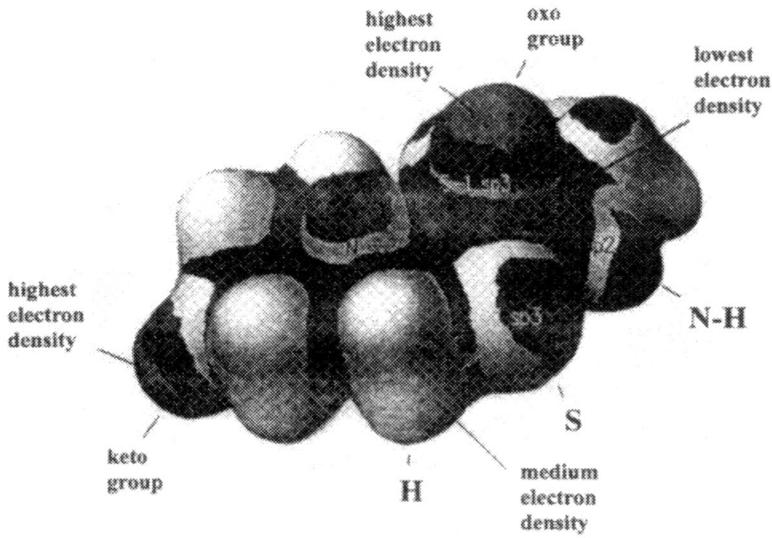

Figure 11. A complex of Tc(V)O similar to that in Figure 10, but with some of the organic part removed (the methyl and hydroxyl groups) to simplify the calculation. The program ZINDO[23,24] was used to generate the electron density on the complex. In the original the electron density is colour coded. It is sufficient here to point out that the electron density on the oxo group of the Tc is about as high as that on the keto group of the complex, which may affect the molecular recognition properties of the complex.

References

1. Brubaker GR, Johnson DW. Molecular Mechanics in Coordination Chemistry. Coord. Chem. Rev., 1984; 53:1-57.
2. Hancock RD. Molecular Mechanics Calculations as a Tool in Coordination Chemistry, Progr. Inorg. Chem., 1989; 37:187-291.
3. Hay BP. Methods for Molecular Mechanics Modeling of Coordination Compounds. Coord. Chem. Rev. 1993; 126: 177-236.
4. Comba P. The Relation between Ligand Structures, Coordination Stereochemistry, and Electronic and Thermodynamic Parameters. Coord. Chem. Rev. 1993; 123: 1-48.
5. Comba P, Hambley TW. Molecular Modelling of Inorganic Compounds. VCH Publishers: Weinheim, 1995.
6. Anderson C.J. John CS, Li Y, Hancock RD, McCarthy TJ, Martell AE, Welch MJ. N,N'-Ethylenedi-L-cysteine (EC) and its complexes with Ga(III) and In(III). Molecular Modelling, Thermodynamic Stability, and *in vivo* Studies. J. Nucl. Med. Biol. 1995; 22: 165-170.
7. Wieghardt K, Kleine-Boymann M, Nuber B, Weiss J. Macrocyclic Complexes of Indium(III): Novel m-hydroxo and m-oxo Bridged Complexes. Crystal Structure of {$L_2In(m\text{-}OH)_6](S_2O_6)_3.4H_2O$. Inorg. Chem. 1986; 25: 165 4-1659.
8. Bossek U, Hanke D, Wieghardt K, Nuber B. Crystal Structure of Indium(III) with 1,4,7-tris(mercaptoethyl)-1,4,7-triazacyclononane. Polyhedron, 1993; 12: 1-5.
9. LiY, Martell AE, Hancock RD, Reibenspies JH, Anderson CJ, Welch MJ, N,N'-Ethylenedi-L-cysteine and Its Metal Complexes: Synthesis, Characterisation, Crystal Structures, and Equilibrium Constants. Inorg. Chem., 1996; 35: 404-414.

10. Clark M, Cramer RD, van Opdenbosch N. Validation of the General Purpose Tripos 5.2 Force Field. J. Comput. Chem. 1989; 10: 982-1012.
11. Allinger NL. Conformational Analysis. 130. MM2. A Hydrocarbon Force Field Utilizing F_1 and F_2 torsional terms. J. Amer. Chem. Soc. 1977; 99:8127-8134.
12. Hancock RD, Reichert DE, Welch MJ. A Molecular Mechanics Force Field for Modeling Technetium(V) Complexes. Inorg. Chem. in the press.
13. Zuckman SA, et al. Preparation and X-ray Structure of trans-Dioxo(1,4,8,11-tetraazacyclotetradecane)technetium(V) Perchlorate Hydrate. Inorg Chem. 1981; 20: 2386-2389.
14. Rochon FD, Melanson R, Kong PC, Rearrangement of Tetramethyl-thiourea to Dimethyldithiocarbamate, and Crystal Structure of $[Tc(O)(C_5H_{12}N_2S_2)_2[(CH_3)_2NCSS)](PF_6)_2$. Inorg. Chim. Acta. 1992; 194: 43-50.
15. Abrams, MJ, Larsen, SK., Zubieta, J. Investigations of the Technetium-hydrazido core. Synthesis and structural characterisation of $[n\text{-}C_4H_9)_4N]\{Tc_2(NNPh_2)_2(C_6Cl_4O_2)_4].CH_2CL_2.2CH_3OH$, a Tc(V)/Tc(VI) catecholate complex with the hydrazido ligands adopting the unusual η^1 briudging mode. Inorg.Chem., 1991: 30:2031-2035
16 Bandoli G, Mazzi U, Roncari E, Deutsch E. Crystal Structures of Technetium Compounds. Coord. Chem. Rev. 1982; 44:191-227.
17. Davison A. et al. Synthesis and Characterisation of Hexakis(alkyl-isocyanide) and Hexakis(arylisocyanide) Complexes of Technetium(I). Inorg. Chem. 1983; 22: 2798-2800.
18. Martell AE, SMith RM. Critical Stability Constants. Plenum Press, New York, 1974-1985.
19. Cram DJ, et al. Host-Guest Complexation. 35. Spherands, the First Completely Preoranized Ligand System. J. Am. Chem. Soc. 1985; 107: 3645- 3657.
20. Sun Y, et al. Indium(III) and Gallium(III) Complexes of Bis(amino-ethanethiol) Ligands with Different Denticities: Stabilities, Molecular Modeling, and in vivo Behavior. J. Med. Chem. 1996; 39: 458-470.
21. Agre VM, Kozlova NP, Trunov VK, Ershova SD. Crystal Structure of trisodium[ethylenediaminetetraacetate sulfitoindium(III)]tetrahydrate. Zh. Struct. Khim. 1979; 22: 138-146.
22. Chi,DY., O'Neil, PO., Anderson, CJ., Welch, MJ., Katzenellenbogen, JA. Homodimeric and hetrodimeric bis(amniothiol) oxometal complexes with Rhenium (V) and Technetium (V). Control of heterodimeric complex formation and an approach to metal complexes that mimic steroid hormones. J.Med.Chem. 1994; 37: 928-937.
23. Bingham RC, Dewar MJS, Lo DH. Ground States of Molecules. XXVI. MINDO/3 Calculations for Hydrocarbons. J. Am. Chem. Soc. 1975; 97: 1294-1301.
24. Stewart JJP. Optimization of Parameters for semi-empirical Methods. 1. Method. J. Comp. Chem. 1989; 10: 209-264.
25. Zerner MC, Loew GH, Kirchner RF, Mueller-Westerhoff UT. An Intermediate Neglect of Differential Overlap Technique for Spectroscopy of Transition Metal Complexes. J. Am. Chem..Soc. 1980; 102: 589-599.
26. Anderson WP, Cundarai TR, Drago RS, Zerner MC. Utility of the Semiempirical INDO/1 method for the Calculation of the Geometries of Second Row Transition Metal Species. Inorg. Chem. 1990, 29, 1-3.

MICROAUTORADIOGRAPHY

Philip J Blower

Introduction

In nuclear medicine both diagnosis and dosimetry are based on the macroscopic distribution of radiotracers in the body with a resolution of several millimetres. However, knowledge of the underlying distribution at the microscopic level (cellular and sub-cellular, henceforth referred to as microdistribution), is essential to understand the uptake mechanisms of radiopharmaceuticals and the biological effects of their emitted radiation.

A compelling reason to study microdistribution of radionuclides, whether diagnostic or therapeutic, is the prediction of the effect of their emissions on genetic material. While "pure" γ-emitters such as Tc-99m are selected for imaging because they lack harmful particulate nuclear emissions, the effects of secondary electrons (Auger electrons etc.) must be taken into account. These "high LET" electrons usually have very limited range (< 1 μm), but if deposited within cell nuclei, they have the ability to inflict genetic damage because the local dose is very high. This effect can be exploited in the design of therapeutic radiopharmaceuticals (e.g. using I-125 or I-123-labelled steroid hormones or nucleoside analogues that target nuclei), but is undesirable in diagnosis. Thus, it is important to be able to show that a high-LET radionuclide used for therapy is accumulated in cell nuclei, while one used for imaging is not. The quantification of radiation dose to organelles such as nuclei is the aim of microdosimetry, which provides the link between microscopic distribution of radioactivity, and its biological effects. Several model frameworks for microdosimetry have appeared recently, applicable at various levels from the subcellular (1 μm) to the lower limit of scanner resolution (several mm) [1-3]. Various radionuclides are modelled, including Auger emitting diagnostic nuclides, β-emitters with a range of energies, and α-emitters, in the context of various cell and tissue geometries and various limiting model microscopic distributions. The inherent value of these model calculations is that they identify the problem that macroscopic dosimetry is no guide to radiation doses to nuclei if the microscopic distribution is non-uniform. Their potential in helping to solve the

S. J. Mather (ed.), Current Directions in Radiopharmaceutical Research and Development, 219–232.

problem through application in the clinical situation remains unrealised until the model microscopic distribution of radionuclides in tissues is replaced by real data. A recent example of the combination of experimental sub-cellular distribution information with an anatomical/microdosimetric model to estimate radiation dose rates to cell nuclei is given in ref. 4.

A second reason for investigating microdistribution is that a greater understanding of the targeting mechanisms of radiopharmaceuticals will contribute to better diagnosis through a fuller biochemical interpretation of scans. This is the basis of the tissue characterisation approach to diagnosis. A good starting point for the necessary mechanistic studies is the identification of the anatomical site of uptake in the tissue at the microscopic level. Pinpointing this site (intracellular/extracellular, membrane bound, nuclear, cytoplasmic etc.) will then permit hypotheses to be advanced and explored at a molecular level.

Methods for determining microdistribution

THE MULTI-CELLULAR LEVEL

Whole body autoradiographic techniques (macroautoradiography) can provide resolution at the 100-200 μm level. It involves cryosectioning whole animals [5-7] or organs [8] and placing the sections in contact with an X-ray film (e.g. Agfa-Gevaert Structurix D-7). For dosimetry at this level, methods have been developed for measuring dose distribution (rather than radioactivity distribution) in tissue using thin strips of thermoluminescent material implanted in the tissue. These are useful for measuring absolute doses at different depths in tissues, and the devices can be used in vivo. However, there is no correlation with tissue structure information, and it is not always certain that the devices do not perturb the radioactivity field [9,10].

THE CELLULAR/SUB-CELLULAR LEVEL

There are two main types of approach for determining the cellular and sub-cellular target sites of radiopharmaceuticals. One is sub-cellular fractionation of homogenised tissue. The other comprises a variety of direct imaging techniques: electron microscope methods, secondary ion mass spectrometry (SIMS), and microautoradiography.

Sub-cellular fractionation. Homogenisation and sub-cellular fractionation of tissues is probably the most common method of determining sub-cellular distribution. The homogenised cell fragments are separated by density gradient centrifugation. The location of the tracer is determined by assaying the various fractions for radioactivity. It is usual to monitor the purity of the fractions by assaying for enzymes known to be selectively located in the various organelles; reports that do not include these assays have diminished credibility. Used in isolation, this technique can yield misleading results: it is inherently disruptive and can disturb the sometimes labile interaction of radiotracers with binding sites. Another disadvantage of this technique is that it does not differentiate between cell types within the tissue or account for extracellular targeting.

Secondary ion mass spectrometry (SIMS). SIMS is a technique for imaging the spatial distribution of elements (rather than radioactivity) in materials [11]. It has recently been used to map the microdistribution of radionuclides used in diagnostic imaging [12,13]. Briefly, some of the atoms at the sample surface are ionised and vaporised by an ion beam and analysed mass spectroscopically to reconstruct an image of their spatial distribution in the sample surface. The main disadvantage of the technique is low sensitivity: isotopes at the no-carrier-added level appear to be only just within the detection limit - and then only by identifying the more abundant daughter product. A second disadvantage is the high instrumentation cost. SIMS has been used [12] to map Tc-99 in leucocytes labelled with Tc-99-HMPAO, and Tc-99 was found in equal concentration in cytoplasm and nuclei, in agreement with previous cell fractionation studies. The same group applied the method to meta-iodobenzylguanidine (MIBG) in a human neuroblastoma cell line xenograft in nude mice. MIBG was found to be absent from the cell nucleus [13].

Electron microprobe analysis. Electron microscope methods are similar to SIMS in that detection is not related to radioactivity but to the presence of the element, so they suffer from the same lack of sensitivity compared to autoradiography. Interaction of the electron beam with atoms in the sample causes emission of X-rays and back-scattered electrons, each with a spectrum characteristic of the element. These can be analysed to determine the concentration of heavy elements in selected sub-cellular regions. The method has been used to study of the sub-cellular location of carrier Tc-99-MIBI in freeze-dried frozen sections of cultured chick heart cells. Technetium concentration in mitochondria was shown to be 1000-fold higher than in cytosol[14].

Microautoradiography. Microautoradiography is discussed in detail below.

Microautoradiography techniques

Microautoradiography (MAR) is defined here as a range of autoradiographic methods for studying the cellular and sub-cellular distribution of radiolabelled compounds [15,16]. Radiolabelled tissue is placed in contact with a layer of radiosensitive emulsion. A typical procedure is summarised in Fig. 1. Particulate emissions are recorded by their interaction with silver bromide crystals suspended in the emulsion. The tissue and superimposed developed emulsion are then viewed under the microscope. The application of autoradiography to biological molecules and pharmaceuticals labelled with C-14 or H-3 is well established. However, it has seen surprisingly little use in nuclear medicine research.

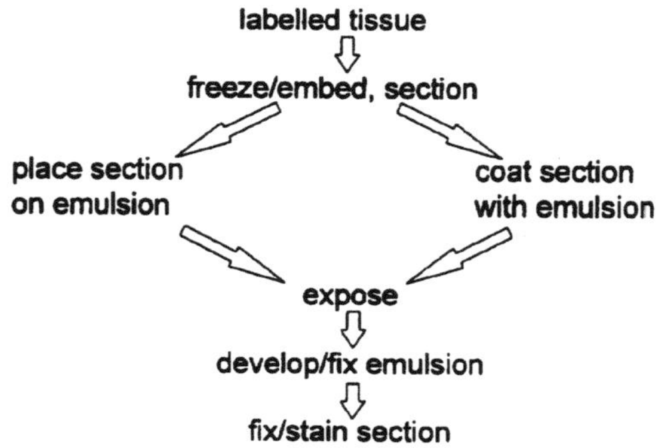

Figure 1. Generalised procedure for microautoradiography.

The following sections address the actual and perceived problems of applying MAR to study diagnostic and therapeutic radiopharmaceuticals.

AUTORADIOGRAPHIC PROPERTIES OF MEDICAL RADIONUCLIDES

Compared to tritium, which is very widely used for MAR, imaging radionuclides are non-ideal. A comparison between Tc-99m and tritium illustrates the problems.

Table 1. Extra-nuclear electron emissions from technetium-99m decay.

electron energy (KeV)	emissions per disintegration	range in emulsion (μm)	range in water (μm)
142.2	0.0011	85	192
140.0	0.0039	85	187
139.8	0.0035	80	187
137.7	0.0018	80	182
121.5	0.0088	66	148
119.4	0.0913	66	144
17.8	0.0055	2.2	5.3
15.4	0.0152	2.0	4.3
1.9	0.1093	<0.2	<0.2
1.6	0.9860	<0.2	<0.2
0.4	1.2359	<0.2	<0.2

Tritium-labelled samples can be exposed for months because of the long half-life, ensuring abundant silver grains even with low-activity samples. With Tc-99m, exposures longer than 24 h are pointless, and much higher initial activities are required to achieve similar grain densities. Some workers have therefore employed the longer half-life analogues Tc-95m and Tc-96 for MAR. The β-emission of tritium has low energy and a narrow energy range, ensuring uniform penetration and good resolution.

Tc-99m has no β-emission, and autoradiography depends on secondary emission of electrons (Auger and internal conversion electrons) which have a broader energy spectrum than the tritium β-particle (Table 1). The lower energy Auger electrons, however, are of similar energy to the tritium β-particle, and of greater abundance per disintegration. They also outnumber the higher energy electrons, and emulsions are more sensitive to them.

These factors can contribute to excellent quality autoradiographs with resolution within 1 μm [17] if simple precautions are taken. These are: using thin emulsion layers (to minimise detection of high energy electrons); using thin sections (to minimise the ratio of high-energy to low-energy electrons reaching the emulsion); and ensuring that the grain density does not approach saturation (again, to minimise the ratio of high energy to low energy electrons detected). Resolution (usually expressed as the distance from the edge of a uniform radioactive source at which the silver grain density drops to half of the value over the source) better than 2 μm has been confirmed experimentally for Tc-99m and several other medical radionuclides (Table 2).

Table 2. Resolution values obtained for medical radionuclides in microautoradiography, measured as half-distance values from uniform planar sources (distance from edge at which grain density falls to half the value over the source).

nuclide	Tc-99m	In-111	Sr-89	Re-188	I-131	F-18	I-125
resolution (μm)	<2.1	0.6 (ref. 17)	3.1	3.9	2.7	<2.1 (ref. 18)	2.0

Compared with Auger electrons, the β-emitters used in radiotherapy have the disadvantage of high β-energies, and the advantage of longer half-lives. The high energy β-particle is unwieldy for autoradiography. The rate of energy loss of the particle is low at the point of emission, and the range is longer (up to several millimetres) resulting in lower resolution. Nevertheless, with suitable precautions (i.e. using the thinnest emulsion layers and samples practicable) even the higher energy β-emitters (e.g. Re-188) can readily be traced to individual cells. Positron emitters (e.g. F-18, see Table 2) [18] can usefully be studied by MAR, although the extremely short half-life of many of them imposes practical limitations.

An elementary but important point is that at the microscopic level as well as the macroscopic level, the grain density (grains per unit area) is directly proportional to the radioactive concentration as long as saturation is not reached. MAR can therefore be used quantitatively as a measure of tissue radioactive concentration.

SAMPLE PREPARATION METHODS

Tissue and cell samples may be presented to the autoradiographic emulsion either as smears of whole cells, or as sections of tissue or cell suspensions. Each has its own advantages in different circumstances, although, in general, sections are most appropriate. Sections offer an important advantage over smears of cells in quantitative interpretation of autoradiographs: provided the section is in close contact with the emulsion, the radioactivity in the layer of the section immediately adjacent to the emulsion will be accurately represented in the autoradiograph, and all sub-cellular structures in this plane will be equally represented. With whole cells, in contrast, radioactivity within internal sub-cellular structures will be shielded from the emulsion, while cell-surface radioactivity will be in close contact with the emulsion and will be disproportionately represented in the autoradiograph. Section thickness should be minimised, for reasons outlined earlier. For most tissues a thickness of < 1 μm is impractical, but this is sufficiently thin to achieve sub-cellular resolution for most Auger emitters.

Conventional tissue fixation methods, followed by dehydration, clearing and wax-embedding, are often used in MAR. This has the advantage that very thin sections can be cut, and histological clarity is good. Nevertheless, the results from this method must be interpreted with caution. Many radiopharmaceuticals are small soluble molecules that are not necessarily tightly bound at their target sites in vivo. Fixing and embedding methods are chemically disruptive, and so are generally only suitable for 'fixable' substances (such as proteins or nucleic acids) and cannot be applied to diffusible compounds without risk of redistribution or loss of radioactivity. Furthermore, these methods are protracted which limits their use with short half-life isotopes.

Several methods exist for the study of diffusible compounds. All share the initial step of freezing tissue to preserve the in vivo distribution of the radiotracer. Most techniques involve sectioning frozen tissue directly. Tissue may be frozen in liquid propane, isopentane or similar high specific heat capacity coolant, cooled with liquid nitrogen, and sectioned with a microtome in a cryostat. The sections can be freeze dried for 24 h, then placed on a pre-formed emulsion layer and exposed in a moisture free environment [19]. A method adopted in our laboratory is an adaptation of the Appleton method [20]. Tissue is frozen as before and sections are cut in a cryostat and mounted directly onto the pre-chilled (< -30°C) nuclear emulsion. No deliberate steps are taken to freeze dry the sections, but there is evidence that this occurs nonetheless, while the frozen section is in contact with the emulsion. This method is rapid and effectively immobilises soluble radioactivity. Drawbacks include the difficulty of routinely cutting sections less than 5 μm thick, and reduced histological quality compared with conventionally fixed and embedded material. The main cause of this damage is ice recrystallisation within the tissue section during exposure [16]. For this reason the exposure temperature should be kept below -80°C. Frozen sections are more liable to produce chemographic artefacts [16] (chemically induced sensitisation/de-sensitisation of the emulsion) than fixed sections, although Appleton found that chemography could be reduced by lowering the exposure temperature[20].

While all these methods have their respective advantages and disadvantages, no single method has all the desirable characteristics to ensure complete confidence in the results, and in many instances it is most appropriate to apply several methods, the results of which will be complimentary to one another. In our own work on leucocytes labelled with radioactive colloid, for example [21-23], the interpretation of results was aided by using both frozen sections of unfixed cells, and whole cell smears of glutaraldehyde-fixed cell suspensions.

EMULSION PREPARATION

Some of the available nuclear emulsions and films are summarised in Table 3. Appropriate emulsions are available for either electron microscope or light microscope MAR. The autoradiographic emulsion may be presented for exposure in a variety of forms, the choice between which depends on individual circumstances. Usually an emulsion is supplied as a gel which must be melted, diluted if necessary, and applied to the sample in one of several ways. It may be spread on a coverslip by dipping, allowed to set and dry [20]. This gives a robust, rigid layer of uniform and controlled thickness, which is convenient to use and can be stored. Frozen samples can be applied to it without risk of thawing. The disadvantage of this method is that uneven samples may not adhere evenly to it, so that contact may not be uniformly intimate. This problem can be overcome by the widely used alternative method of applying the molten emulsion directly to the sample.[24] This ensures intimate contact but may allow soluble radioactive species to diffuse within the section or into the emulsion. Various methods of forming the emulsion into a thin film, using either wire loops [25] or blowing a bubble,[26] have been developed in attempts to solve these problems. The thin films dry rapidly immediately before contact with the frozen sample, and are flexible, giving a good chance of intimate contact. Dry emulsion layers are also available commercially as stripping films, which may be removed from their glass base and applied to frozen or freeze dried sections.[15] Another approach that has been tried is coating the sample with an impermeable layer, such as collodion or carbon deposited from the vapour [27], before applying the molten emulsion.

Table 3. Some commercially available nuclear emulsion and their properties.

Manufacturer	Crystal diameter (μm)	Sensitivity[a] (0 - 5)
Ilford	0.27 (G series)	5
Ilford	0.20 (K series)	0, 1, 2, 5
Ilford	0.14 (L series)	4
Kodak (UK)	0.20 (AR10*)	2
Eastman-Kodak	0.34 (NTB-3)	5
Eastman-Kodak	0.29 (NTB)	2
Eastman-Kodak	0.26 (NTB-2)	3
Eastman-Kodak	0.05 (129-01)	2

*Available as stripping film only. [a]High sensitivity: 5; low sensitivity: 0. A high sensitivity emulsion is recommended for high energy β-emitters because the rate of energy transfer close to the origin is low. For low energy emitters the low sensitivity emulsions are recommended because sensitivity to background radioactivity is low.

The thickness of the emulsion layer can be controlled by altering the viscosity of the molten emulsion by dilution. The thickness is selected depending on the range of the emissions and on whether "track autoradiography" or "grain density autoradiography" is to be performed (Fig. 2). In the former technique, a thick (> 5 μm) layer of emulsion is used, so that a charged particle of high energy sensitises several silver bromide crystals along its path, resulting in the formation of an identifiable track. The appropriate emulsion thickness depends on the emission energy of the isotope. For example, a 60 μm thick layer is suitable for the high-energy β-emitter P-32 [15]. The origin of the track is determined by tracing it through the developed emulsion. An advantage of track autoradiography is the ease of distinction of the tracks from background grains [28]. Disadvantages are the time taken to identify the origin of each track, and the lack of amenability to computer image analysis (see below). Also, the time required for development, fixation, and histological staining is necessarily increased to allow diffusion of the reagents through the tissue or emulsion layer [15]. Another difficulty is that the region of tracks close to their origin can be faint or invisible due to weak interaction between the high-energy electron and the emulsion. These tracks can be visualised by applying a gold-latensification process immediately before development of the exposed emulsion [28].

In the grain density method, a thin emulsion layer is used (1-5 μm). The passage of a charged particle through the emulsion results in the sensitisation of only one or two silver bromide crystals. The particle giving rise to the silver grain is assumed to originate from the tissue directly beneath it, unless the grain density is so high that the emulsion may be saturated (Fig. 2). At such levels, the less abundant longer-range electrons may be registered distant from their origin in significant numbers, and this assumption breaks down. Consequently, for grain density autoradiography, resolution must be maximised by using a thin emulsion layer (and, as discussed above, a thin tissue section), and avoiding saturation of the emulsion, to minimise the number of long range electrons detected compared to short range electrons. In the author's opinion, the grain density method is more generally desirable than the track method, particularly for quantitative work. If very low activity samples are to be studied (e.g. human biopsies), track autoradiography may be preferable, to maximise sensitivity at the expense of resolution.

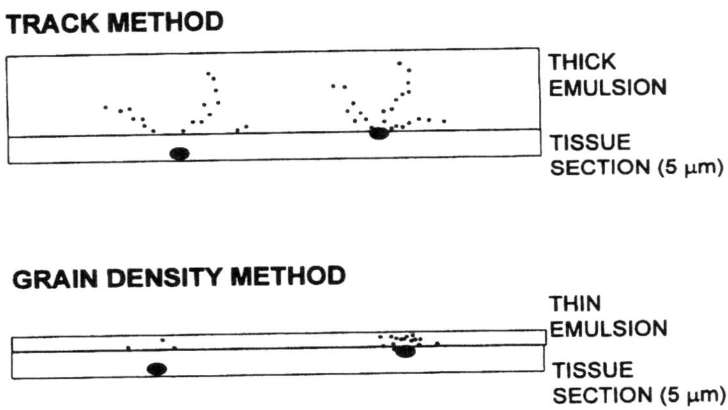

Figure 2. Thick and thin emulsions for track and grain density autoradiography, respectively.

An interesting double-isotope technique has been developed to compare the localisation patterns of F-18-labelled tracer and H-3 thymidine (used as an indicator of cell proliferation) [29]. Because of the short half-life of F-18, this method depends on use of frozen sections, which are mounted on pre-chilled slides coated with emulsion, to detect F-18. After a four-hour exposure, the emulsion layer was developed and the tissue fixed. After complete decay of F-18, a stripping film was applied to the other face of the tissue sections, and exposed for a further three weeks to detect tritium. Thus, the tissue section is sandwiched between two emulsion layers, one for each isotope. Despite the elegance of the dual tracer technique, it is restricted to isotopes with a large difference in half-life.

Ultimately the choice of autoradiographic technique depends on the isotope and the chemical nature of the radiopharmaceutical. Again, it may be advantageous to use complimentary approaches.

INTERPRETATION OF AUTORADIOGRAPHS

The problems of interpretation of microautoradiographs are often not given sufficient consideration, and this may well be a cause of disappointment in the results. Consequently, MAR is not used to its potential in nuclear medicine research. Unlike macroscopic autoradiography, at the microscopic level individual silver grains have to be identified with histological structures, rather than using densitometry (measuring the level of fogging) as a measure of radioactive concentration in a region. Direct qualitative visual interpretation, the most attractive feature of any imaging technique, is only applicable at very high grain densities, because the eye is not sufficiently competent at distinguishing small (several-fold at best) variations in grain density when individual grains are visible. High grain densities introduce additional, more serious problems: the emulsion may become saturated, with loss of linearity of response and loss of resolution. In addition, the greatest advantage of autoradiography -- the ability to view superimposed tissue and autoradiograph -- is lost because the underlying tissue can be obscured beyond identification. Even if it is desirable, high grain density is often impractical to achieve with medical radionuclides because of the non-ideal decay properties (unless very large initial activities are employed). It is therefore essential to count grains individually in the regions of interest. When performed manually with a graticule micrometer, as has usually been the case, this is time-consuming, error-prone, and subject to lack of objectivity. Many fields of view have to be examined because of the small numbers of grains (perhaps tens or less) in each. Fortunately, the arrival of computer image analysis (IA) has greatly enhanced autoradiograph quantification and consequently, interpretation [30]. An analogue image, obtained by attaching a video camera to the microscope, is digitised into "grey levels". This approach has been routinely used for many years in analysis of macroautoradiographs using densitometry. In MAR, the grey levels are not used to determine grain densities directly, but to distinguish grains from underlying tissue [21,22,30]. Silver grains are identified by selecting an appropriate threshold grey level, a process termed thresholding. The slight difference in focal plane between the tissue section and the silver grains can be exploited to assist visualisation of the tissue and grains: each can be viewed while the other is out of focus [21]. Under conventional bright-field illumination conditions it is sometimes difficult to distinguish silver grains from the underlying tissue (Fig. 3a). Use of dark-field illumination during automatic grain counting can solve this problem (Fig 3b) [21,30]. Sample regions of interest are delineated and stored under bright-field (Fig. 3a); then, under dark-field, silver grains (which are more reflective/diffractive than the tissue and appear as bright spots on a dark background -- see Fig. 3b), are thresholded and counted automatically. This permits rapid and reproducible grain quantification. Large sample areas and grain numbers can be quantified compared with visual methods, greatly increasing the accuracy and statistical significance of the results. Consequently, grain densities that are only fractionally above background (much lower than apparent to the eye) can be detected (e.g. less than one grain per 100 μm2 above background) [30].

The other important advantage of computer IA is that precise area measurements, required for grain density determination, can be obtained from pixel counts within non-uniform structures (e.g. cell nuclei and other tissue components) by generating regions of interest (ROI, Fig. 3a), either manually using a graphic input device such as a mouse, or automatically by thresholding differentially stained tissues

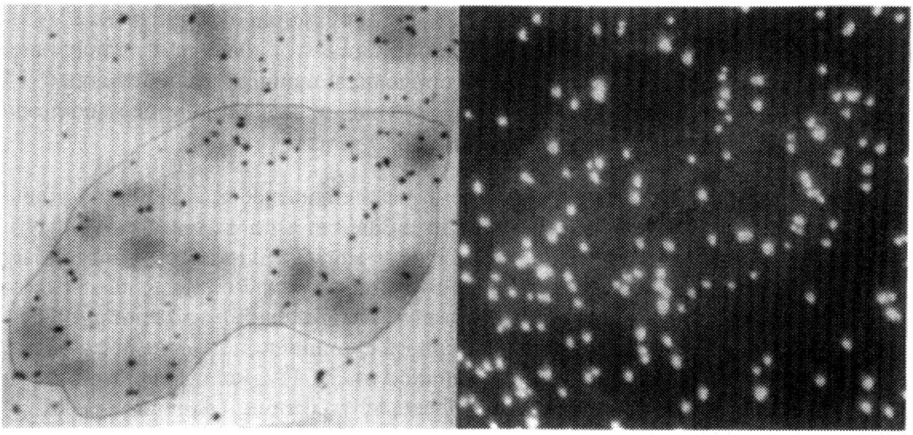

a) b)

Fig. 3. (a) microautoradiograph of a section of mouse renal cortex after injection with Tc-99m-DMSA, with a region of interest (renal tubule cross section) outlined, bright field illumination. (b) the same area of tissue under dark-field illumination, showing the relative ease of identifying silver grains.

At the extreme of resolution of the light microscope, and routinely with electron microscope autoradiography, the problem arises that the distance between the silver grain and the radionuclide that gave rise to it is significant, compared to the size of organelles, even for the shortest range emission. It must then be appreciated that the grain location does not represent the actual point of emission, but only a probabilistic indication of it (see below).

A common problem with interpretation of microautoradiographs arises from chemography. This may be positive (grains formed by chemical influences) or negative (grains removed, or prevented from forming, by chemical influences). Various tissues have differing capacity to cause chemography, and so do various microscopic tissue components. This can seriously mislead, and controls should be performed on all samples by allowing some of the tissue sample to decay completely in liquid nitrogen storage before autoradiography. Several tissues have been characterised in their chemographic behaviour [26]. A particular problem with Tc-99m agents is the presence of stannous reducing agents which can cause serious chemography.

ELECTRON MICROSCOPE AUTORADIOGRAPHY

MAR at the light microscope level is capable of distinguishing nuclear from cytoplasmic targeting, or whether the tracer is bound to the plasma membrane. However, to determine localisation patterns at the ultrastructural level, i.e. to specific sub-cellular organelles or regions of the nucleus, requires the use of the electron microscope. As noted above, analysis of EM autoradiographs is complicated by the high degree of image spread relative to the resolution limit of the electron microscope. To aid interpretation in these circumstances, mathematical models were developed [31] which predicted silver grain distributions arising from sources with defined geometries or calculated a best fit to the observed distribution of grains.

Currently, application of EM autoradiography for the study of diffusible compounds is limited by the lack of sample preparation methods that both preserve the in vivo radioactivity distribution and are compatible with electron microscopy. Particularly problematical is the need to apply emulsion in liquid form directly to the ultrathin tissue section. Baker and Appleton [27] addressed this problem by evaporating a layer of carbon onto the section prior to application of the emulsion. At present however, the main limitation of the frozen section method at the EM level appears to be the unacceptable loss of ultrastructural detail caused by freezing. Applications of EM autoradiography in a nuclear medicine context have been very few to date [32].

Conclusions

Information about microdistribution of radionuclides is an essential part of understanding the targeting mechanisms, dosimetry, and radiobiology of radiopharmaceuticals. The most direct and generally applicable means of obtaining this information is by microautoradiography. Visual inspection of autoradiographs cannot, in general, lead to a complete picture, and indeed usually leads to disappointment and provides no useful information at all. Full quantitative analysis by counting grains in regions of interest corresponding to tissue structures of measured cross sectional area is essential, and computer image analysis is essential for this. Resolution is sufficient to identify whether sub-cellular uptake is nuclear or not, permitting sub-cellular dosimetry to be based on real distributions rather than model ones. A variety of methods of sample and emulsion preparation provides complimentary information leading to greater confidence in the results. This review has described the techniques, and their advantages and disadvantages. A compilation of examples of use of the techniques in the study of radiopharmaceuticals is provided elsewhere [33].

Acknowledgement

The author is indebted to Dr M R B Puncher for his contribution to the installation and development of these techniques at the University of Kent.

References

1. Humm JL, Macklis RM, Bump K, Cobb LM, Chin LM. Internal dosimetry using data derived from autoradiographs. J Nucl Med 1993;34:1811-1817.
2. Farragi M, Gardin I, de Labriolle-Vaylet C, Moretti J-L, Bok B. The influence of tracer localization on the electron dose rate delivered to the cell nucleus. J Nucl Med 1994;35:113-119.
3. Humm JL, Cobb LM. Nonuniformity of tumor dose in radioimmunotherapy. J Nucl Med 1990;31:75-83.
4. Blower PJ. Microdosimetry in labelled leucocytes. In: Cox PH, Buscombe J, eds. The imaging of infection and inflammation. Kluwer, Dortrecht (in press).
5. Yonekura Y, Brill AB, Som P, Bennett GW, Fand I. Quantitative autoradiography with radiopharmaceuticals, part 1: digital film-analysis system by videodensitometry: concise communication. J Nucl Med 1983;24:231-237.
6. Som P, Yonekura Y, Oster ZH, et al. Quantitative autoradiography with radiopharmaceuticals, part 2: applications in radiopharmaceutical research: concise communication. J Nucl Med 1983;24:238-244.
7. Ullberg S. The technique of whole body autoradiography. Science Tools (special issue) LKB-Produkter AB, Stockholm.
8. Willis KW, Martinez DA, Hedley-White ET, Davis MA, Judy PF, Treves S. Renal localisation of 99mTc-stannous glucoheptonate and 99mTc-stannous dimercaptosuccinate in the rat by frozen section autoradiography. Radiat Res 1977;69:475-488.
9. Yorke ED, Williams LE, Demidecki AJ, Heidorn DB, Roberson PL, Wessels BW. Multicellular dosimetry for beta-emitting radionuclides: autoradiography, thermoluminescent dosimetry, and three-dimensional dose calculations. Med Phys 1993;20:543-550.
10. Griffith MH, Yorke ED, Wessels BW, DeNardo GL, Neacy WP. Direct dose confirmation of quantitative autoradiography with micro-TLD measurements for radioimmunotherapy. J Nucl Med 1988;29:1795-1809.
11. Burns MS. Biological microanalysis by secondary ion mass spectrometry - status and prospects. Ultramicroscopy 1988;24:269-282.
12. Fourre C, Halpern S, Jeusset J, Clerc J, Fragu P. Significance of secondary ion mass spectrometry microscopy for technetium-99m mapping in leukocytes. J Nucl Med 1992;33:2162-2166.
13. Clerc J, Halpern S, Fourre C, et al. SIMS microscopy imaging of the intratumor distribution of metaiodobenzylguanidine in the human SK-N-SH neuroblastoma cell line xenografted into nude mice. J Nucl Med 1993;34:1565-1570.
14. Piwnica-Worms D, Kronauge JF, Davison A, Jones AG, Ingram P, LeFurgey M, Lieberman M. Mitochondrial localization of Tc-MIBI in cultured chick heart cells by electron probe X-ray microanalysis. J Nucl Med 1990;31:748 (abstract).
15. Baker JRJ. Autoradiography: a comprehensive overview. Oxford University Press/Royal Microscopical Society 1989.
16. Rogers AW. Techniques of autoradiography, 3rd edn. Elsevier North Holland Biomedical Press, NY, 1979.
17. Morrell EM, Tompkins RG, Fischman AJ, et al. Autoradiographic method for quantitation of radiolabeled proteins in tissues using indium-111. J Nucl Med 1989;30:1538-1545.
18. Kubota R, Yamada SY, Kubota K, Ishiwata K, Ido T. Micro-autoradiographic method to study [18F]FDG uptake in mouse tissue. Nucl Med Biol 1993;20:183-188.
19. Stumpf WE, Roth LJ. Dry-mounting high-resolution autoradiography. In Isotopes in experimental pharmacology ed. Roth LJ, pp. 133-143. University of Chicago Press, Chicago 1965.
20. Appleton TC. Autoradiography of soluble labelled compounds. J Royal Microsc Soc 1964;83:277-281.

21. Puncher MRB, Blower PJ. Autoradiography and density gradient centrifugation of technetium-99m-Exametazime (HMPAO) lebelled leucocytes reveals selectivity for eosinophils. Eur J Nucl Med 1994;21:1175-1182.
22. Puncher MRB, Blower PJ. Frozen section microautoradiography in the study of radionuclide targeting: application to indium-111-oxine-labaled leukocytes. J Nucl Med 1995;36:499-505.
23. Puncher MRB, Blower PJ. Labelling of leucocytes with colloidal technetium-99m-SnF2: an investigation of the labelling process by autoradiography. Eyr J Nucl Med 1995;22:101-107.
24. Flitney E. Autoradiography. In: Theory and practice of histological techniques, 3rd Edn. Ed: Bancroft JD, Stevens A. Churchill Livingstone NY, 1990.
25. Caro LG, Van Tubergen RP. High resolution autoradiography. 1. Methods. J Cell Biol 1962;15:173-188..
26. Kawamoto T, Shimizu M. A method for preparing whole-body sections suitable for autoradiographic, histological and histochemical studies. Stain Technol 1986;61:169.
27. Baker JRJ, Appleton TC. A technique for electron microscopic autoradiography (and X-ray microanalysis) of diffusible substances using freeze-dried fresh frozen sections. J Microscopy 1976;108:307-315.
28. Wirquin E, Masse R, Meignan M, Galle P. Microautoradiography of (-emitters: interest of latensification process. Int J Appl Radiat Isot 1984;35:489-493.
29. Kubota R, Yamada S, Ishiwata K, Kubota K, Ido T. Active melanogenesis in non-S-phase melanocytes in B16 melanomas in vivo investigated by double-tracer microautoradiography with 18F-fluorodopa and 3H-thymidine. British J Cancer 1992;66:614-618.
30. Schnitzer JJ, Morrell EM, Colton CK, Smith KA, Stemerman MB. Absolute quantitative autoradiography of low concentrations of 125I-labeled proteins in arterial tissue. J Histochem Cytochem 1987;35:1439-1450.
31. Blackett NM, Parry DM. A simplified method of "hypothetical grain" analysis of electron microscope autoradiographs. J Histochem Cytochem 1977;25:206-214.
32. Davis HH, II, Senior RM, Griffin GL, Kuhn C, III. 111Indium-labeled human alveolar macrophages and monocytes: function and ultrastructure. J Immunological Methods 1980;36:99-107.
33. Puncher MRB, Blower PJ. Radionuclide targeting and dosimetry at the microscopic level: the role of microautoradiography. Eur J Nucl Med 1994;21:1347-1365.

INDEX

Developments in Nuclear Medicine

1. P.H. Cox (ed.): *Cholescintigraphy*. 1981 ISBN 90-247-2524-0
2. P.H. Cox (ed.): *Progress in Radiopharmacology*. Selected Topics. Proceedings of the 3rd European Symposium (Noordwijkerhout, The Netherlands, April 1982). 1982 ISBN 90-247-2768-5
3. M.H. Jonckheer and F. Deconinck (eds.): *X-Ray Fluorescent Scanning of the Thyroid*. 1983 ISBN 0-89838-561-X
4. K. Kristensen and E. Nørbygaard (eds.): *Safety and Efficacy of Radiopharmaceuticals*. 1984 ISBN 0-89838-609-8
5. A. Bossuyt and F. Deconinck: *Amplitude/Phase Patterns in Dynamic Scintigraphic Imaging*. With a Foreword by A. Bertrand Brill. 1984 ISBN 0-89838-641-1
6. M.R. Hardeman and Y. Najean (eds.): *Blood Cells in Nuclear Medicine, Part I*. Cell Kinetics and Bio-distribution. 1984 ISBN 0-89838-653-5
7. G.F. Fueger (ed.): *Blood Cells in Nuclear Medicine, Part II*. Migratory Blood Cells. 1984 ISBN 0-89838-654-3
8. H.J. Biersack and P.H. Cox (eds.): *Radioisotope Studies in Cardiology*. 1985 ISBN 0-89838-733-7
9. P.H. Cox, G. Limouris and M.G. Woldring (eds.): *Progress in Radiopharmacology 1985*. 1985 ISBN 0-89838-745-0
10. P.H. Cox, S.J. Mather, C.B. Sampson and C.R. Lazarus (eds.): *Progress in Radiopharmacy*. 1986 ISBN 0-89838-823-6
11. H. Deckart and P.H. Cox (eds.): *Principles of Radiopharmacology*. 1987 ISBN 0-89838-774-4
12. W.-D. Heiss, G. Pawlik, K. Herholz and K. Wienhard (eds.): *Clinical Efficacy of Positron Emission Tomography*. 1987 ISBN 0-89838-898-8
13. G.B. Gerber, H. Métivier and H. Smith (eds.): *Age-related Factors in Radionuclide Metabolism and Dosimetry*. 1987 ISBN 0-89838-953-4
14. K. Kristensen and E. Nørbygaard (eds.): *Safety and Efficacy of Radiopharmaceuticals 1987*. 1987 ISBN 0-89838-986-0
15. C. Beckers, A. Goffinet and A. Bol (eds.): *Positron Emission Tomography in Clinical Research and Clinical Diagnosis*. Tracer Modelling and Radioreceptors. 1989 ISBN 0-7923-0254-0
16. M. De Schrijver: *Scintigraphy of Inflammation with Nanometer-sized Colloidal Tracers*. 1989 ISBN 0-7923-0272-9
17. Ch. Kessler, M.R. Hardeman, H. Henningsen and J.-N. Petrovici (eds.): *Clinical Application of Radiolabelled Platelets*. 1990 ISBN 0-7923-0729-1
18. H.J. Biersack and P.H. Cox (eds.): *Nuclear Medicine in Gastroenterology*. 1991 ISBN 0-7923-1074-8
19. R.P. Baum, P.H. Cox, G. Hör and G.L. Buraggi (eds.): *Clinical Use of Antibodies*. Tumours, infection, infarction, rejection and in the diagnosis of AIDS. 1991 ISBN 0-7923-1424-7

Developments in Nuclear Medicine

20. J.C. Baron, D. Comar, L. Farde, J.L. Martinot and B. Mazoyer (eds.): *Brain Dopaminergic Systems: Imaging with Positron Tomography.* 1991 ISBN 0-7923-1476-X
21. M.K. Dewanjee: *Radioiodination.* Theory, Practice, and Biomedical Application. 1991 ISBN 0-7923-1491-3
22. P.A. Schubiger and G. Westera (eds.): *Progress in Radiopharmacy.* 1992 ISBN 0-7923-1525-1
23. B.M. Mazoyer, W.D. Heiss and D. Comar (eds.): *PET Studies on Amino Acid Metabolism and Protein Synthesis.* 1993 ISBN 0-7923-2076-X
24. G. Stöcklin and V.W. Pike (eds.): *Radiopharmaceuticals for Positron Emission Tomography.* Methodological Aspects. 1993 ISBN 0-7923-2340-8
25. P.H. Cox and M. Pillay (eds.): *The Clinical Applications of SPET.* 1995 ISBN 0-7923-3187-7
26. D. Comar (ed.): *PET for Drug Development and Evaluation.* 1995 ISBN 0-7923-3716-6
27. R.M. Lambrecht: *Biological Models in Radiopharmaceutical Development.* 1996 ISBN 0-7923-3836-7
28. R. Bares and G. Lucignani (eds.): *Clinical PET.* 1996 ISBN 0-7923-4160-0
29. R. Duncan (ed.): *SPECT Imaging of the Brain.* 1996 (forthcoming) ISBN 0-7923-4186-4
30. S.J. Mather (ed.): *Current Directions in Radiopharmaceutical Research and Development.* 1996 ISBN 0-7923-4254-2

Kluwer Academic Publishers - Dordrecht / Boston / London

MIX
Papier aus verantwortungsvollen Quellen
Paper from responsible sources
FSC® C105338

If you have any concerns about our products,
you can contact us on
ProductSafety@springernature.com

In case Publisher is established outside the EU,
the EU authorized representative is:
Springer Nature Customer Service Center GmbH
Europaplatz 3, 69115 Heidelberg, Germany

Printed by Libri Plureos GmbH
in Hamburg, Germany